Susan ♡ P9-CBW-282

Measuring Functioning and Well-Being

Measuring Functioning and Well-Being

The Medical Outcomes Study Approach

With a foreword by Alvin R. Tarlov

Anita L. Stewart & John E. Ware, Jr., Editors

Duke University Press   Durham and London   1992

Third printing in paperback, 1993
© 1992 The RAND Corporation
All rights reserved
Printed in the United States of America
on acid-free paper ∞
Library of Congress Cataloging-in-Publication Data
appear on the last printed page of this book.

Contents

VI Summary, Discussion, and Future Directions

Tables

Foreword

Alvin R. Tarlov, M.D.

The wide adoption of a system to measure the outcomes of health services and to valuate those outcomes against costs possibly could do more to improve the cost-effectiveness of health care than any other innovation. This volume on the Medical Outcomes Study (MOS) using functioning and well-being measures is a step that could help advance those assessments from research tools to instruments for improved clinical practice and more cost-effective health care.

The health status of a population is conventionally measured by morbidity and mortality rates and by life expectancy. The health of an individual ordinarily is measured using biological metrics pertaining to the disease or the organ system affected, that is, milligrams percent blood sugar in diabetes or ejection fractions in heart disease. Both the population and the individual health appraisal systems, in effect, tend to regard each person or organ as an independent self-contained entity reactive only to itself ignoring the influences on health of the social environment. Neither system is adequately concerned with the effects that a disease or treatment have on a person's performance in everyday activities with family, friends, neighbors, and colleagues at home, work, and in his or her community. Neither system reports on the patient's view of their health in general or on a patient's appraisal of his or her own well-being. Yet maintaining or returning to normalcy those elements of health-related quality of life is the real fundamental purpose of medical care.

Thus, we have neither adequate measures of the health of the nation nor satisfactory knowledge of what is being accomplished by health care. With $813 billion spent on health in 1992, 14 percent of the gross national product, we lack the means to valuate the investment. The salient characteristics of the M OS from which long-term importance might derive are its broadened conceptual framework of health, its emphasis on obtaining a patient's perspective on his or her health status, and the use of relatively brief and efficient information collection systems that can be broadly applied. In addition to measuring the biological state of a chronic disease, a measure of the cost of care, and the level of satisfaction with care, the M OS also asks patients how well they are doing in their everyday activities, how they feel, and how they rate their health. The broadened conceptual framework of health provides a much-needed sharper instrument for monitoring the results of health care under different systems of care, different payment methods, different medical specialties, different styles of doctor-patient interaction, and different rates of use of health care resources.

This volume hopefully will advance the date when large numbers of individuals and organizations can begin using routinely the M OS methodology. Broad application across the country in different systems, both public and private, can lead to evaluation, improvement, and perhaps adoption of new ways to gauge health services. The greatest ambition expected from advances in health status measurements is that widespread application will lead to improved outcomes from health services and better health for the nation. This book is an early step toward achievement of that ambition.

Preface

Traditionally, medical scientists have measured the outcomes of medical care through mortality rates and in terms of morbidity, described as the extent and severity of the pathology of a disease as measured by laboratory reports and pathologists. Since the 1970s, however, the emphasis in America on what patient outcomes to measure to determine health status has been shifting. The focus on the outcomes of medical care is now shifting to the assessment of functioning, or the ability of the patients to perform the daily activities of their lives, how they feel, and their own personal evaluation of their health in general.

This shift in emphasis is timely because of major changes that are occurring in health policy evaluations, clinical trials, clinical decision-making, and in health services research. The health care financing debate, long dominated by cost-containment issues, is expanding its focus beyond costs to health care outcomes. Outcome assessments in clinical trials and in clinical practice increasingly include the patients' point of view regarding functional status and well-being in addition to the traditional biomedical parameters. Patient-completed health status measures have become tools of health services research. This book attempts to meet the needs of the recent shift to patient-based assessments of medical outcomes by explaining advances in health status measurement.

Methodological advances in the MOS are presented to help meet the increasing demand from several health sectors for information about the measurement of health from the patient's point of view, the availability of practical and useful health indicators, the methods for evaluating and choosing among indicators, and the interpretation of results. Another of the aims of the book is to clarify measurement research for health professionals not trained in psychometric theory and methods.

Measuring Functioning and Well-Being: The Medical Outcomes Study Approach is a book that concentrates not on the history, evaluation, or interpretation of the significance of the medical outcomes approach, but on the description of a large-scale study that used both standardized patient surveys and clinical evaluations as measures of health status, now defined to combine three parameters: clinical status, functioning, and well-being. The book summarizes some of the important features of the Medical Outcomes Study (MOS), a quasi-experimental study of variations in physician practice styles and patient outcomes in different health care delivery systems (Tarlov, Ware, Greenfield, et al., 1989).

The MOS is distinctive for two major reasons. The MOS measures clinical status, functioning, and well-being in parallel initially and longitudinally. In assessing the effects of medical care with a particular emphasis on functioning, disease severity and other indicators of clinical status were controlled for in the MOS. The MOS is the first large-scale study in which patients with different medical and psychiatric conditions completed the same measures of patient functioning and well-being.

The MOS, which spans the decade of the 1980s and continues, evaluated improved health status surveys in several samples drawn from over 22,462 patients from 523 medical practices in three large cities in the United States. A subsample of 11,242 patients completed a 20-item survey of functioning and well-being at the time of a doctor visit. A subsample of 3,053 patients with one or more chronic conditions completed a more extensive follow-up survey, which is the primary focus of this book. A subsample of 2,349 of those is being followed longitudinally.

Measuring Functioning and Well-Being presents specific methodological advances of the MOS, which include increased understanding of some widely used survey measures; improvements in existing survey measures in terms of validity and ease of use; the construction of new measures to replace old; and the attempt to measure new health concepts. The MOS expresses a new philosophy of measurement, one that calls for increasing standardization of generic health surveys across studies and populations. Most importantly, the MOS demonstrates the feasibility of using self-administered questionnaires. These advances have broad applications to other health studies. The greatest ambition expected for these advances in health status measurement is that widespread application will lead to improved outcomes from health services and better health for the nation. This book is a first step toward accomplishing this goal.

The focus of the book is on the MOS patient survey measures of functioning and well-being; data from medical histories and clinical examinations and measures of patient satisfaction are not described. The measures documented are comprehensive, reflecting a full range of concerns of patients, and are based upon a conceptual framework that incorporates a broad spectrum of health concepts and a full range of levels of functioning and well-being.

The text is organized into six parts, each focusing on a different aspect of the outcomes approach: Health Assessment, Creation of Databases on the Health of Individuals, Generic Health Concepts and Measures, Short-Form Measures, Validity of MOS Measures, and Future Directions.

The two chapters in part I, "The New Era of Health Assessment," provide an overview of the MOS. Chapter 1 characterizes the state of the art of health assessment and identifies some of the advances necessary to meet the needs of various applications of health surveys. The importance of improved standards for selecting appropriate measures is also discussed. Chapter 2 introduces a new, comprehensive, conceptual framework of health that incorporates patient health surveys and other data sources.

Part II, "Creation of Databases on the Health of Individuals," presents information on the manner in which the MOS sample was obtained and the methods for collecting health status data in the physician's office and in periodic surveys.

In part III, "Generic Health Concepts and Measures," the introductory chapter explains psychometric theory and methods in constructing health measures and presents the methods used in the MOS. Chapters 6–15 cover the conceptual and methodological issues unique to the health concepts, including physical functioning, psychological distress/well-being, cognitive functioning, health perceptions, energy/fatigue, health distress, social functioning, role functioning, pain, sleep, and physical/psychophysiologic symptoms.

Each chapter in part III is divided into five sections, corresponding to the processes underlying measurement development: (1) issues of definition and measurement; (2) content and measurement strategy; (3) construction and evaluation of scales; (4) characteristics of measures;

and (5) resolution of issues and future directions. The chapter on sleep is slightly different because it required a detailed rationale for its relevance in a comprehensive battery. A review of its relationship to other health status measures is included.

Part IV reports advances in the development of short-form measures. Chapter 16 introduces advances in developing short-form multi-item health scales and illustrates the use of those measures in assessing the health of the general U.S. population. Finally, in chapter 17 a newly developed set of single-item general measures of six health concepts is described and their use in patient populations is illustrated.

Part V begins with an explanation of empirical methods for validating health measures generally and the MOS measures specifically (chapter 18). Chapter 19 illustrates the logic of construct validity for the purposes of improving understanding of how to interpret scores for MOS health measures. The introduction to part V condenses journal articles, previously published in *The Journal of the American Medical Association (JAMA)*, that illustrate clinical applications of MOS measures, namely, comparing the burden of chronic medical and psychiatric conditions.

Part VI presents a recommended core set of MOS measures of functioning and well-being and summarizes findings about their use and interpretation. Chapter 20 summarizes the MOS measures and discusses their similarities and differences relative to other widely used health surveys. The appendix provides copies of the two survey questionnaires discussed in part III.

The audience for the book might include health investigators, policymakers, physicians, nurses, behavioral and social scientists, and students in health disciplines. Parts of the text are directed to clinical investigators, both those interested in using survey measures of patient outcomes for evaluating drugs, technology, and other interventions and those interested in evaluating general health benefits. Other parts are directed to the health practitioner who wishes to apply health assessment in daily clinical practice. Managers of health care systems and policymakers concerned about the quality and cost of care could also benefit from the book.

The MOS has been sponsored by grants from the private sector, including three foundations active in improving health care in America: the Henry J. Kaiser Family Foundation, The Robert Wood Johnson Foundation, and the Pew Charitable Trusts. The MOS has also been

supported by agencies in the public sector, including the Agency for
Health Care Policy and Research, the National Institute on Aging, and
the National Institute of Mental Health. Additionally, The RAND
Corporation and the New England Medical Center have supported the
MOS from their research funds. Grant support to date has been roughly
evenly divided between the public and private sectors. The total financial support equals approximately fourteen million dollars.

Planning for the MOS began in summer 1981, under the leadership
of Alvin R. Tarlov, M.D., then a physician at the Department of
Medicine at the University of Chicago and now at the Health Institute,
New England Medical Center, Boston. The multidisciplinary planning
team included Edward Perrin, PH.D., a statistician from the Department of Health Services Research at the University of Washington; John
E. Ware, Jr., PH.D., a psychometrician, then at The RAND Corporation, Health Sciences Program, and now at the Health Institute; Mi-
chael Zubkoff, PH.D., an economist at Dartmouth Medical School;
and Eugene Nelson, PH.D., a health services researcher at the Hospital
Corporation of America in Nashville, Tennessee. In 1984, John E.
Ware, Jr., became the principal investigator. He was joined by Sheldon
Greenfield, M.D., an internist and health services researcher from the
University of California at Los Angeles (UCLA) and The RAND Corporation, who became the medical director of the MOS. Kenneth B. Wells,
M.D., a psychiatrist on staff at UCLA and The RAND Corporation and
a recognized expert in mental health services, became director of the
psychiatric component of the MOS. William H. Rogers, PH.D., a senior
statistician at The RAND Corporation, assumed responsibility for
sampling and general study design. Sandra H. Berry, PH.D., Director of
the RAND Survey Group, assumed responsibility for self-administered
survey data collection and Maureen Carney, M.S., assumed responsibility for health examination and face-to-face survey data collection.

Anita L. Stewart, PH.D., a social psychologist, then at The RAND
Corporation, and Cathy D. Sherbourne, PH.D., a sociologist at The
RAND Corporation, coordinated measurement development for base-
line surveys and longitudinal surveys, respectively. Other MOS staff
and consultants, who contributed to the success of the study but did not
author chapters, include: Audrey Burnam, PH.D., Marcia Daniels,
M.D., Toshi Hayashi, Sherrie H. Kaplan, PH.D., Willard G. Manning,
PH.D., Lynn Ordway, Judith Perlman, and Barbara Rose, PH.D.

Several committees provided project oversight. The Clinical Liaison
Committee, which assisted with the recruitment of participating clini-

cians, included representatives; Robert McGinnis, M.D., and Claudene Clinton, PH.D., from the American Academy of Family Physicians; Robert Haggerty, M.D., and Janet Perloff, PH.D., from the American Academy of Family Physicians, and Gretchen Fleming, PH.D.; Boy Frame, M.D., and Robert Moser, M.D., from the American College of Physicians; Steven Sharfstein, M.D., Harold Pincus, M.D., and Boris Astrachan, M.D., from the American Psychiatric Association; and Gary VandenBos, PH.D., from the American Psychological Association.

The Clinical Advisory Committee, which assisted in designing the study and implementing data collection in office practices, included family physicians David Frechette, M.D., and William Gillanders, M.D.; internists Edwin Overholt, M.D., and Robert Tyson, M.D.; pediatricians Birt Harvey, M.D., and Lawrence Nazarian, M.D.; psychiatrists Steven Green, M.D., and Ronald Mintz, M.D.; and psychologist Gary VandenBos, PH.D.

Technical advisory committees formed by the sponsoring foundations included: Jeremiah Barondess, M.D., Mark Blumberg, M.D., Theodore Cooper, M.D., David Cornfeld, M.D., Karen Davis, PH.D., Howard Freeman, PH.D., John Geyman, M.D., Benjamin King, PH.D., Harold Luft, PH.D., Herbert Pardes, M.D., Steven Schroeder, M.D., Anne Scitovsky, M.A., Walter Spitzer, M.D., and Gail Wilensky, PH.D. Lewin and Associates assisted in selecting study sites.

Participating HMOs also helped in the Medical Outcomes Study, including Charles G. Hertz, M.D., and William Rollow, M.D., of the ANCHOR Organization for Health Maintenance in Chicago; B. Ross Landess, M.D., from the CIGNA Healthplans of Southern California; and Stephen Schoenbaum, M.D., and Donald M. Berwick, M.D., of the Harvard Community Healthplan in Boston. Local medical societies and representatives of various mental health specialty professional associations assisted with the recruitment of clinicians in other group and solo practices at each site.

Invaluable to the preparation of this book was the editorial work of Marie Kirchner Stone, PH.D., and the assistance of Kathleen Clark, who coordinated the production of the manuscript, including management and presentation of the numerous tables and materials. The Henry J. Kaiser Family Foundation contributed directly to the preparation of this book through funding of Dr. Stewart to supervise preparation of the initial draft of the book and through funding for professional editing of the book.

Administrative support to the MOS was also provided by Sandra Blau and Mary Anderson. The secretarial support of Irene Hayes, Nelie Gill, Patti Thompson, Kim Wong, Patrick Henderson, and Rebecca Voris is also appreciated.

Last, but not least, we acknowledge the time and effort of over 523 physicians and health care providers and over 22,000 of their patients. They were asked to do something very different, to tell us what life is like as a patient and about the outcomes of their medical care in terms of their functioning and well-being.

I

The New Era of Health

Assessment

1. Measures for a New Era of Health Assessment

John E. Ware, Jr.

A Change in Emphasis

During the past decade, one of the more important developments in the health care field has been recognition of the centrality of the patient's point of view in monitoring the quality of medical care outcomes (Geigle and Jones, 1990). A medical outcome has come to mean the extent to which a change in a patient's functioning or well-being meets that patient's needs or expectations. This sentiment was well expressed in the medical literature much earlier in this century (Codman, 1914; Lembcke, 1952). Nearly forty years ago, Lembcke wrote: "The best measure of quality is not how well or how frequently a medical service is given, but how closely the result approaches the fundamental objectives of prolonging life, relieving distress, restoring function and preventing disability." More recently, these objectives have been echoed by those arguing that the goal of medical care for most patients is the achievement of a more effective life (McDermott, 1981) and the preservation of functioning and well-being (Cluff, 1981; Schroeder, 1987; Tarlov, 1983; American College of Physicians, 1988; Ellwood, 1988). Although the patient is the best source of information regarding the achievement of these goals, information from patients about their experiences of disease and treatment has not been routinely collected in clinical research or medical practice. Since this information is not a part of the medical record, it is unavailable for analysis in the current health care database.

In the new era which America is now entering, information about functioning, well-being, and other important health outcomes is being added to the health databases. This information is being used by policy analysts, who compare the costs and benefits of competing ways of organizing and financing health care services, and by managers of health care organizations, who seek to produce the best value for each health care dollar. It is also utilized by clinical investigators evaluating new treatments and technologies, and practicing physicians and other providers trying to achieve the best possible patient outcomes. The primary source of new information on health outcomes is rapidly becoming standardized patient surveys and other measurement tools that have been serving research effectively during the past decade.

Several advances in methods for assessing patient perspectives about functioning, well-being, and other important health care outcomes have been presented during the past decade. These advances have been the subject of numerous conferences (Wenger, Mattson, Furberg, et al., 1984; Lohr and Ware, 1987; Katz, 1987; Lohr, 1989). Some significant advances are an improved understanding of the major dimensions of health and the validity of specific measurement scales in relation to those dimensions (Hays and Stewart, 1990; Ware, Brook, Davies, et al., 1981; Liang, 1986); demonstration of the usefulness of standardized health surveys in clinical trials (Croog, Levine, Testa, et al., 1986; Fowler, Wennberg, Timothy, et al., 1988; Bombardier, Ware, Russell, 1986); health policy evaluations (Patrick, Bush, and Chen, 1973; Brook, Ware, Rogers, et al., 1983; Ware, Brook, Rogers, et al., 1986); general population health surveys (Bergner, Bobbitt, Carter, and Gilson, 1981; Stewart, Hays, and Ware, 1988, 1989; Ware, Brook, Rogers, et al., 1986); and medical practice (Nelson and Berwick, 1989). Until now, it has been impractical to use most of these assessment methods on a large-scale basis. Questions remain regarding the appropriateness of these methods for use among patients with chronic conditions and for patients in all age ranges.

The Improvement of Health Status Surveys

The use of standardized surveys to assess functioning and well-being can be traced back over 300 years. Methodologic interest, however, has been greatest during the last half of this century (Katz, Ford, and Moskowitz, 1963). Most health measures used prior to the 1970s were not based upon methods of scale construction. The psychometric techniques of scale construction, now more widely used in the health field, have been available for most of the past century (Thurstone, 1928; Likert, 1932; Guttman, 1944). In the past fifty years, psychometric techniques have been used successfully in constructing numerous health status scales (DiCocco and Apple, 1958; Williams and Lindern, 1976; Ware, 1976; Berki and Ashcraft, 1979; Dupuy, 1969).

Not only the techniques but also the content of measures have changed. The earlier focus of measures was limited to the presence or absence of negative health states, functional limitations, symptoms of disease, and acute and chronic problems. Some health measures still focus exclusively on the latter negative content (Kaplan, 1989). During the last half of this century, the changing content of published measures of functioning and well-being has been well documented (Stewart, Ware, and Brook, 1978; Ware et al., 1978; Ware, Johnston, Davies-Avery, et al., 1979; Wenger, Mattson, Furberg, et al., 1984; McDowell and Newell, 1987).

One of the most extensive applications of psychometric theory and methods to the development and refinement of health status surveys took place during the Health Insurance Experiment (HIE) (Brook, Ware, Rogers, et al., 1983; Ware et al., 1986; Valdez, Ware, Manning, et al., 1989). The goal in the HIE was to construct the best possible scales for measuring a broad array of functioning and well-being concepts for nonaged adults and for children. That work was summarized in an eight-volume set of RAND technical reports and in *Medical Care* (Brook, Ware, Davies-Avery, et al., 1979; Eisen and Grob, 1979; Eisen, Donald, Ware, et al., 1980). The HIE clearly demonstrated the potential of scales constructed from self-administered surveys as reliable and valid tools for assessing changes in health status for both adults and children in the general population. The HIE left two basic questions unanswered: can methods of data collection and scale construction such as those used in the HIE work in sicker and older populations? and can more efficient scales be constructed? The answer to these questions was the challenge for the Medical Outcomes Study (MOS).

The MOS provided the opportunity for a large-scale test of the feasibility of self-administered patient questionnaires and generic health scales for adults with chronic conditions, including the elderly. For each of twelve major health concepts, the task of constructing MOS scales began with the choice of selecting or adapting available survey questionnaire items rather than constructing new items and scales. The options and the theoretical and methodological issues were unique to each of the conceptual areas: physical, role, and social functioning; mental health; physical symptoms; health perceptions and energy/ fatigue; sleep; and pain.

The MOS surveys, like the HIE surveys, were based on a multidimensional model of health. These patient surveys are comprehensive, assessing a breadth of physical and mental functioning and well-being outcomes. The more than three dozen scales, identified in part III, that were constructed for the MOS represent components of twelve major health concepts and various levels of aggregation across scales.

In the MOS, assessments of the most frequently studied and important health concepts are advanced in several different ways. Some new health concepts represent attempts to fill in gaps in the HIE surveys and in the field in general (chapters 10, 11, and 14). For other health concepts, the focus of measurement changes to distinguish better the impact of physical versus mental conditions (chapter 12). For still other health concepts, the choice among MOS measures follows traditional practices, such as pain measures in studies of arthritis, functional status in studies of rehabilitation medicine, and measures of psychological distress in studies of psychiatric disorders. For the six important health concepts, the MOS is testing a family of measures, ranging from the simplest and shortest single questionnaire item to a full-length multi-item scale.

The core set of MOS health measures is referred to as generic because it assesses health concepts that represent basic human values and are relevant to everyone's health status and well-being (Ware, 1987; 1990). These measures are called generic not only because they are universally valued but also because they are not specific for any one age, disease, or treatment group. Generic health measures assess health-related quality of life outcomes, namely, those known to be most directly affected by disease and treatment.

The standardized patient survey of generic health concepts is one of the key features of the MOS for monitoring the results of care. Prior to the MOS, a comprehensive array of generic functioning and well-being measures had not been shown to be suitable for use across diverse populations and health care settings. As a result, the opportunity to describe differences in functioning and well-being for the sick and the well was lost. Little was known about how patients suffering from one chronic medical or psychiatric condition differ from each other in terms of functioning and well-being. One noteworthy exception is the Sickness Impact Profile (Bergner, Bobbitt, Carter, and Gilson, 1981). The

MOS generic health measures provide a common yardstick to compare those patients with chronic health problems with those sampled from the general population (chapters 17 and 18).

The generic health measures are neither designed nor intended to serve as substitutes for traditional measures of clinical endpoints. To the contrary, the greatest advances in this field during the next decade are likely to come from studies that field generic health measures in parallel with clinical measures. The potential of such comparisons is illustrated in the profiles of functioning and well-being for MOS patients with different medical and psychiatric conditions and in contrast to the general U.S. population (part V). These comparisons serve at least two important purposes. The comparisons test the validity of generic scales in describing groups of patients known to differ in functioning and well-being. These comparisons also facilitate under-standing among clinicians of the meaning of differences in generic functioning and well-being concepts because these diagnostic groups are familiar to them. The MOS also documents the widespread impact of chronic disease and the kinds of revelations possible when the same comprehensive assessment of generic health concepts is used to compare different medical and psychiatric conditions (part V).

For all health concepts, a new standard of evaluation is being applied. The MOS is evaluating the relative choices among the measures in terms of their performance judged by formal tests using clinical criteria. The external criteria for evaluation of these concepts includes their validity in discriminating among diagnostic groups known to differ in morbidity and predictive tests of validity in relation to subse-quent utilization of health care resources.

New standards of measurement evaluation were necessary because the old standards addressed the wrong questions for the MOS ap-proach. Traditional tests typically show that longer measures are more reliable and more valid (Manning, Newhouse, and Ware, 1982). The best tests, however, are those most clearly approximating the intended use of the measure (Ware, 1990). The new direction in the assessment of outcomes calls for new standards formulated in answers to two ques-tions: which concepts should be measured? and how much measure-ment is enough for a particular purpose (McHorney, Ware, Rogers, et al., 1992)?

For the MOS, gains in measurement efficiency were necessary be-cause the same standardized questionnaires were administered to over 20,000 people in over 500 clinical practice settings and to over 2,000 people in a general population survey. As insight is gained regarding which generic health concepts are most important across purposes and populations and which scales prove to be most useful, attention can be focused on the construction of more efficient scales. Such scales can be enumerated from a subset of the best questionnaire items and with reduced respondent burden.

Considerations of respondent burden and of the costs of data collection caused rethinking of measurement goals and, accordingly, the criteria used in constructing and evaluating standardized health surveys. For a battery of health measures to excel in relation to traditional psychometric standards of reliability, validity, and precision is no longer adequate. The highest level of traditional psychometric standards is no longer the goal. Today's new opportunities to measure health status routinely and on a large scale demand the best compromise between traditionally defined psychometric elegance and the new standard of feasibility and practicality. The MOS attempted to achieve reductions in respondent burden without sacrificing measurement precision below the critical level. This reduction can be accomplished by constructing scales from more efficient items. In the HIE, for example, twenty-five items were necessary to define seven levels of physical functioning (Stewart, Ware, and Brook, 1978). The MOS Physical Functioning Scale required only ten questionnaire items to define twenty levels of functioning (chapter 7).

The MOS surveys and measurement scales are more practical because they are shorter than many in the field. Lengthier research tools served as a point of departure in developing a new generation of MOS short survey tools. The MOS tested short- and long-form measures that differed greatly in respondent time and in the cost of collecting and processing data. Users of MOS measures have choices among the health concepts they choose to measure and the precision of measurement for each concept.

The MOS survey and measurement scales are also practical because for the great majority of respondents, MOS surveys can be self-administered. The reliance on self-administration as the primary mode of data collection, even for surveys with more than 250 questions, was based in part on the successful use of relatively lengthy self-administered questionnaires in the HIE (Ware, Brook, Davies-Avery, et al., 1980). However, the MOS population was much older and much sicker than the HIE population. Half of those in the MOS longitudinal panel were aged sixty years or older, about 40% were eligible for

Medicare, and all suffered from one or more chronic conditions. Self-administered surveys were adopted on the strength of MOS pilot studies fielded before the formal MOS. Self-administration worked well using standard survey methods (chapter 4). Only rarely was a telephone interview or face-to-face interview necessary.

Applications of Health Surveys

Among the many potential applications of health surveys containing generic measures of patient functioning and well-being, four are pressing: (1) health care policy studies to evaluate alternatives for organizing and financing health care services; (2) clinical trials of new interventions and technology; (3) monitoring the health of the general population; and (4) clinical decision-making in medical practice.

The first application is pressing because the medical care system in the United States is being restructured to contain rising health care expenditures. Those implementing cost-containment strategies such as diagnosis-related groups (DRGs), prepaid health plans, preferred provider organizations, and professional review organizations have directed little attention to the effects of the strategies on patients. A policy of accountability is now leading policymakers to demand information about the effects of different cost-containment strategies on patient health outcomes (Tarlov, 1983; Ellwood, 1988; Roper, Winkenwerder, Hackbarth, et al., 1988). The MOS was designed specifically to explore the effects of cost containment on patient outcomes (Tarlov, Ware, Greenfield, et al., 1989), including a broad array of outcomes from the patient's point of view. This approach serves as a measurement model for the "effectiveness initiative" and for "outcomes management" (Roper, Winkenwerder, Hackbarth, et al., 1988; Ellwood, 1988). Both require a consideration of outcomes and a transition from a narrower set of clinical endpoints, traditionally measured for purposes of evaluating medical efficacy and treatment effectiveness, to the broader set of health outcome measures described in this book. The MOS approach represents a transition from measures of outcome in terms of biologic phenomena to human phenomena (Lohr, 1989).

The second pressing application of the health surveys is to evaluate clinical trials of new interventions and technology. Outcome standards, like those documented in the text, traditionally have not been used to evaluate alternate treatments and health care technologies. The effect of treatment on patient functioning or well-being has only rarely been thoroughly assessed, although there have been some noteworthy recent exceptions (e.g., Bombardier, Ware, Russell, 1986; Croog, Levine, Testa, et al., 1986; Fowler, Wennberg, Timothy, et al., 1988). It is increasingly becoming accepted that alternative treatment regimens and health care technologies in general should be evaluated in terms of their impact on patient functioning and well-being in addition to traditionally defined medical endpoints and their dollar costs (Chobanian, 1987). One reason for this position is that a treatment might represent a trade-off between an improvement of some clinical parameter and a decrement in quality of life. Another reason is that two drugs that are equally efficacious in terms of biologic functioning (e.g., blood pressure control) might differ in their impact on quality of life. A further reason is that new strategies for improving patient functioning and well-being are necessary to meet the needs and expectations of the American public.

A third application of the health survey is in monitoring the health of the general population, which cannot be well understood from analyses of treatment survival rates or from population mortality statistics. Survival rates, even when available by medical procedure, provide information about outcomes which can be misleading because the rates apply for only a minority of patients. For example, since 95–98% of patients who undergo heart surgery typically survive, rates of restoration of functioning and general well-being must be evaluated in addition to survival rates of competing systems of health care delivery. Population mortality statistics tell little about the health of the general population in well-developed countries (Elinson, 1984). Standardized measures of functioning and well-being like those described in this book could be relied upon for purposes of monitoring the health of the general population (National Center for Health Statistics, 1981). The resulting norms can, in turn, serve as benchmarks in interpreting health status data for specific groups.

A fourth application relates to clinical decision-making. Standardized health surveys have the potential to become the new "laboratory tests" of medical practice. At best, patient functioning, well-being, and other aspects of quality of life that are affected by disease and treatment are discussed informally during the medical history. Changes in functioning and well-being over time are not enumerated systematically as are other important clinical parameters. The American College of Physicians has called for the standardization of assessments of functional status and well-being in everyday medical practice (American College of Physicians, 1988). Such routine assessments would be useful in detecting and explaining decreased functional capacity, keeping track of changes in functioning over time, making it possible to consider the patient's total functioning better in choosing among therapies, guiding the efficient use of community resources and social services, and predicting more accurately the course of chronic disease. Patients and physicians cannot make informed choices between alternative treatments if the clinical and functional trade-offs involved are not well understood (Fowler, Wennberg, Timothy, et al., 1988). Only good data regarding the differences in functioning and well-being can inform these choices.

For the improvement of health practice numerous other applications have been suggested by others (e.g., American College of Physicians, 1988; Bergner and Rothman, 1987; Steinwachs, 1989; Ware, Brook, Davies, et al., 1981) such as for purposes of a needs assessment in areas where people need help, an assessment of the quality of care, an examination of the benefits of health promotion activities, and an evaluation of models of the predictors of optimal functioning and well-being. For many applications of importance, MOS measures are appropriate. For example, to promote optimal functioning and well-being, it is essential to understand better the factors that predict functioning and well-being, including social support, stressful life events, compliance, coping styles, will to function, health knowledge, exercise, smoking, body weight (and overweight), eating habits, and alcohol use. Health status measures can also be used to forecast the demand for health care services (Manning, Newhouse, and Ware, 1982; Ware, Manning, Duan, et al., 1984; Connelly, Philbrick, Smith, et al., 1989).

A major factor limiting the rate of progress with all of these applications has been the absence of general health measures that are easily administered and well documented. This book represents an attempt to bridge this gap.

2. The Medical Outcomes Study Framework of Health Indicators

Anita L. Stewart

The World Health Organization (WHO) defines health as "a state of complete physical, mental, and social well-being and not merely the absence of disease or infirmity" (WHO, 1948). Few attempts have been made to define physical, mental, or social well-being, making the WHO definition an outline utilized as a basis for many operational definitions or measures of health. The WHO definition calls attention to the multidimensionality of health (Ware, 1987). The multiple dimensions include not only the physical, mental, and social dimensions specified by the WHO, but also multiple types of indicators of those dimensions such as functioning, symptoms, emotional status, and various diagnoses.

Few would disagree with the dimensions of physical and mental health, but whether social health is equivalent conceptually to these two dimensions is controversial (Ware, 1986). Physical health pertains to the body, including anatomical, physical, and physiologic elements. Mental health, which pertains primarily to the mind, including emotional and intellectual components, can also pertain to other concepts such as perception of reality, self-awareness, integration of the personality, adjustment, range of interests, social effectiveness, and self-actualization (Bradburn, 1969; Dupuy, 1984; Endicott, Spitzer, et al., 1976; Jahoda, 1958; Taylor and Brown, 1988; Vaillant, 1977; Ware, Johnston, Davies-Avery, et al., 1979). Social health is usually defined in terms of people's ability to engage in normative social interactions or to function within the community (Greenblatt, 1976; Renne, 1974; Spitzer, 1987; Donald, Ware, Brook, et al., 1978). The MOS assumed two dimensions of health, physical and mental, and incorporated social functioning primarily as an indicator of those dimensions.

Indicators of Health

Many attempts have been made to organize specific health measures into a few conceptual categories or types of indicators, which can be considered as one way of identifying the multiple dimensions of health. Elinson is credited with the once popular "five D's": death, disease, disability, discomfort, and dissatisfaction (Sanazaro and Williamson, 1968). The Human Population Laboratory defines physical health in terms of energy level, symptoms, chronic conditions, impairments (sensory or loss of limb), disability, and perceptions of health in general (Breslow, 1972; Berkman and Breslow, 1983). In the Vital and Health Statistics series, the National Center for Health Statistics (1974) defines health in terms of acute conditions, chronic conditions, chronic activity limitations, chronic mobility limitations, physical impairments, physiological measurements, and psychological measurements. Jette provides a three-component scheme: symptoms/feeling states (not observable by others), observable signs, and performance or functioning (Jette, 1980).

Bergner defines five types of indicators: genetic foundation (basic structure on which other aspects of health status must build); biochemical/physiologic/anatomic condition (including disease states, whether obvious or not); functional condition (performance of usual activities of life, including social/role, physical, and cognitive performance); mental condition (mood, feelings, affect); and health potential (longevity, prognosis, functional potential) (Bergner, 1985). Ware defines six health concepts: physical functioning, mental health, social well-being, role functioning, general health perceptions, and symptoms (Ware, 1986).

Patrick and Elinson propose five categories (besides death): disease, physical well-being, psychological well-being, social well-being, and general quality of life (Patrick and Elinson, 1984). Liang suggests three major approaches: the physical definition or medical model, the functional model or social definition, and the psychological model or subjective evaluation (Liang, 1986). Starfield suggests six dimensions: resilience, achievement, disease, satisfaction (health perceptions), comfort (symptoms and feelings), activity, and longevity (Starfield, 1974).

The diversity of schemes is notable. Only one category, functioning or behavior, is included in all schemes. Most include a psychological category, only Bergner and Starfield include future indicators, and only Bergner includes genetic foundation.

Many schemes confuse the underlying theoretical dimensions of physical and mental health with the types of health indicators (Liang, 1986). For example, mental health is often given an equivalent status with functioning or symptoms. It would seem more useful to consider that symptoms or limitations in functioning could be indicative of either physical or mental health.

MOS Framework of Health Indicators

The MOS framework, taking these concerns into account, consists of five categories of indicators of physical and mental health: (1) clinical status, (2) physical functioning and well-being, (3) mental functioning and well-being, (4) social/role functioning and well-being, and (5) general health perceptions (Table 2–1). Functioning pertains to the ability to perform various daily activities and functions (e.g., walking, performing household tasks, working). Well-being refers to more subjective internal states not observable by others such as symptoms or feelings.

The MOS framework emphasizes that two important underlying or theoretical dimensions of health, physical and mental, can each be defined in terms of a wide variety of indicators or measures. Some specific MOS indicators primarily reflect physical health (e.g., physical functioning), others reflect primarily mental health (e.g., psychological distress), and still others reflect both physical and mental health (e.g., energy/fatigue, sleep problems).

The MOS framework reflects the decision to consider problems in social and role functioning as indicators of mental health problems such as feeling depressed as well as physical health problems. A third underlying dimension, social health, therefore, is not defined.

Clinical Status This category includes information on the presence and severity of various diseases or conditions, either chronic or acute (e.g., the presence of a virus, infection, or chronic heart condition, the severity of a psychosis). Impairments are also included. The National Center for Health Statistics defines impairments as chronic or permanent defects resulting from disease, injury, or congenital malformation (Jackson, 1973; Givens, 1979). The WHO (1980) defines impairments as abnormalities of body structure, organ function, or system function (such as visual and hearing loss, paralysis, and the absence of extremities). The clinical status category incorporates the WHO reference to

Table 2–1 The MOS Framework of Indicators of Physical and Mental Health

Category/Indicator	UNDERLYING DIMENSION	
	Physical Health	Mental Health
Clinical status		
Presence/severity of physical conditions and impairments	x	
Presence/severity of mental illness		x
Physical functioning and well-being		
Physical functioning	x	
Mobility	x	
Pain	x	
Energy/fatigue	x	x
Sleep problems	x	x
Physical/psychophysiologic symptoms	x	x
Mental functioning and well-being		
Cognitive functioning		x
Psychological distress		x
Depression/behavioral-emotional control		x
Anxiety		x
Psychological well-being		x
Positive affect		x
Feelings of belonging		x
Health distress	x	x
Social/role functioning and well-being		
Social activity limitations due to health[a]	x	x
Role limitations due to health	x	x
Role limitations due to physical health	x	
Role limitations due to emotional problems		x
Marital functioning[a]		
Family functioning[a]		
Sexual functioning[a]	x	x
General health perceptions and satisfaction		
Current health perceptions	x	x
Health outlook	x	x
Prior health	x	
Satisfaction with physical functioning	x	

Note: Each indicator is hypothesized to measure primarily physical health, primarily mental health, or both (indicated by an *x* in the appropriate column).
[a] Could also represent a social health factor—see text.

health as "the absence of disease or infirmity" (WHO, 1948) and includes most of the disease-specific indicators traditionally used to describe health. Such indicators comprise what has been referred to as the "medical model" of health (Engel, 1976). The term "clinical status," used because most of the information depends on clinical judgment, is nearly identical to physiologic health in the Health Insurance Experiment (Lohr, Kamberg, Keeler, et al., 1986) and similar to Bergner's biochemical/physiological/anatomic category. In addition to clinical signs, clinicians use information about patients' functioning, symptoms, and feelings to judge particular diagnoses. But the thing that distinguishes the clinical status category from the others and on which it partially depends is that such judgment requires a synthesis of information and that the pattern of elements fits some predetermined criteria for each condition.

Several well-known systems exist for classifying both physical and mental conditions and impairments according to specified criteria. The International Classification of Diseases (ICD) (U.S. Dept. of Health and Human Services, 1980) classifies both physical and mental disorders. The National Center for Health Statistics uses the ICD system to report on the prevalence of various acute and chronic conditions in their Series 10 (e.g., Ries, 1979). The American Psychiatric Association (1980) has developed a classification scheme for mental disorders, the Diagnostic and Statistical Manual (DSM-III), that is widely recognized. The World Health Organization has specified an international classification scheme of impairments, disabilities, and handicaps (WHO, 1980).

In the Health Insurance Experiment, operational definitions for the presence and severity of fifteen chronic conditions and impairments are provided based on patient reports and clinical assessments of a representative sample of a general population (Lohr, Kamberg, Keeler, et al., 1986).

An indicator used for designating hospital costs, the Diagnosis Related Groups (DRGs), classifies individuals being discharged from hospitals in terms of their disease or problem (Fetter, Shin, Freeman, et al., 1980; Thompson, Fetter, and Shin, 1978). Although groups are not diagnostically homogeneous, each DRG represents a group presumably requiring similar services from a hospital.

Diagnoses are made with varying levels of certainty, and different levels of severity can be defined within a diagnosis. Severity is typically defined in terms of signs and symptoms of a particular condition, which combine to form an indicator of the stage of the diagnosis, comorbidity, complications that develop in conjunction with a condition, and response to treatment (e.g., Horn, Sharkey, and Bertram, 1983; Gonella and Goran, 1975). Severity has also been defined in terms of functional levels (Goldman, Hashimoto, Cook, et al., 1981; Berman, Brook, Lohr, et al., 1981) and risk factors. Thus, severity definitions incorporate many types of indicators. In the Health Insurance Experiment, many indicators of chronic conditions incorporated both certainty and severity information into one indicator (e.g., Berman, Brook, Lohr, et al., 1981).

Physical Functioning and Well-Being Physical functioning and mobility are both clear indicators of physical health because they pertain to the body and because these limitations are most likely to be caused by physical health problems (Stewart, Ware, and Brook, 1982). The reason sleep problems are indicative of either physical or mental health is that both physical health problems and depression or anxiety cause sleep problems. Symptoms that are expressed physically can also indicate either physical or mental health problems. Some primarily indicate physical health (e.g., fever, sore throat). Others, psychophysiologic symptoms, can indicate either physical or mental health (e.g., fatigue, appetite loss, upset stomach). Pain is considered as mainly indicative of physical health because it is usually perceived in terms of a specific physical location. Fatigue has been regarded as primarily a component of physical health (Belloc, Breslow, and Hochstim, 1971) and as primarily a component of psychological well-being (McNair, Lorr, and Doppleman, 1971; Dupuy, 1984). However, Ware, Brook, and Davies-Avery (1980) found a measure of vitality (energy and fatigue) to be indicative of both physical and mental health.

Mental Functioning and Well-Being The category of mental functioning and well-being includes both cognitive and affective components, which are the most direct indicators of mental health. Cognitive functioning pertains to memory, concentration, perception, psychomotor ability, attention span, confusion, comprehension, problem solving and judgment, and orientation in time and space (Kane and Kane, 1981). Diagnosed cognitive disorders (e.g., Alzheimer's disease) are included in the clinical status category. Many people experience variations in confusion and forgetfulness, however, that are important to everyday functioning and well-being. These variations are what the MOS is interested in as part of the patient's perspective on functioning and well-being. Positive and negative affect have long been considered basic components of psychological well-being (Bradburn, 1969). Key dimensions of these include depression, anxiety, anger, positive affect, and feelings of belonging (Menninger, 1945; Dupuy, 1984; Jahoda, 1958; Ware, Johnston, Davies-Avery, et al., 1979; Bradburn, 1969). Psychological distress that is attributed specifically to health problems (e.g., worry about health) can be defined, in which case the distress may be indicative of physical health as well as mental health.

Although feelings of distress and well-being have typically been considered the core of mental health (Ware, Johnston, Davies-Avery, et al., 1979), there is some debate as to whether the occurrence of more positive and fewer negative feelings should be considered as indicative of better mental health. Feelings are often a product of the environment (Kane and Kane, 1981). Because life presents countless opportunities to feel appropriately anxious or depressed, the absence of anxiety and depression should not necessarily be a sign of mental health (Vaillant, 1977; Jahoda, 1958). However, psychological distress for whatever reason can lead people to seek help from the medical care system and is a relevant component of the MOS definition of health because reduction of distress is one goal of health care.

Social/Role Functioning and Well-Being Limitations in the ability to perform daily social and role activities because of health problems have long been considered health indicators. The National Center for Health Statistics' measure of activities limitations has been widely used for decades. This category of indicators is one in which the social consequences of diagnosed conditions and of problems in physical and mental functioning and well-being become the indicators of health.

Because social/role functioning can be affected by many things other than health, to use this functioning as a health indicator necessitates defining limitations that are due to health or to a particular condition. Bergner, Bobbitt, Carter, and Gilson (1981) refer to this as "health-related" dysfunction. One problem with attributing limitations to health is that a health-related cause might be unclear to the individual (e.g., a person may not know that an underlying health problem is causing sexual problems). Also, if the problem is due to a side effect of a treatment (e.g., impotence caused by antihypertensive medications), people might not attribute the problem to their health. Thus, in some instances it is preferable to define functioning per se without asking for a health attribution. Not obtaining one, however, can be an even bigger problem, because a concept might be defined that contains information on much more than health, making it less valid as a health indicator.

Limitations in social and role activities can be caused by both physical and mental health problems, in contrast to most physical functioning limitations, which are likely to be caused only by physical health problems. For example, problems working or interacting socially can be caused by such mental health problems as depression. Social and role limitations due to mental health problems, therefore, can be considered an indicator of mental health. The MOS approach to assessing social/role functioning and well-being is focused on health-related limitations, including limitations due to emotional problems.

By defining physical or mental health in terms of limitations in role and/or social functioning, information on social well-being as specified in the WHO definition of health can be incorporated. That is, if physical or mental conditions are interfering with a person's role or social functioning, this is important information about health. However, in this approach, limitations in social functioning not caused by health problems are not defined as health.

The MOS measures of marital and family functioning are not considered indicators of either physical or mental health. If the MOS had hypothesized an underlying dimension of social health, this type of measure could represent that dimension. Although social functioning problems are not considered indicators of mental health, such problems are commonly treated by mental health specialists. Thus, the line between mental health and social functioning is unclear.

General Health Perceptions and Satisfaction Perceptions of health are personal judgments and evaluations of one's own health status. Health perceptions are one way information about different components such as disease, functioning, symptoms, and feelings can be integrated. Such perceptions reflect actual physical and mental health as well as the person's values, cultural background, and personal beliefs about what constitutes health. People's own experience of their health might be discordant with their "objective" diseases, symptoms, or functioning. Because people value various aspects of health differently, some feel "healthy" in the face of a chronic disease or other health problems, and others feel "sick" without any disease or illness. How people perceive their own health is as important as the other indicators, because it is how they think about health that makes them decide whether or not to stay home from work or to visit a doctor.

What can be even more important than people's self-reports of their levels of health is whether they are satisfied with their health status. One person may be satisfied with a level of health which another person would be dissatisfied with. For example, a person with no interest in participating in vigorous sports might be completely satisfied with a level of physical functioning that does not allow such participation. Thus, people's preferences for different health states are an important additional component of health status that can be assessed.

Positive Health

The WHO definition emphasizes the importance of defining health in terms of positive states, not simply the absence of disease and infirmity. Dubos (1965) considers the concept of perfect and positive health a "utopian creation of the human mind," a point toward which medical science can chart its course but not a state or goal that anyone should expect to attain. Dubos suggests that positive health is a moving target, and that over time people have become "less willing to accept the infirmities, pains, and blemishes, the catarrhs, coughs, and nauseas that used to be regarded as inevitable accompaniments of life." Herzlich (1973) suggests that when one is in good health, health is not thought about; health is essentially an "unawareness" of the body. Herzlich probably agrees that positive health can be defined as the absence of problems or limitations. Twaddle (1974) suggests that there is a range of less than perfect health which is considered normal or at least acceptable to the individual. Hinkle (1961, cited in Dolfman, 1973) notes that even the healthiest people sometimes have colds and accidents or become anxious or depressed. Thus, healthy people simply have less disease or illness than unhealthy people.

If, as presented in the framework, we accept that health includes not only concepts of clinical status but also concepts of how people feel, function, and think about their health, and if we determine that a person has no disease, feels fine, has no limitations in functioning, and thinks he or she is healthy, is positive health defined? Must the definition extend into yet more positive states such as feeling vital, joyful, and energetic, or functioning extraordinarily well? What if a person is functioning poorly physically but feeling well (e.g., the wheelchair-bound paraplegic happy with work and family)? Two major questions regarding the meaning of positive health are posed: how positive do definitions have to be before well-being or positive health are defined? and must a person be at the extreme "healthy" end of all indicators to achieve positive health?

Because of the multidimensional nature of health, it might be more important to define positive health separately for each individual component or indicator of health. Each type of indicator has a different approach to defining positive health. The most positive state defined by each type of indicator in general is summarized in the list below.

Clinical status	Absence of conditions, impairments
Physical functioning and well-being	Absence of physical limitations Absence of symptoms, pain Absence of sleep problems No difficulty doing strenuous activities Presence of energy, pep
Mental functioning and well-being	Absence of cognitive problems Absence of psychological distress Presence of psychological well-being
Social/role functioning and well-being	Absence of health-related limitations Absence of sexual problems Presence of good family functioning
General health perceptions and satisfaction	Positive health perceptions Satisfaction with physical abilities

For some types of indicators, the optimal condition is the absence of problems; for others, more positive states can be defined. One could argue that we are simply perpetuating the medical model, viewing health as the absence of problems, and only adding some dimensions on which to look at problems. However, if the practice of medicine could be advanced to focus on achieving the breadth of positive health status defined by the MOS indicators, giant steps will have been taken.

A Single Health Indicator

There is a continual demand and search for summary indicators of overall health (Berg, 1973; Bergner, 1985; Chen and Bryant, 1975). Such an overall index would have to represent some composite or integration of physical and mental health dimensions across all types of indicators. How to combine information across health concepts has been addressed (Ware, 1984; Kaplan and Anderson, 1987), but presents many problems. For example, how can an overall health score be assigned to a person with a serious chronic disease, such as diabetes, who feels well and functions as a productive person with no role or social limitations? Any method of doing so requires understanding the different values or preferences of the individuals for different health states (Bergner, 1985; Bush, Anderson, Kaplan, et al., 1982).

Although some operational definitions of health are intended to capture overall health (e.g., health perceptions), they do so only partially. For example, the common item "How would you rate your health in general?" is intended to capture people's own overall evaluation of their health, but can only reflect their subjective experience, taking into account their own values and preferences. It cannot adequately reflect the entire framework of concepts.

Sullivan (National Center for Health Statistics, 1966) describes an idea proposed by Sanders (1962) concerning a type of aggregate index. Sanders suggested an index of the number of years in which the person fulfilled the appropriate social role requirements, which he referred to as effective life years. This idea has been refined into the concept of "quality adjusted life years" in which information on length and quality of life are combined (Kaplan and Anderson, 1987; Weinstein and Stason, 1977; Weinstein, 1980). However, such an index should be used with caution because its derivation and limitations are not fully understood (Smith, 1987).

Conclusions Regarding the Framework

The types of indicators interrelate and affect one another. The clinical judgment of physicians and mental health specialists may be influenced by patients' functioning and well-being. How people perceive their health depends on their clinical status, functioning, and well-being. Similarly, their functioning depends on their clinical status and feeling states. Thus all of the indicators combine to define the underlying constructs of physical and mental health.

Mental health indicators are underrepresented in many of the general approaches to assessing health, perhaps because most health assessment studies have been primarily concerned with the description of physical health, and most evaluation studies have been concerned with the evaluation of medical care rather than mental health care.

Mental health is increasingly considered an essential part of health; mental health care is beginning to be evaluated in terms of outcomes in the same way that medical care has been. The definition of mental health will need to become more sophisticated in response to these changes. For example, the inclusion of a measure of self-esteem, which could be considered an important outcome of mental and nonmental health care, might be the first to be added. Some have already included self-esteem in their health definitions (Parkerson, Gehlbach, Wagner, et al., 1981). The addition of more indicators of mental health for the purposes of evaluating mental health care may require the incorporation of social health or social functioning as a third dimension, which we rejected for this study. Social functioning for such purposes would include all limitations in social functioning whether or not they were caused by health problems. This would take into account the fact that many general definitions of mental health pertain to social adjustment. For example, people's ability to get along with others would be an extremely relevant outcome of mental health care for people with chronic mental disorders.

MOS Concepts of Functioning and Well-Being

Table 2–2 presents the definitions and operational strategy for the twelve major MOS concepts of functioning and well-being and indicates the chapter describing the measures of each concept.

Table 2–2 Definitions and Operational Strategies for Twelve Major Concepts of Functioning and Well-Being Assessed in the Medical Outcomes Study

Concept	Chapter	Definition	Operational Strategy
Physical functioning	6	Performance of physical activities such as self-care, walking, climbing stairs, and vigorous activities	Extent of limitations in physical activities due to poor health; satisfaction with physical abilities
Mobility	6	Getting around in the community	Need for help in getting around; confinement to the house

Table 2–2 (*Cont.*)

Concept	Chapter	Definition	Operational Strategy
Role functioning	12	Performance of usual role activities such as working at a job, housework, child care, community activities, and volunteer work	Limitations in role activities (such as took frequent rests, had difficulty, or accomplished less than wanted) due to physical health and to emotional problems; inability to work or do housework due to health
Social functioning	9–11	Functioning in normal social activities with family, friends, neighbors; marital functioning; sexual problems	Limitations in social activities due to health problems; changes in social activities due to changes in health. Satisfaction with marital functioning; general family functioning; extent of sexual problems
Psychological distress/well-being	7	Positive and negative psychological states including anxiety, depression, behavioral-emotional control, loneliness, positive affect, feelings of belonging	Frequency and intensity of psychological states
Cognitive functioning	7	Cognitive problems such as forgetfulness, difficulty concentrating	Frequency of cognitive problems
Health perceptions	8	Personal evaluations of health in general including current and prior health, health outlook, resistance to illness	Extent of agreement with evaluative statements about health
Health distress	8	Psychological distress due to health	Frequency of feelings of distress due to health
Energy/fatigue	8	Feelings of energy, pep, fatigue, tiredness	Frequency of feelings of energy/fatigue
Sleep	14	Quantity, disturbance, adequacy of sleep	Frequency of sleep problems; average amount of sleep; ratings of adequacy of sleep
Pain	13	Subjective feelings of bodily distress or discomfort such as headaches or backaches	Severity of pain in general; extent to which pain affects daily activities and mood
Physical/psychophysiologic symptoms	15	Subjective perceptions about the internal state of the body, such as stiffness and coughing	Frequency of general (non-disease-specific) physical and psychophysiologic symptoms

II

Creation of Databases on the Health of Individuals

The two chapters that comprise part II describe the collection of health data on the individuals who make up the MOS. Part II also describes the respondent composition, burden, and cooperation. Many data collection instruments were administered to the MOS respondents; for most of these, only general information is provided. For two instruments, the Initial Screening Form by Patients and the Patient Assessment Questionnaire, descriptions are provided in greater detail because they are the source of data for the health measures described in this book.

Chapter 4 describes the survey methods of data collection, including short screening forms administered to patients in doctors' offices and questionnaires that were mailed to respondents. Respondent burden and lessons learned about how to gain cooperation from both the patient and the provider are also discussed in terms of the problems and the solutions. The problems and solutions are applicable to many large-scale studies.

Chapter 3 discusses the sampling goals and methods. The selection of study sites and systems of care as well as some characteristics of the providers in solo and small group practices, multispecialty groups, and health maintenance organizations are described. A description of the representation of provider specialties is also presented. An important feature of the MOS sampling strategy was the selection of patients for follow-up according to the tracer conditions: hypertension, diabetes, depression, and heart disease as defined by a recent myocardial infarction or congestive heart failure.

3. Methods of Sampling

_William H. Rogers, Elizabeth A. McGlynn,
Sandra H. Berry, Eugene C. Nelson, Edward Perrin,
Michael Zubkoff, Sheldon Greenfield,
Kenneth B. Wells, Anita L. Stewart,
Sharon B. Arnold, and John E. Ware, Jr._

Goals of Sampling

The sample design for the MOS responded to multiple and sometimes competing needs. The study had a large cross-sectional component designed to fulfill multiple purposes: to describe the impact of chronic diseases on patient functioning, to estimate selection effects by describing case-mix differences across clinician specialty groups and systems of care, and to describe the style of care of study clinicians. The longitudinal panel study was designed to describe changes in health status over time and to explain these and other outcomes in terms of system of care, provider specialty, style of practice, and other factors that influence utilization of health care resources.

In implementing the design, it was necessary to find a balance between the most generalizable sample to maximize external validity and cases that best met tracer condition criteria in order to allow a comparison of outcomes over time. Additional design considerations included obtaining patient and provider cooperation and maintaining it over time and the cost of including cases of various kinds in the sample.

Overview of Sampling Methods

The basic sample design for the MOS involved a five-stage process: (1) identification of appropriate geographic sites in which to conduct the study; (2) selection of health maintenance organizations (HMOs) and

multispecialty group practices (MSGS) within those sites; (3) selection
of physicians and other providers within each practice type; (4) selection of patients within those practices for the cross-sectional survey;
and (5) selection of patients for the longitudinal panel. Patients were
selected for a cross-sectional survey during an office visit to a study
clinician. Those patients eligible for the longitudinal portion of the
study, determined from information on the cross-sectional survey, were
interviewed by telephone, and those who met further eligibility criteria
were asked to participate in the panel. Respondents who accepted and
completed the baseline instruments comprised the baseline sample
pool. Because the baseline sample pool was larger than was needed for
the longitudinal analysis, the final panel was sampled from the pool.

Stages One and Two: Selection of Sites and Group Practices

The sampling unit for sites was Standard Metropolitan Statistical Areas
(SMSAS) because they are designed to represent different economic
market areas. SMSAS with mature forms of the three systems of care
were identified. The 1984 InterStudy HMO Census and the Membership Directory of the Medical Group Management Association
(MGMA) were used to identify sites with the systems of care of interest.
Initially, sixty sites were considered, thirty were evaluated, and twelve
were judged acceptable. The four major criteria for site selection were:
geographic diversity; presence of an HMO with a minimum of 100,000
enrollees and in operation at least three years; presence of MSGs with at
least ten physicians, in operation at least three years, and a mixture of
prepayment and fee-for-service; and willingness of HMOs and MSGs to
participate in the study.

The original intent was to include a rural site in the study, but the
forms of organized medical practices in the rural areas were substantially different from those found in major metropolitan areas. The
inclusion of a rural site would have reduced the possibility of a
meaningful combined-sites analysis. The MOS could not afford to
include a rural site with sufficient numbers of physicians and patients to
analyze separately.

The Medical Group Management Association membership directory and information obtained by the MOS on other MSGs in each of the
sites was used to identify appropriate groups. These groups were

arrayed on two key MSG dimensions: number of providers and percent-age of prepayment. MSGs were selected that had patients with both fee-for-service and prepaid insurance arrangements and that were of moderate to large size. The average group size was forty clinicians. The minimum group size considered was ten members. In all sites, more than one MSG was asked to participate. Health maintenance organiza-tions were chosen to provide diversity in markets served and organiza-tional structure. The three first-choice HMOs agreed to participate.

Stage Three: Selection of Clinicians

To ensure that each system was adequately represented, the process of identifying and enrolling clinicians differed slightly by system of care. Clinicians were selected in the specialties of family practice, general internal medicine, cardiology, endocrinology, psychiatry, and clinical psychology because they treat the MOS tracer conditions: hyperten-sion, diabetes, heart disease (recent myocardial infarction or congestive heart failure), and depression. HMO providers also included nurse practitioners and master's-level mental health providers, because they are responsible for patient care in that setting. Physicians were required to be between the ages of thirty-one and fifty-five; board certified, board eligible, or (in clinical psychiatry) licensed for independent practice in their specialty; primarily involved in office-based patient care; and primarily in nongovernmental practice (e.g., not employed by the Veterans Administration or military). In addition to these criteria, clinicians who had been in their current practice location at least one year and who had a sufficiently large patient panel to make sampling efficient were preferred. Clinicians with a large non-English-speaking patient load were excluded because the survey instruments were only available in English. The major purpose of these eligibility criteria was to ensure the enrollment of comparable clinicians who were likely to be treating patients with the MOS tracer conditions and to facilitate meaningful specialty comparisons in the fee-for-service system.

Selecting Solo and Small Group Practitioners For the purpose of sampling, a small group was defined as having seven or fewer clinicians practicing together. Three sources of information were used to identify solo and small group providers in the three sites: (1) a sample of physicians who appeared to meet MOS criteria from the AMA Masterfile; (2) a list of board-certified family practitioners from the American Academy of Family Practice; and (3) a list of licensed clinical psychologists from the American Psychological Association. The actual sample frame was constructed to exclude clinicians known to practice in HMOs or in large MSGs. From the remainder, a subsample practicing in the same zip codes or in demographically similar nearby zip codes as the enrolled HMOs or MSGs were selected.

Selecting HMO and MSG Clinicians In the HMOs and MSGs, the upper level management was contacted to obtain their cooperation in participating in the MOS. The HMO or MSG then provided the MOS with a list of eligible clinicians based on the inclusion criteria discussed above. Eligible clinicians were contacted and enrolled individually by MOS field representatives. A major difference between the providers enrolled in the HMOs and those enrolled in the solo practices is the inclusion of mid-level providers in the HMO sample (e.g., nurse practitioners).

Representativeness of MOS Clinicians Obtaining the cooperation of individual clinicians, especially in the fee-for-service sector, was critical for the MOS. Very high participation rates are taken as prima facie evidence that a study has achieved a representative sample. Another indicator of representativeness is the similarity of those who participated and those who did not along key dimensions of interest.

The multistep approach for solo and small group practices was designed to build a workable, long-term relationship with the clinicians. After the demanding data requirements were explained to them (and also for other reasons), many elected to drop out at various stages.

It is difficult to calculate a response rate for fee-for-service providers that accurately reflects the proportion who accepted an invitation to participate because enrollment was explored in stages. Some clinicians who refused at an early stage to participate might well have been ineligible had they accepted. Further, not all eligible providers were asked to participate because quotas were established for each specialty and enrollment was discontinued when the quota was met. A participation rate can be reported at each stage and compared with rates from similar research. Assessed in this way, the MOS compares favorably. The multiplicative effect of nonparticipation across stages means, however, that only about one-third of the fee-for-service providers identified as eligible and asked to participate actually did so.

In the HMOs and MSGs, where the method of enrollment differed substantially and the number of steps to enrollment was reduced, the participation rates for the eligible providers were much higher (67% for

MSGS, 87% for HMOs). By collecting data about the providers at several steps, the MOS had the opportunity to evaluate possible bias at later steps using the data from earlier steps. The HMO and MSG clinicians are likely to be representative because of the high participation rates. For solo and small group practices, where participation rates were lower, refusal to proceed was not related to practice characteristics available to us, except for specialty.

Representativeness of Solo and Small Group Practitioners From an initial sample of 2,216 potentially eligible solo clinicians, 1,373 (62%) ten-minute screening interviews were completed. In comparison, Gunn and Rhodes (1981) obtained a 58% response rate for a thirty-minute telephone interview of physicians without incentive payments. Berk and Meyers (1980) reported a 66% response rate for a fifteen-minute telephone interview with physicians as part of the National Medical Care Expenditures Survey.

Across the three sites, 41.7% of providers in Los Angeles refused to participate, 36.8% in Boston, and 40.1% in Chicago. Based on the data on background characteristics from the AMA Masterfile, the clinicians who were not interviewed (nonrespondents) had similar demographic characteristics to the clinicians who completed the interview (Table 3–1).

With respect to specialty, however, there were some differences in response rates. The most important difference was that psychologists were much more likely to participate than physicians. About 80% of the psychologists completed the interview compared with about 42% of the cardiologists, 57% of the general internists, 59% of the family practitioners, 63% of the psychiatrists, and 64% of the endocrinologists.

Of the 1,373 providers who completed telephone interviews, 895 (65%) were determined to be eligible. Of the 895 eligible clinicians, 709

Table 3–1 Characteristics of Clinician Selection Survey Respondents/Nonrespondents

Characteristic	Respondents (N = 1,373)	Nonrespondents (N = 843)
Mean Age	40.3	40.0
Female (%)	16.8	13.3
Foreign medical graduate (%)	25.9	24.5

(79%) were contacted by local physician leaders in their community ("encouragers"). The remaining 186 (21%) either could not be contacted or were not approached because their specialty quota had been met.

Of the 709 clinicians who were contacted by encouragers, 124 (17%) were ineligible. Of the 585 remaining clinicians, 491 agreed to be contacted by an MOS field representative to discuss participation. Of the 491 who agreed to be contacted, 298 (61%) actually enrolled and completed the patient screening process. The 298 participating providers represent 51% of the 585 eligible solo and small group clinicians.

Possible response bias was evaluated based on the 491 solo and small group clinicians who agreed to consider participation (see Table 3–2). Across the different sites, the rate of participation was 55% in Los Angeles, 67% in Boston, and 61% in Chicago. None of these differences is statistically significant.

At this stage of the process, specialty did not appear to be an important factor in the decision to participate. Seventy percent of the family practitioners, 64% of the cardiologists, 63% of psychologists, 58% of endocrinologists, 57% of psychiatrists, and 56% of the general internists completed patient screening. These differences were not significant.

The best comparison with these rates is the National Study of Medical and Surgical Specialties, carried out in 1976–78 by Robert Mendenhall, M.D., and his associates. In this study, fee-for-service providers were asked to complete logs of their patient encounters

Table 3–2 Comparison of Solo and Small-Group Clinician Participants and Nonparticipants after Agreeing to Consider Participating

Characteristic	Nonparticipants ($N = 193$)	Participants ($N = 298$)
Mean age	41.4	40.4
Female (%)	13.3	16.8
Foreign medical graduate (%)	22.9	23.0
Patient load (per week)	52.7	53.4
Fee-for-service (%)	93.3	91.5
Number of locations of practice	1.5	1.5

Table 3–3 Comparison of Multispecialty Group Practice Clinician
Participants and Nonparticipants

Characteristic	Participants	Nonparticipants
Average number of clinicians in organization	11.7	9.5
Mean age	39.0	40.0

without patient involvement. These providers reported overall cooperation rates of 55% for all of the twenty-four specialties included in the
study. A direct comparison by the specialties included in the MOS
shows rates of 37% for general practitioners, 57% for cardiologists,
82% for endocrinologists, 50% for psychiatrists, and 53% for general
internists.

Representativeness of Multispecialty Group Practices Multispecialty
groups were initially chosen because they served in areas similar to the
HMOs. Approximately one-half of the MSGs approached agreed to
participate in the study. The MSGs served a substantially smaller
market share than the HMOs or the solo and small group providers. The
twelve MSGs selected practiced in twenty-five separate clinical locations. Of the 118 MSG clinicians approached, thirty-one (26%) were
ineligible. Of the remaining eligible clinicians, sixty-eight (78%) agreed
to participate and subsequently screened patients, and nineteen (22%)
declined to participate. The differences between these two groups were
not statistically significant (Table 3–3). MSGs showed somewhat different participation rates across specialty groups and sites ($P < .05$). All of
the cardiologists and family practitioners participated, whereas only
two of the six eligible psychologists (33%) participated. In Boston 33%
refused, in Los Angeles 16% refused, and in Chicago none refused.

Representativeness of Health Maintenance Organizations Each HMO
had both a "flagship" or central clinic and several satellite offices. The
three flagship offices had about 36% of the sample. The twenty-three
satellite offices contained the other 64%.

Among the 296 clinicians whose names were provided by the HMOs
as potential participants, 116 (39%) were ineligible. Of the remaining
180, 157 (87%) agreed to participate and screened patients. The other
twenty-three (13%) refused. The eligible clinicians who participated
and refused are compared in Table 3–4. Only the percentage at flagship

Table 3–4 Comparison of Health Maintenance Organization Clinician Participants and Nonparticipants

Characteristic	Participants	Nonparticipants
Average number of clinicians per practice location	27.3	35.6
Mean age	40.1	41.6
Percentage at flagship HMO	38.2	66.9

HMOs was significantly different ($P = .05$). HMOs showed somewhat different participation rates across specialty groups. The participation rates across sites were similar.

Clinician Sample Description As a result of the above procedures, the MOS clinician sample consists of 298 clinicians from solo and small group practices, 68 from MSGs, and 157 from HMOs, for a total of 523. Some of the solo and small group practice clinicians were reclassified based on their response to questions about group structure and size. The number of providers is broken down by specialty and by this system of care classification (see Table 3–5).

By design, the demographic characteristics of clinicians participating in the MOS differed from those of the general U.S. physician population. The average age of participating clinicians was forty, and about 94% were between thirty and fifty years old, as expected on the

Table 3–5 Number of Clinicians by Specialty and System of Care

Specialty	SYSTEM OF CARE			Total
	SOLO	MSG	HMO	
Medical Specialties				
Cardiology	31	7	2	40
Endocrinology	19	2	3	24
Family practice	61	8	22	91
Internal medicine	78	42	74	194
Nurse practitioner	0	0	13	13
Mental health specialties				
Psychiatrist	55	7	14	76
Psychologist	46	6	22	74
Mental health masters	0	4	7	11
Total	290	76	157	523

basis of our selection criteria. About 21% of the clinicians were women. While the majority of clinicians were white (85%), there was representation from blacks (4%), Latinos (3%), and Asians (7%). Clinicians in the different systems appear to be somewhat different. For example, in addition to certain demographic differences, clinicians in the solo and small group category were more sensitive to issues of cost. McGlynn (1991) also reported different levels of job satisfaction between physicians practicing in different systems of care.

Stage Four: Selection of Patients for Cross-Sectional Survey

Each patient completed one of two versions of the Initial Screening Form by Patient (sp). Data on demographic characteristics, presence of the tracer conditions, and other key concepts were collected on both forms. One version of the patient screener included information on comorbid conditions as well as general health status measures (Health Status form; see introduction to part IV). The other version collected information on utilization, style of care, and patient satisfaction (Style form).

Table 3–6 Demographic Characteristics of MOS Participating Clinicians by Revised System of Care (in percentages)

Characteristic	SYSTEM OF CARE			Total
	SOLO	MSG	HMO	
Age				
31–40	53.1	63.2	65.0	57.8
41–50	44.4	23.5	24.1	36.2
51–60	2.5	10.3	11.0	5.9
Gender				
Female	17.3	22.0	22.4	21.0
Male	82.7	78.0	77.6	79.0
Race				
White	86.0	84.8	83.1	84.8
Black	1.7	6.1	5.2	3.7
Latino	1.7	1.5	5.2	2.9
Asian	8.7	7.6	5.9	7.5
Other	1.7	0.0	0.7	1.1

Table 3–7 Percentage of Eligible Patients Completing Screening Forms by Clinician Specialty and System of Care

Specialty	SYSTEM OF CARE			Total
	SOLO	MSG	HMO	
Cardiology	67.4	73.9	84.2	69.4
Endocrinology	65.0	85.8	88.6	69.8
Family practice	67.2	79.5	71.8	69.8
Internal medicine	64.2	73.3	76.4	71.4
Nurse practitioner	—	—	81.2	81.2
Psychiatrist	57.9	60.9	66.4	60.2
Psychologist	67.8	78.8	68.2	68.7
Mental health masters	—	68.4	68.0	68.1
Total	65.2	74.2	75.1	70.2

The percentage of eligible patients completing screening forms, broken down by specialty and system of care, is based on the data compiled from logs kept by each clinician (see Table 3–7). Based on practice logs for patients of the 523 clinicians, complete screening data were available for about 75% of the eligible patient visits in HMO and MSG practices. In solo and small group practices about 65% of eligible patients completed screenings. The lower rate reflects differences in the field staffing strategy. Patients in HMOs and MSGs were generally approached by MOS field staff, whereas in solo and small group practices we relied upon office staff, who had other duties as well.

A total of 22,462 Initial Screening Forms by Patient (SP) were collected, of which 11,336 were the Health Status form (see part IV) and 11,126 were the Style form. The clinician was asked to fill out the Initial Screening Form by Clinician (SD) for each patient. A total of 22,120 such forms were filled out. Some mismatches—patients who filled out a form when their clinician did not and vice versa—occurred. As a result, there are 21,481 matched pairs of SP and SD forms (see Table 3–8).

The cross-sectional analysis sample consists of 11,186 of the 11,336 Health Status questionnaires (150 forms came in after the measurement development analyses were performed).

The demographic characteristics for each of the cross-sectional or screening sample groups are presented in Table 3–9. There are no

Table 3–8 Results of Patient Screening for the MOS

Patient Form Completed?	CLINICIAN FORM COMPLETED?		Total
	Yes	No	
Health Status	10,838	498	11,336
Style	10,643	483	11,126
No	639	0	639
Total	22,120	981	23,101

Table 3–9 Demographic Characteristics of Cross-Sectional Screening Sample by Sample Group

Patient Characteristic	SAMPLE GROUP	
	Health Status ($N = 11,336$)	Style ($N = 11,126$)
Age	47.1	46.9
Male (%)	38.4	37.5
Married (%)	54.1	54.0
Working (%)	65.7	65.3
Caucasian (%)	79.1	78.9
Education (years)	13.7	13.7
Adjusted 1985 Income ($1,000)	24.0	24.1

Note: Sample sizes for each individual measure are smaller, depending on response rates for the desired items.

significant differences in demographic characteristics between the two halves of the screening sample.

Stage Five: Selection of Patients for Longitudinal Portion of the MOS

Patients with both the SP and SD questionnaires who appeared to have one of the tracer conditions and were not otherwise excluded advanced to the next stage of the selection process, the Tracer Condition Interview (TCI). The purpose of the TCI was to determine whether the patient had major depression and to enroll patients with one of the three medical tracers or major depression. During the course of the TCI, the definition of depression was expanded to include some patients with prior major depression, dysthymia, or depressive symptoms without identifiable disorder.

Each enrolled patient was sent a packet of material, including a Patient Assessment Questionnaire, a Calendar Diary, and an invitation to the Health Exam. Based on returns from these instruments, contact with the RAND Survey Research Group, and the patient's level of disease, a longitudinal subsample of patients was chosen.

Eligibility for Tracer Condition Interview Information obtained from both the Patient and the Clinician Initial Screening Forms was used to identify patients who appeared to have at least one of the four MOS tracer conditions and who met other criteria of eligibility for the longitudinal study. This subset of patients received a telephone-administered interview (TCI) designed to obtain more details about the tracer condition and to enroll these patients in the longitudinal study.

Exclusion criteria were applied to identify persons with an unstable relationship with the MOS clinician or with medical conditions, other than MOS tracer conditions, associated with severe limitations in functioning. These exclusion criteria were applied separately for each tracer:

cancer: diagnosed within the last three years except skin cancer
mental deficit: clinician indicated that the patient had a mental deficit that would interfere with completing a self-administered question-naire
unstable treatment relationship: two of these three conditions were met: visit was for a consult only, clinician did not treat most of the patient's medical and/or personal problems, and first time the patient had seen the clinician
heart attack: clinician said that the patient had a myocardial infarction (MI) in the previous twelve months but that another physician provided the majority of care for that condition
in bed: patient indicated that he or she spent twenty or more days in bed in the last month
insulin: patient was taking insulin injections or was a diabetic diagnosed before age thirty
pacemaker: patient said he or she had a pacemaker
paralysis: patient said he or she had major paralysis or neurologic

problems, including stroke, multiple sclerosis, and muscular dystro-
phy

specialty: clinician was a diabetologist or endocrinologist and the patient
did not have diabetes or depression or congestive heart failure; or
clinician was a cardiologist and the patient did not have hypertension
or MI; or clinician was a mental health provider and the patient did
not have depression

stroke: clinician said patient had a post-stroke residual neurologic deficit

surgery: clinician said patient had major surgery (e.g., colectomy, pneu-
monectomy) in the previous six months, except heart disease patients
who had coronary artery bypass graft or angioplasty

untreated condition: patient or clinician indicated that patient had high
blood pressure but was not being treated for it

unmatched screener: only the patient or clinician screener was available

youth: under age eighteen.

Eligibility for each of the four tracer conditions was fairly broad at
this stage of sampling. Later, as patients were actually selected into the
baseline sample and the panel, more stringent criteria were sometimes
applied. This information documents the sampling stages and should
not be used to determine the definitions of the four tracer conditions.
The final definitions of the tracer conditions depended on a variety of
sources of information and varied according to the particular analysis.

For diabetes, case-finding at this stage consisted of screening for type
II, adult onset or non-insulin-dependent diabetes cases. Patients who
developed their diabetes after the age of thirty were considered to have
type II diabetes even if they were insulin-dependent at the time of
screening. Insulin dependency was determined from the patient screening form and age of onset was taken from either the patient or clinician
form, with a preference for patient data.

Hypertension was diagnosed using systolic and diastolic blood
pressure. At this stage, patients with hypertension were identified from
clinician reports.

For heart disease, case finding consisted of screening for patients
with recent myocardial infarction or congestive heart failure as identified by the clinician on the screening form.

Case finding for the depression tracer was more complex than for the
medical tracers. The MOS began with the well-documented assumption
that general medical clinicians could not be relied upon for such
diagnoses. Further, self-assessment of depressive symptoms was also
not a definitive way of diagnosing major depression. In order to reduce

study costs and respondent burden, a two-stage procedure was designed to identify patients with major depression based on previous work. The first stage used a self-assessment measure of depressive symptoms to identify patients with a high likelihood of major depression and/or dysthymia.

The first stage screener is based on the CES-D scale (Radloff, 1977), modified as described in Burnam, Wells, Leake, et al. (1988). The second stage used a structured interview to confirm a current major depressive episode or dysthymic disorder. The second stage screener was a telephone-administered version of the depression section of the Diagnostic Interview Schedule (DIS) of the National Institute of Mental Health (Robins, Helzer, Croughan, Ratcliff, 1981), which allows diagnoses to be assigned consistent with DSM-III criteria. A two-stage process has also been used by Schulberg et al. (1985) and others.

The number of patients who met MOS criteria for each tracer condition but who were excluded from further consideration are shown by tracer condition in Table 3–10. For depression, the number who met MOS criteria and who were excluded refer to the first-stage depression screener only (i.e., depressive symptoms). The reasons for exclusion are unique. That is, if more than one reason disqualified a patient, the patient is counted only in the "multiple" reason category. Many patients have more than one tracer; therefore, it was possible to be excluded for one tracer but included for another. For example, a depressed diabetic could be sampled in a mental health practitioner's office. The patient would be included for depression but not for diabetes, since the mental health clinician was not the primary provider for diabetes. Although the numbers in the "not excluded" row add to 9,876, this represents only 8,040 individuals because some have multiple tracers. The most common combinations were patients with diabetes and hypertension and patients with one of the medical tracers and depression.

Of the 8,040 patients with at least one tracer condition and not otherwise excluded, 7,335 cases (91%) that were eligible for enrollment into the longitudinal patient panel were passed to the telephone center for the TCI. The remaining 695 (9%) either did not complete or sign the required stage two authorization or provided insufficient information for making a second contact.

For the medical tracers, any patient contacted for the TCI was eligible, so the MOS attempted to enroll them at the beginning of the interview. If patients refused to enroll, the interview was not completed.

Table 3–10 Numbers of Patients Excluded from TCI Panel Eligibility
by Reason and Medical Tracer Conditions

	TRACER CONDITION			
Reason	Hypertension	Heart Disease	Diabetes	Depression
Met criteria for				
tracer condition	5,736	909	3,218	4,813
Not excluded	3,926	677	1,610	3,663
Excluded for:				
Cancer	79	21	32	—
Mental deficiency	34	16	15	42
Unstable treatment				
relations	50	19	28	166
Heart attack	9	—	12	14
In bed	33	—	27	—
Insulin	—	—	282	—
Pacemaker	36	—	—	—
Paralysis	74	15	52	109
Amputee	170	—	—	—
Specialty	135	26	134	—
Stroke	40	10	13	13
Surgery	121	31	60	103
Untreated				
condition	265	—	166	291
Unmatched	125	35	90	148
Youth	40	8	12	30
Multiple	599	51	685	234

For patients with depressive symptoms, the MOS needed to assess whether their depression met the DIS standard. Since these patients needed to be interviewed before eligibility could be determined, those who met DIS criteria were enrolled after the interview.

Of the 7,335 cases that were passed to the telephone center, 5,341 (73%) completed the TCI. A completion meant that either the patient was eligible for a medical condition tracer and agreed to be in the longitudinal study, or the patient had depressive symptoms (CES-D positive) and agreed to be interviewed further.

Description of Baseline Sample

Of the 5,043 cases with a medical tracer condition, 3,513 (70%) agreed to enroll and completed the TCI regarding their medical condition. Of the 3,663 cases with depressive symptoms, 2,262 (62%) agreed to be interviewed and completed the TCI. Between the start of the TCI and enrollment in the MOS panel, patients with depression had several opportunities to discontinue the enrollment process. Similarly, the MOS had several opportunities to decide whether or not to include them in the panel. Of the 2,262 patients interviewed, 1,801 were enrolled. Of these, 1,037 were unique depression cases (had no medical tracer condition) and 764 had depression in addition to one of the medical tracers. This group of 764 is part of the 3,513 cases who agreed to enroll. An additional 292 unique depression cases, from the previously interviewed depression cases, were enrolled in a second phase of selection.

There were three possible reasons why eligible patients were not enrolled: (1) patients did not provide the necessary authorization or information to be recontacted, (2) patients could not be reached for the TCI, or (3) patients were contacted but refused further participation.

Of the 4,842 patients who agreed to enroll, 3,445 (71%) completed Form A of the Patient Assessment Questionnaire (PAQ). Of these, 3,053 were available at the time of the analysis, thus comprising the PAQ baseline sample on which the health measures reported here were developed.

Because enrollment procedures differed in important ways for those with medical conditions and depressive symptoms, two separate analyses of bias are presented: one for the patients with medical tracers

Table 3–11 Distribution of Medical and Depression Patients Enrolled in the MOS

Depression only	1,037
Medical and depression	764
Medical only	2,749
Additional depression	292
Total	4,842
Depression	1,801
Medical	3,513

Table 3–12 Demographics of 5,043 Medical Tracer Patients by Tracer Condition Interview (TCI) Completion Status

Characteristic	No TCI (N = 1,530)	Took TCI (N = 3,513)
Age	62.3	59.4a
Education (years)	12.3	12.9a
Nonwhite (%)	25.6	24.4
Employed (%)	43.9	50.3a
Married (%)	55.7	61.6a
Male (%)	42.0	42.4
Adjusted 1985 Income ($1,000)	19.6	22.0a

a$p<0.001$

Table 3–13 Demographics of 3,513 Enrolled Medical Tracer Patients by Patient Assessment Questionnaire (PAQ) Completion Status

Characteristic	No PAQ (N = 1,229)	Returned PAQ (N = 2,284)
Age	60.0	59.0
Education (years)	12.5	13.1
Nonwhite (%)	29.1	21.8a
Employed (%)	49.1	50.9
Married (%)	56.5	64.4a
Male (%)	39.3	44.1b
Adjusted 1985 Income ($1,000)	20.5	22.8a

a$p<.001$
b$p<.01$

and one for those with depressive symptoms. Tables 3–12 and 3–13 describe the medical tracer patients, and Tables 3–14 and 3–15 describe the depression tracer patients. Table 3–12 shows that there were some important differences between enrolled and nonenrolled medical tracer patients. Patients who took the TCI were younger, somewhat better educated, had a higher income, and were more likely to be married and employed.

The next step after enrollment and completion of the TCI was completion of the PAQ, which was returned by 65% of the medical tracer patients. Table 3–13 contrasts the patients who returned this form with those who did not. This table also shows some important biases in the medical tracer sample that returned the PAQ. This sample was considerably more likely to be white, married, male, and to have higher incomes.

For the patients who were selected for the depression tracer, there were fewer significant differences. The sample that did not complete the TCI was somewhat less educated, more likely to be male, and less likely to be married. Almost no differences in PAQ returns exist among depressed subjects.

The overall return rates of the PAQ for depression tracer patients (58%) were substantially lower than for the medical tracers (65%).

Table 3–14 Demographics of Selected Depressive Symptoms Patients by Tracer Condition Interview (TCI) Completion Status

Characteristic	No TCI (N = 1,401)	Took TCI (N = 2,262)
Age	44.3	44.6
Education (years)	13.1	13.5[a]
Nonwhite (%)	23.4	23.4
Employed (%)	61.8	62.4
Married (%)	39.3	47.1[a]
Male (%)	31.4	27.7[a]
Adjusted 1985 Income ($1,000)	21.8	21.1

[a]$p<.01$

Table 3–15 Demographics of 1,801 Enrolled Depression Patients by Initial Patient Assessment Questionnaire (PAQ) Completion Status

Characteristic	No PAQ (N = 750)	Returned PAQ (N = 1,051)
Age	45.3	45.7
Education (years)	13.2	13.5
Nonwhite (%)	22.4	20.5
Employed (%)	60.6	59.7
Married (%)	44.9	49.2
Male (%)	26.2	26.6
Adjusted 1985 Income ($1,000)	20.7	21.4

Recall that these were partial returns—that is, they reflect the subset of 3,053 (out of 3,445) PAQs returned at the time of the MOS measurement development analyses reported here.

Although the differences between those who completed the TCI or the PAQ and those who did not were statistically significant in many cases, this probably does not affect the work in this book. The medical tracer sample that completed the PAQ was not appreciably different from the general chronic disease sample initially screened. For example, the largest sampling biases were about two-tenths of a standard deviation, so there was a substantial overlap between patients who did and did not return the PAQ. Similar findings were true for the TCI. These biases can be offset in analysis by appropriate sample weighting schemes.

Biases were consistent across specialty groups and systems of care. Thus, the comparisons which the MOS (as opposed to the book) was designed to address should not be affected.

With respect to the book, we point to the conventional wisdom that relationships are rarely altered by including sampling probabilities. If one item is correlated with another, it will remain correlated whether or not the questionnaire is completed by relatively younger or relatively older people.

Summary of Sample Characteristics by System and Site

The number of clinician and patient participants by system and site is shown in Table 3–16.

The characteristics of the final baseline sample are shown in Tables 3–17 and 3–18. The average age of the sample was 54 and the range in ages was considerable (18–98). More than one-third of the sample was elderly. The proportion of women and nonwhites was higher than their prevalence in the population. Income and education levels suggest a lower SES population.

The distribution of tracer conditions reflects the high proportion of patients with hypertension and diabetes. The two heart disease tracers contributed 9%; major depression was diagnosed among 13%. Most of the sample had one or two tracers; about 12% had a medical tracer and major depression or depressive symptoms.

Table 3–16 Number of Study Participants by System and Site

| System | Clinicians | PATIENTS | |
		Cross-Sectional	Baseline
HMO			
Los Angeles	46	2,178	387
Boston	68	3,711	321
Chicago	43	2,094	374
Subtotal	157	7,983	1,082
Multispecialty groups			
Los Angeles	31	1,834	205
Boston	31	1,596	153
Chicago	14	685	113
Subtotal	225	4,115	471
Solo and small groups			
Los Angeles	92	2,922	518
Boston	95	3,127	459
Chicago	103	3,306	518
Subtotal	290	9,355	1,495
Total	523	21,453	3,053

Table 3–17 Demographic Characteristics of MOS Baseline Sample (N = 3,053)

Characteristic	
Age	
Mean	54
Range	18–98
Over 65 (%)	28
Over 75 (%)	8
Gender (%)	
Male	39
Female	61
Race (%)	
White	79
Nonwhite	21
Household income (1985 adjusted)	$22,975
Education (mean in years)	13

Table 3–18 Tracer Status Characteristics of M O S Baseline Sample
(N = 3,053)

Characteristic	%
Tracer conditions	
Congestive heart failure	6
Diabetes	22
Hypertension	58
Major depression	13
Myocardial infarction	3
Number of tracers	
None	3
One	67
Two	24
Three	5
Four	1
Medical condition and major depression	3
Medical condition and major depression/depressive symptoms	12

4. Methods of Collecting Health Data

Sandra H. Berry

Health Data Collected

The purposes of collecting data from MOS patients were threefold: (1) to determine their eligibility for the longitudinal portion of the study; (2) to provide information about their health, health behaviors, demographic characteristics, the style of care practiced by their provider, their satisfaction with the care provided, and utilization of services; and (3) to obtain information about their relationship with the provider during the study. Data were also collected from clinicians to determine their eligibility for the MOS to obtain information regarding their personal background, training, and practice style, and to learn their perspective on the health of each of their participating MOS patients.

Several sources were used to collect these data: self-reports by patients about themselves and their providers; direct measurements of patients, such as their blood pressure; ratings by trained clinicians of the patients, such as the Hamilton Interview; provider reports of their patients' health status; and provider self-reports of their own characteristics, behavior, and opinions.

Four methods of data collection—self-administered questionnaires, face-to-face interviews, telephone interviews, and health exams—were used to collect data from patients and providers, as described in Table 4–1.

Table 4–2 shows the specific instruments that were administered by these methods to patient and clinician populations in the MOS. The first MOS instrument was the Clinician Selection Survey, administered by telephone to fee-for-service clinicians. This instrument was used to

Table 4–1 Methods Used to Collect Various Types of MOS Health Data

Source/Type of Data	METHODS USED			
	Self-administered questionnaires	Face-to-face interviews	Telephone interviews	Health exams
From Patients				
Self-reports of health status, behavior, and attitude	x	x	x	
Physical status				x
From Providers				
Reports of patient status	x			
Self-reports of behavior and opinions	x		x	

select the sample of fee-for-service clinicians (chapter 3). After clinicians were selected and enrolled, including those in practices, groups, and fee-for-service, they were asked to complete the Clinician Background Questionnaire, a self-administered questionnaire that described the clinicians and their practices. Providers who refused to enroll were asked to complete a Clinician Background Questionnaire for evaluation of provider noncooperation patterns.

As part of patient screening, both the providers and the patients completed self-administered instruments (the Initial Screening Form by Patient and the Initial Patient Screening Form by Clinician). Both forms, which described the patient's medical conditions, were completed in the providers' offices at the time of patient visits. Once an eligible baseline enrollment sample of patients was selected, patients were given the Tracer Condition Interview by telephone to obtain their consent to enroll them in the longitudinal portion of the study and to obtain more background information about their medical conditions. These patients were also asked to participate in the Health Examination, which included physical and laboratory tests.

At the same time, patients were sent their first Patient Assessment Questionnaire (PAQ) and monthly Calendar-Dairy, containing the Health Care Report and the Medical Visit Report Form by Patients. These items were used to report visits to providers during the first six months of the study and to report the details of the content of visits to MOS providers. For four years, PAQs were sent to patients at six-month intervals. Patients enrolled in the depression tracer were given repeat

Table 4–2 Overview of M OS Clinician and Patient Instruments and Samples

Instrument	Method	Instrument Completed by
Clinician Selection Survey	Telephone Interview	Clinician
Clinician Background Questionnaire	Self-administered	Clinician
Initial Screening Form by Patient	Self-administered	Patient
Initial Patient Screening Form by Clinician	Self-administered	Clinician
Tracer Condition Interview	Telephone Interview	Patient
Clinical Assessment	Face-to-face Interview, physical exam, labora- tory tests	Technician staff
Patient Assessment Questionnaire	Self-administered	Patient
Health Care Report (Diary)	Self-administered	Patient
Medical Visit Report Form by Patient	Self-administered	Patient
Medical Visit Report Form by Provider	Self-administered	Provider

a In item counts each field that could be filled in by the respondent counts as one field. In most cases the actual number of items completed is less than the total number of items due to skip patterns.

telephone Tracer Condition Interviews to document depressive episodes at approximately twelve months and twenty-four months after enrollment. At the end of two years, participants were asked to take part in a second in-person health exam similar to the initial one.

Sample	Purpose	# Items/Time[a]
Potential FFS physicians on AMA tape; lists of physicians in each pre-paid group	Screen FFS physicians for eligibility	24 items (5 min)
Enrolled clinicians	Describe enrolled MOS clinicians' background characteristics and style of care	95 items (15–20 min)[b]
Screening sample (first cross-sectional sample; first screening for MOS panel)	Screen patients for possible tracer conditions; establish preliminary eligibility for panel	Version A = 60 items Version B = 80 items (10–15 min)
Screening sample of patients	Cross-sectional database; describe style of care of physicians	66 items (5–10 min)
Medical tracers: eligible patients; depression: patients to be screened for depression	Confirm tracer conditions; establish final eligibility for panel; describe style of care of providers	356–556 items (20–45 min)
Longitudinal panel	Disease severity measure	323–844 items (1–3 hr)
Longitudinal panel	Ongoing health assessment every 6 months	Average 250 items[b] 30 minutes
Longitudinal panel	Disability days, utilization-monthly	32 items
Longitudinal panel	Describe medical visits	87 items (15–30 min) for entire monthly diary[b]
Longitudinal panel	Describe medical visits	100 items (5–10 min)[b]

[b] Estimates derived from pretests only. Actual completion of the form could not be observed directly.

Providers were given lists of their enrolled patients and asked to complete a Medical Visit Report Form by Providers, describing each visit those patients made during the first six months of the study. Forms were distributed to providers by MOS field representatives and returned by mail.

Methods of Data Collection

Self-Administered Questionnaires Self-administered questionnaires were used extensively for providers and patients because they are less expensive than other data collection methods, offer respondent flexibility and privacy to complete at a convenient time, and reduce or eliminate possible interviewer bias. Self-administered forms can be administered by mail, delivered to groups of people, or presented to an individual by a study representative, who might or might not remain with the respondent during completion of the questionnaire. Several variations were used in the MOS. During the screening phase of the study, self-administered forms for providers and patients were delivered in batches to the providers' offices. In the larger group practices, MOS field representatives were stationed in waiting rooms during the screening period to enroll patients and to ensure that the patients and providers completed their forms describing the patients. In smaller practices, providers' receptionists were asked to distribute the forms to patients. Field representatives were sent to screen patients in only a few cases where receptionists were unsuccessful. However, even when the providers' staffs handled enrollment, the field representatives visited the offices daily at the beginning of the screening period and every few days throughout the screening period to answer questions and encourage the providers and receptionists to continue participation. MOS providers kept a brief log of all patients seen in their offices during the screening and enrollment period. The logs were records of the age and sex of the patient, whether or not patients were asked to participate in the MOS, and if not, the reason. These logs allowed the MOS to calculate the percentage of eligible patients who when asked to participate agreed.

During the screening period, patients were made aware of the study as they entered the waiting rooms through such devices as posters, stating "We are Participating in the Medical Outcomes Study," hanging in the waiting rooms, large buttons for the office staff to wear during the screening period, and smaller buttons for patients to wear after they completed enrollment. All enrolled patients received a copy of their consent form and a booklet, "Questions and Answers about the Medical Outcomes Study," to take home for reference.

Once patients were enrolled, forms were sent to them by mail. Nonrespondents were followed up extensively and were important in achieving acceptable final response rates. Normal procedures for a PAQ were an initial first-class mailing of a personalized cover letter, the instrument with an identification label, and a five-dollar check. One week later a reminder card, thanking those who completed the questionnaire and urging those who did not, was sent. The reminder card provided a name and telephone number to contact if the questionnaire was not received. Three weeks after the initial mailing, a reminder letter to nonrespondents and an additional questionnaire were sent, followed by a telephone call timed to occur at about the time the second questionnaire arrived. If the respondent indicated at the time of the call that both copies of the questionnaire were lost or had been discarded, another copy was mailed. As a last resort, a short-form version of the PAQ was sent, followed by a final telephone call. These procedures resulted in response rates of about 85%.

For providers, self-administered questionnaires were used for background interviews describing the provider and his or her practice (Clinician Background Questionnaire), patients during the screening visit (Initial Screening Form by Clinician), and patient visits (Medical Visit Report Form by Providers) in the first six months of the longitudinal study. The Clinician Background Questionnaire and the Initial Screening Form by Clinician were distributed and collected in person by MOS field representatives during the screening period. The Medical Visit Report Forms were delivered in person by the MOS field representative, who assisted the provider and office staff with devising an appropriate "tickler" system to ensure the enrollment of all patients seen in the office. In some cases, this procedure was as simple as placing the forms in the patients' records. In other situations, it involved programming a message into the computer system which appeared whenever the patients' records were accessed. Thereafter, additional blank Medical Visit Report Forms were mailed to the providers and the completed forms were returned by mail.

Telephone Interviews Telephone interviewing for the MOS was completed using RAND's Computer Assisted Telephone Interviewing (CATI). The CATI system, instead of pencil-and-paper interviews, was selected because of the complexity of the skip patterns required to collect the data required by the MOS, including information on from one to four tracer conditions for any one patient. Another reason for using CATI was to make the data available for analysis in a timely way. In addition, the CATI system was linked directly to the Record Management System and used for tracking the status and whereabouts of patients and clinicians. These data could be easily transferred back and forth to facilitate fieldwork and to update records based on field experience.

Two MOS questionnaires were completed by telephone: the Clinician Selection Survey, administered as part of the sample selection of fee-for-service physicians to determine eligibility, and the patient Tracer Condition Interview (TCI), which was done at the time of enrollment to determine eligibility for the depression tracer and to provide additional information about all patients. The TCI was used to enroll patients in the longitudinal portion of the study and to schedule initial appointments for the Health Exam, using a computer-linked appointment calendar program. A special version of the TCI for depression tracer patients was completed annually following enrollment to update the patient's status with regard to depressive episodes.

Health Examinations and Face-to-Face Interviews Health examinations of MOS participants were undertaken to provide standardized and therefore comparable measures of clinical status for MOS tracer conditions (e.g., blood pressure, blood sugar) and to provide certain measures not commonly used by MOS providers (e.g., fundus photographs for diabetes patients). Health exams also included, depending on the tracer condition involved, taking background measures such as height and weight, a physical exam, a medical history interview, lab tests of blood and urine, an EKG, an inventory of medication use, a Diagnostic Interview Schedule (DIS), and a Hamilton Interview.

The medical history, medications use, depression screening (DIS), and Hamilton Interview portions of the health exam were administered through in-person interviews conducted at the exam centers. Interviewers were trained nurses or physicians. Patients who did not come into the exam centers were interviewed by telephone, using the same instruments and the same interviewers.

Initial health examinations were administered to MOS participants as soon as possible after enrollment. These exams required patients to come to the exam center in each site for exams that lasted from one to three hours, depending on the tracer condition or combination of tracers that applied to the patient.

Since the purpose of the health exams was to provide reliable measures of clinical status, special attention was given to reliability of testing procedures and laboratory analysis or other interpretation of results. This emphasis was handled as part of training, where inter-rater reliability was routinely tested until an acceptable level was reached. The exam protocols included taking multiple measures (e.g., blood pressure or blood samples) from each patient and blindly retesting a designated portion of the patients. Reliability was also handled in interpretation by consolidating testing or by sending all samples to one person or laboratory for evaluation and by incorporating split samples with "dummy" identifiers into the testing procedures.

Problems of Data Collection

Respondent Burden Minimizing respondent burden was a difficult goal to meet. In a large and expensive study, there is a strong desire to answer all the interesting questions and to obtain as much data as possible "since we are talking to them anyway." Practical and budgetary constraints operated as a brake on respondent burden, dictating the allowable length of key instruments, as shown in Table 4–2.

Practical constraints dictated that screening instruments should take no longer than ten to twelve minutes for patients to complete. The MOS found in the initial pilot studies that if they were longer patients could not complete them while waiting, in addition to reading the basic study materials and signing the informed consent. To deal with this time constraint in data collection, the screening instrument was constructed in two alternative forms, each containing the same core set of variables required for all patients. Alternative forms, however, contained half of the additional information required. One-half of the sample, selected at random, received one of the forms and the other half the alternative form. Respondent burden was reduced by about one-third while still providing the minimum database required for the cross-sectional study.

The PAQs were mailed and self-administered at the patient's home, so practical concerns were less obvious. PAQs were budgeted at preset levels based upon two factors: mailing costs, based on the number of pages, and data processing costs, based on the number of data items to be checked, edited, and entered. Draft instruments were checked against these guidelines and cuts were made as required. In the case of the initial PAQ, the number of baseline items was so large that the instrument had to be divided into Part A and Part B, which were administered separately in each of two months.

Another aspect of reducing burden was the development of short-form PAQs, designed as a final measure in follow-up of nonresponse and administered by mail or telephone in cases where the respondents indicated that they were too ill to complete the regular form. In a longitudinal health study, it is important to prevent the loss of the sickest people from the panel since it introduces a serious bias. Thus, measures that address that problem are valuable even if their development and administration cost seem disproportionately high for the number of patients involved.

The health exam represented a special burden on patients since it required them to visit the exam centers. This visit represents a greater psychological barrier than simply filling out a form and mailing it in or responding to questions on the telephone. Many respondents were reluctant to submit to an examination by anyone other than their regular provider, even though the examiners were trained nurses or physicians and the exam centers were friendly and reassuring places. Others simply did not feel that they had three to five hours to devote to travel and to the exam.

For many respondents the exam represented a physical barrier, since their mobility was reduced by age and illness. To be effective, often it required that someone assume the responsibility for transporting patients to and from the exam center. The exam centers were located centrally in urban areas that comprised each site. Nonetheless, many participants had to drive long distances to the center. Despite the fact that maps were provided for reaching the centers by public transportation and by private car and for adequate safe parking, coming into the center of the city was an unfamiliar experience for many participants. These problems led to a high rate of rescheduling of appointments, cancellations, and no-shows. Once participants were persuaded to come into the exam center, however, they not only provided valuable information about their health but also received a personal exposure to the study staff. Their impressions were positive and seemed to carry through at least the early stages of the longitudinal study.

Respondent Cooperation The magnitude of the data collection agenda raised a number of general issues centering around two main problems: how to obtain complete and high-quality data and how to obtain maximum efficiency from data collection in the interest of controlling costs.

Respondent characteristics that can affect cooperation include: for patients, age, education, and health status; for clinicians, medical specialty and practice locations; and for both, compliance orientation and accessibility to researchers. Unfortunately, the actual impact of these characteristics is poorly understood, and the concept of compliance orientation is poorly articulated and measured. For example, the common wisdom about age and illness runs in both directions: on the one hand, older and/or sicker people may be considered to have more free time and to be more likely to be interested in taking part in research; on the other hand, older people may be considered to be more conservative and suspicious, and sicker people to be physically or mentally incapacitated, and therefore less likely to take part in research. Both may be true, and there is limited information about in what circumstances they apply.

While respondent characteristics are of interest, in practical terms they are usually not entirely subject to the researcher's control. The design of a particular study simply requires a study population with given characteristics. Certain subsets of the general population of interest might be included or excluded on the basis of the difficulty in gaining cooperation (i.e., the frequent exclusion of nursing home patients from health studies). In most cases, researchers must shape study characteristics to maximize the cooperation of available respondents.

For both patients and providers, respondent cooperation is dependent on the perceived loss or gain from having the study conducted at all and the perceived personal loss or gain from participating. The perceived loss or gain from having the study conducted at all depends on several factors: the domain in which the study is likely to have effects, the size of these effects, and whether the results are likely to be positive or negative in terms of the respondent's interests. If the study is expected to have major effects in a domain of importance to the respondent and these effects are likely to be negative, respondents are unlikely to participate. If the study is likely to have positive effects in a domain of importance, the respondent will be disposed to take part, assuming the loss to them of participating is not too high. If the perceived loss or gain from having the study conducted at all is small, this will probably be a neutral factor in the decision and the gain or loss from personal participation will determine the outcome.

The losses from participating include costs in terms of time and effort, direct monetary costs of participating, loss of income from unreimbursed time spent on the study, and loss of privacy. Benefits include positive feelings about participating such as feeling honored to be asked to participate, feeling that participation is in aid of some goal the respondent feels is important, and positive feelings through interactions with interviewers and study staff.

While these factors are similar for patients and providers, the specifics operate somewhat differently. Providers were aware of the potential importance of major studies like the MOS in shaping government, third-party payer, and other policies. Providers were also aware of the direct and indirect costs to them of participating in studies (e.g., the cost of their own time, the time of their office staffs, and the goodwill of their patients). Many patients were also aware of how larger issues in health care affected them, particularly in light of the policies being implemented by government and private insurers limiting their coverage for health care and decreasing their range of choice by emphasizing prepaid or preferred provider plans. Patients were also concerned about the time and effort required to satisfy the extensive data collection agenda for the study.

Provider Cooperation

The MOS structured and presented the study in such a way that respondents felt that having the study conducted would be either neutral or beneficial to them. The MOS also attempted to make perceptions of personal gain or loss come out on the positive side by obtaining cooperation in several ways.

Approach to Providers From the early phases of planning for the MOS, it was felt that establishing the credibility of the study to providers was the key to obtaining high levels of provider and patient cooperation because patients are inclined to trust their provider's judgment. From the outset, the MOS involved provider specialty groups in the planning of the MOS. High-level representatives of the American College of Physicians, the American Academy of Family Practice, the American Psychiatric Association, and the American Psychological Association participated in planning, and their interests and concerns were made part of the initial design of the study. Three of these organizations formally endorsed the study, and all provided formal and informal support in identifying and contacting providers in their specialties.

Representatives of these organizations served on a Liaison Committee, which worked on insuring that providers would understand MOS goals and view the conduct of the study as a positive or at least neutral element in the medical politics arena. This advisory committee served as a communication link by bringing the concerns of the provider specialty groups into the MOS planning process on an ongoing basis and keeping the specialty groups aware of the progress of the MOS. The committee members also served as the nucleus for the development of a provider encouragement network. The MOS planners also consulted with a Clinical Advisory Committee, which included practicing physicians of each specialty group, who operated in the domain of how best to increase the direct gain to providers and minimize the cost through design of incentives and study procedures. The Clinical Advisory Committee was influential in shaping the data requirements for the study by commenting on the kind and level of burden they would impose on practicing clinicians. This committee was instrumental in establishing the upper limit on the length of provider-completed forms. It also suggested the need for local staffs of MOS field representatives in each site and indicated ways of providing suitable nonmonetary incentives for providers and the most effective ways of informing practicing clinicians about the MOS.

Information about the MOS was conveyed to the providers by the promotion of general awareness of the study though information to editors of national and local specialty and society newsletters and at appropriate local and national meetings of providers. To establish and maintain among participants a clear identity for the study, an attractive logo was designed, which appeared on all written study materials and on incentives given to encourage participation.

Selection of Providers The second phase involved the selection of the individual providers practicing in groups and in private practice. Within groups, the effort was directed at selecting and enrolling the providers at the group level. The main avenue for enrolling groups was through the managers of the group. To improve the quality of presentation and reduce the cost, a videotape describing the study was presented to key study staff. Once the group agreed to participate, the MOS selected individual providers within the group based on MOS eligibility criteria. These providers were approached separately by MOS field representatives to address individual concerns. This process was complicated in some HMOs that had main and satellite offices. Provider enrollment and patient screening was carried out in several locations for each HMO.

In the solo and small group portion of the sample, the approach to providers was more elaborate and time-consuming. Prior to approaching a provider and asking for cooperation, each selected provider received a letter from the relevant specialty society which introduced the MOS and explained how and why the specialty society was involved in the study. The content of the letters was developed jointly by the MOS and the specialty organization. The letters appeared on the letterhead of the professional organization. In most cases, letters signed by an officer of the specialty organization urged providers to cooperate with the MOS, citing reasons that were relevant to each specialty group. After receiving the letter, a telephone contact for the Clinician Selection Survey was made. With solo and small group providers, the entire effort of enrollment, including gaining access to the provider and explaining the study, had to be repeated for each individual provider. Both the Liaison and Clinical Advisory Committees suggested that a provider encouragement network would help, since providers would be more likely to participate if they were asked personally by someone they knew and respected. Twenty prominent providers in three sites for each specialty were asked to take part in this effort. Their role was to introduce the study, to attest to its importance, and to convey the fact that providers, like the one being approached, were taking part despite the burden. Working with MOS staff to develop a way of contacting their providers, encouragers personalized the process. For encouragers, the most effective method of introducing the MOS was through personal contacts or by telephone. Some encouragers sent letters before or instead of personal contacts, and others contacted providers through professional or special meetings designed to introduce the MOS. Building and maintaining the provider encouragement system was expensive and time-consuming for the project. Encouragers were differentially effective at reaching their providers, but overall they contributed greatly to obtaining the cooperation of physicians.

Approach to Study Staff The final stage of obtaining initial provider cooperation was through direct contact with study staff in the sites. Once the encourager introduced the study and obtained permission for the study to contact the provider directly, an MOS field representative took over to explain the study in more detail and to enroll the provider. The role of the carefully recruited and trained field representatives was crucial. In addition to explaining the study and discussing it intelligently with the providers, field representatives needed to convey both the care with which the study was being conducted and the fact that study procedures were adaptable to different practice settings. A key function of the MOS field representatives was tactfully to train and sometimes coach providers and office staff to carry out patient screening and enrollment effectively, using demonstrations and role-playing.

Incentives for Participation While evidence indicates that even small payments increase cooperation in physician populations (Gunn and Rhodes, 1981; Weber, Wycoff, and Adamson, 1982; Mizes, Fleece, and Roos, 1984; Berry and Kanouse, 1987; Aday, 1989), sponsors felt that paying providers for participation in the MOS would be inappropriate. In contrast, they favored providing small gifts to providers and office staff. Accordingly, the MOS obtained coffee mugs, pads of note paper, paper clip holders, and ballpoint pens imprinted with the MOS logo and the name of the study. These items were distributed by encouragers to MOS providers and office staff.

Many providers, identifying with the goals of the study, found it rewarding to participate in the MOS and were pleased to contribute to the research process. Others found it interesting to be associated with a visible study being conducted in their location. These providers were pleased to be recognized by the MOS and the local encourager as valuable contributors to the research, especially since only the better-trained, board-certified providers in each specialty were selected as participants. The selective aspect of provider participation in the MOS was also emphasized to patients, who seemed suitably impressed, which pleased many providers.

Patient Cooperation

Initial enrollment in the MOS cross-sectional study required minimal informed consent procedures. No payment was offered to patients at the initial enrollment and screening phase. Obtaining patient cooperation was handled initially and effectively through the providers' participation in the study and their explicit endorsement of it in asking their patients to cooperate.

Approach to Patients Selected patients were enrolled in the longitudinal study by telephone in conjunction with conducting the Tracer Condition Interview. At the time patients were asked to enroll in the longitudinal panel, they were reminded that their providers, who were mentioned by name, were participating in the study. Patients also received an informative question-and-answer format brochure explaining the purposes of the study in detail as part of their first mailing of study materials. Patients were offered payments for participating in the longitudinal portion of the study. Checks were included with the initial mailing of each instrument that had to be completed. These payments were made in advance of receiving the completed instrument for several reasons. First, there is evidence that this method is more effective at generating response than payment only for completed instruments (Berry and Kanouse, 1987; Berk, Mathiowetz, Ward, and White, 1987; Dommeyer, 1988). Second, it is simpler to administer since the entire mailing can be prepared at once without additional mailings for checks after the completed instrument is received. The level of payment varied with the instrument to be completed. Five dollars was paid for a semiannual PAQ and two dollars for a monthly Calendar-Diary. Participants in the health exam were paid ten dollars, primarily to cover transportation costs to and from the exam centers. Since the MOS did not incorporate a controlled experiment which tested the effects of payment into the design, it is difficult to assess their value. However, participants often expressed their appreciation for fees, including thank-you notes with their questionnaires. Occasionally checks were returned if patients were unable to complete their questionnaires.

Maintaining Cooperation Over Time Establishing a longitudinal panel in the MOS was clearly a time-consuming and expensive enterprise. It was important that, once selected, both providers and patients be retained in the panel and continue to provide high-quality data on a regular basis. Successful panel maintenance included efforts to identify and personalize the study, to maintain contact with participants, to reduce burden, and to provide for benefits from participation. An additional important element for maintaining contact was an elaborate Record Management System (RMS) to track the current status of MOS providers and patients involved during the cross-sectional and longitudinal phases of the study. The RMS also maintained current contact information for providers and patients in the longitudinal panel. Because both providers and patients were quick to respond to lapses in communication, inconsistencies, and problems not promptly attended to, a sensitive and flexible system was developed. The RMS profiled providers and patients, tracked their participation in the study, and maintained a detailed history of contacts with them. This system was also used for generating personalized letters and other materials used for communicating with study participants. In addition, information from the system was available in a summary form that could be accessed routinely by MOS staff, who were in daily contact with patients and providers. The staff could easily call up a computerized provider or patient record in response to a telephone query from a participant.

Other components of communication related simply to keeping in touch with participants in a positive way. For example, early in the panel period a brochure was sent to patients introducing the key study staff and featuring the people, including a data collection coordinator and one of the interviewers, who would be in closest contact with patients. The brochure provided a telephone number to call collect in case of problems or questions. The telephone was answered by a survey coordinator with access to records about each respondent. In general, the same group of interviewers handled nonresponse follow-up, and many respondents came to know them. The MOS also sent holiday cards to patients; cards and RAND calendars were sent to providers. For providers the MOS developed and mailed a quarterly newsletter informing them of the progress of the study. Longitudinal panel patients, in particular, expressed their satisfaction with taking part in a national study sponsored and carried out by organizations that many of them recognized.

A final key element of maintaining contact is being prompt and aggressive about tracking people who moved residence. All MOS mail was sent with a forwarding address requested. If it was found during follow-up that the participant had moved, tracking was begun immediately through local information, informants at the old address, the names of contacts obtained at the beginning of the study, and the providers who had enrolled the patients into the MOS.

Discussion

The MOS was a complex and difficult study to mount and to manage. Several lessons were learned from the MOS that have resource implications for similar future studies. Considerable resources were spent on the initial enrollment of group practices and on the development of the Provider Encouragement Network. This process took more resources and elapsed time than was anticipated, for several reasons. First, the time required was high-level time. It was necessary for the project management team to meet with directors of groups and, in many cases, with medical staffs in order to obtain their cooperation. Similarly, it required the participation of the senior physicians and psychologists to meet with potential encouragers and obtain their cooperation. Second, the process was slow. In most organizations the decisions were reached after consultation with senior managers, boards of trustees, staff, and/ or legal counsel. This step required availability of personnel to make presentations who had to wait for the appropriate meeting or series of meetings to be held. Third, the process was sequential, necessitating waiting for the decision of a selected group before approaching a replacement. In spite of the elapsed time and increased costs, the result was better cooperation both initially and in the longitudinal portion of the study.

Similarly, the MOS experience demonstrated the value of seeking appropriate advice and pilot testings to achieve a good response. For example, field representatives were not a part of the original MOS design; the task of enrolling providers and facilitating their cooperation was planned as a mail and telephone operation. The adequacy of this plan was questioned by the Clinical Advisory Committee and, therefore, our pilot tests of the enrollment process included field representatives. In retrospect, it seems absurd to think that providers could have been dealt with in any way except in person. Early warnings on this topic were valuable so that this feature could be incorporated into our planning before it was too late. In a number of areas the MOS made investments of considerable resources to improve data quality and response to the study at enrollment and over time.

While there is no set formula for making such decisions, the MOS evolved a process that was useful though difficult to implement. From the onset, the MOS attempted to express its study goals in terms of research questions and to prioritize these questions so that the most important ones were distinct from the subsidiary issues. The MOS related potential costs to the research questions they served to ensure that large costs were not incurred to further subsidiary questions and issues before the primary goals of the data collection were met. Relating resources to research questions provided a useful framework for lively discussion and sometimes painful decision-making.

III

Generic Health Concepts
and Measures

Part III focuses on the twelve health concepts introduced earlier in part II (chapter 2) that are measured in the MOS. For the assessment of two MOS health concepts, psychological distress/well-being (chapter 7) and health perceptions (chapter 8), satisfactory measures were available, requiring only the selection, refinement, and incorporation of them into the final instrument. The MOS is the first large-scale test of these measures among patients with chronic conditions. For physical functioning (chapter 6) and energy/fatigue (chapter 8), the basic questions have been widely used, but revisions were needed to improve the measures. The MOS used a new set of response choices and modified the questions in order to improve the precision of each item. For eight other concepts—health distress (chapter 8), social activity limitations (chapter 9), family and sexual functioning (chapters 10 and 11), role functioning (chapter 12), pain (chapter 13), sleep (chapter 14), and physical/psychophysiologic symptoms (chapter 15), new measures had to be created, necessitating numerous pilot studies.

The specific health measures were usually full-length versions included in the baseline Patient Assessment Questionnaire (PAQ) ($N = 3,053$). This questionnaire was administered to patients eligible for the MOS panel (see chapters 4 and 5). The process for developing measures of each health concept was undertaken in the following eight steps:

(1) define the concept and identify issues to be resolved
(2) determine the content and measurement strategy

(3) collect data by administering pilot questionnaires to pilot study subjects (for selected measures only)

(4) analyze pilot questionnaires (for selected measures only)

(5) select final MOS items

(6) collect data by administering measures to 3,053 MOS patients

(7) construct scales and test scaling assumptions

(8) test reliability and validity of scales

This eight-step MOS process provides the internal organization for each of the ten chapters (chapters 6–15) of part III on the measurement of health concepts. The measures in these ten health chapters are of unequal status. The ten chapters proceed from the older generation of measures to the newest measures. The order in which the chapters are presented reveals information about the significance of the measure and about the meaning of the scores. The two criteria determining the order of the chapters are the centrality of the concept measured in relation to accepted definitions of health and the track record of successful use and validation for each set of measures.

Part III begins with a chapter (chapter 5) describing the methods for constructing health measures. The next ten chapters define the specific health concepts being assessed and explain the manner in which the concept is measured. Chapters 6–8 introduce three generically defined concepts: physical health assessed by measures of physical functioning, mental health assessed in terms of psychological distress/well-being and cognitive functioning, and general health perceptions. Chapter 8 also describes newer measures of energy/fatigue and health distress derived from earlier measures. Chapters 9–12 present MOS advances in the conceptualization and measurement of social and role functioning. Social functioning is differentiated from role functioning and divided into three subcategories: social activities, family functioning, and sexual functioning. Part III concludes with three chapters (chapters 13–15) presenting measures of the three newest health concepts: pain, sleep, and physical/psychophysiologic symptoms.

5. Methods of Constructing Health Measures

Anita L. Stewart, Ron D. Hays, and John E. Ware, Jr.

This chapter summarizes the MOS approach to writing questionnaire items, pretesting measures, constructing multi-item scales, evaluating scale variability, reliability, and stability, and labeling measures. Methods for validating health measures are presented in chapter 18.

In many instances, a single question might be all that is necessary to obtain the desired information. For example, to learn a person's age, sex, or weight, a single question suffices. In research on health and health-related matters, however, the concepts are complex and difficult if not impossible to define by a single item. Multiple items are needed to operationalize adequately each construct. The use of multiple items allows one to "cast light at different angles" (Converse and Presser, 1986). As one example, definitions of depression contain many components such as feeling blue, depressed, and hopeless. Thus, several questions are needed to represent all components of the definition.

Multi-item measures, which were constructed wherever possible, have several advantages over single-item measures: they reduce the number of final scores necessary to define each variable, assuming that separate scores would have been used from the separate items; they increase score reliability by pooling the information that items have in common; they increase validity by providing a more representative sample of information about the concept; they increase score variability and hence sensitivity; they minimize bias caused by individual tendencies to endorse items (acquiescence) or negate them (nay-saying) regardless of content (in cases where both favorably and unfavorably worded items are combined); and they provide the option, if item responses are missing, to estimate scores using other items in the measure, thus reducing missing scores on the multi-item scale.

Writing Items

After a content area was specified, items were written to operationalize each concept. For the MOS, closed-ended questions with a specific set of responses were used. In large-scale studies, open-ended questions are more burdensome and often yield uninterpretable answers, especially from the less educated. Open-ended questions are time-consuming to administer and require experienced coders; thus, they may be unsuitable for self-administered surveys (Dillman, 1978). However, during the pilot phase, some open-ended questions were used to identify any problems missed in structured questions.

Item Content The first step in writing items is to decide precisely what one wants to know. Part of operationalizing the concept being measured includes deciding whether to ask about frequency (how often a symptom occurred—never, occasionally, or often), intensity (how extreme it was—mild, moderate, or severe), or duration (how long it lasted—a few minutes, several hours). With respect to functioning, questions can compare a person's present level with their usual level or with other people their age. Questions about limitations in functioning can ask about limitations due to health, limitations due to a particular condition, or limitations regardless of cause. Questions can ask if people are having trouble doing certain things or need help. These decisions need to be consistent with the definition of the concept and thus warrant considerable preparatory thought to maximize content validity (Ware, 1987).

Item Stems Each item consists of the item stem and the response options. The item stem is the portion of the item that states the issue or question asked of the respondents. Consistent with traditional standards, item stems were short, simple, easy to understand, and restricted to one idea. Double negatives and ambiguous terms were avoided to maximize certainty of meaning. Information on how to write good items can be found in Fowler, 1984, or Converse and Presser, 1986.

Item Response Options The goal in the selection of item response choices was to pick a set of options that would provide approximately interval-level information. To achieve this, three important features of response options were considered: what type of response intervals to use, whether to offer a middle "neutral" category, and what the number of options should be.

Four basic types of response options—endorsement, frequency, intensity, and comparison—were used. Table 5–1 illustrates the three response options that were most frequently used. The endorsement option was used in assessing statements of perceived health such as "I have been feeling bad lately." The frequency option was used to assess various subjective states, such as energy/fatigue and anxiety. The intensity option illustrates a set of verbal choices for rating the severity of a symptom, such as pain. For intensity, a numbered response scale was sometimes used. For example, when asking patients to rate their pain by providing the numbers 1 to 20, endpoints were labeled "no pain at all" and "pain as bad as you can imagine." Whenever possible, similar response choices in different batteries were used so respondents would feel familiar with a limited set of choices.

Although most would agree that the various responses are ordered in terms of increasing levels (i.e., they yield at least an ordinal scale), it is never clear whether such "imprecise quantifiers actually have some common meaning" (Bradburn and Sudman, 1980). As Bradburn and Sudman point out, the meaning depends on the context in which the question is asked (e.g., which types of questions preceded it) and can vary across individuals. Standardized administration procedures minimize differences in interpretation by respondents.

When a final measure is a single item, it is important to understand the intervals between the response categories, because single items tend to have a "custom" set of response choices for which the intervals are likely to be uneven. For example, the difference in health from "excellent" to "very good" may be smaller than the difference between "good" and "fair" and should be reflected in the score. Thus, when a long-form measure of the same concept was available, the distance between categories was sometimes estimated empirically by calculating

Table 5–1 Response Choices Used to Measure Endorsement, Frequency, and Intensity

Endorsement	Frequency	Intensity
1–Definitely	1–All of the time	1–None
2–True	2–Most of the time	2–Very mild
3–Don't know	3–A good bit of the time	3–Mild
4–False	4–Some of the time	4–Moderate
5–Definitely false	5–A little of the time	5–Severe
	6–None of the time	6–Very severe

mean long-form scores for each response level of the single item. This enables the intermediate response levels (i.e., not the extreme levels) to be transformed using interpolation to reflect the intervals observed based on long-form mean values.

With endorsement scales, a neutral (e.g., "don't know") category is often offered to respondents to provide an option for people who have no opinion on a particular question or to provide an additional level of gradation. There is controversy about the usefulness of a neutral category; some argue it should not be offered because people choose it instead of being more committal (Converse and Presser, 1986). The MOS approach was to include it because it provides a valid response.

Regarding the number of item responses, several studies suggest that five to seven well-chosen response categories provide the lower bound necessary for optimal assessment of a measurement domain (Bollen and Barb, 1981; Johnson and Creech, 1983; Johnson and Dixon, 1984). Others note that most people cannot consistently discriminate their feelings beyond a 7-point classification (Osgood, Suci, and Tannenbaum, 1957, cited in Wells and Marwell, 1976), thus suggesting that more than seven categories are unnecessary. Items administered with five to seven response options have been shown to correlate strongly with corresponding items administered with a greater number of response options (Hays and Huba, 1988). Based on these guidelines, five or six options were selected most often.

Writing Multiple Items The optimal approach to measurement, combining several items into a single score, makes it possible to combine a variety of approaches to item content in a set of items. If frequency is chosen as the response option for a set of items, the item stems can reflect a range of severity (e.g., "feeling blue," "thinking about suicide"). If intensity is the response option, questions about usual intensity and intensity at its worst can be asked.

An advantage of combining items that have different response options (e.g., frequency and intensity), is that method effects are reduced. When this is done, it is helpful if the items have the same number of response options in order to enhance the likelihood that they will have equivalent variances and contribute equally to the combined score. A disadvantage of having different response options within one scale is that they cannot easily be administered over the telephone. In selecting psychological distress/well-being items for purposes of a telephone-administered version, many of the item response sets had to be revised to be consistent. If it is more important to retain the different types of response options, respondents can be provided in advance with cards containing the various options that will be read during the interview.

Time Frame A time frame needs to be specified for most questions, especially those asking about intensity or frequency of various states. The time frame needs to be short enough to allow accurate memory for the event being asked about, yet long enough to represent the general time within which the event is likely to occur and to allow for variation across respondents (Fowler, 1984).

For most of the measures, questions were asked about the past four weeks, an interval in which most people could recall health events yet which would provide a reasonably stable sample of those events. This time frame helps to assure the assessment of the average occurrence of various health states rather than daily fluctuations. This interval is most important in the measures of psychological distress/well-being, where a smaller time frame assesses the "mood of the day" rather than the average levels of distress/well-being over a longer period of time.

The MOS rejected wording the items to say "during the past month," because of concern that respondents would think in terms of the last calendar month. Similarly, "the past thirty days" was rejected because thirty days also sounds like a calendar month. One exception to this nomenclature was the psychological distress/well-being items, which refer to the past month in order to maintain comparability with previous research. Because the cognitive functioning items were interspersed with the distress/well-being items, those items also refer to the past month.

Pretesting Items

In developing new items or in modifying existing measures, it is essential to pretest or to pilot test items to assure that they work. One researcher states, "Virtually every questionnaire could be changed in some way to make it easier for respondents . . . to meet the researcher's objectives" (Fowler, 1984). A preliminary pretest, which solves gross administration issues, might consist of a simple survey of a dozen people to judge the clarity of instructions, determine if the questions make sense, and estimate respondent burden. A full-scale pilot study might be conducted using 50–200 people similar to those in the main study. Others discuss what can be gained from adequate pretesting and provide some guidelines (Converse and Presser, 1986).

In a preliminary pretest, the main source of information is a "debriefing" of the pretest subjects to determine which questions are confusing, difficult, or unclear and whether the subject understood the instructions or skip patterns. This method, where subjects are told that it is a pretest and understand that their task is to identify problems, is called a "participating pretest" (Converse and Presser, 1986). In a larger-scale pilot study, information can also be obtained from statistical evaluation of items.

The MOS conducted nine full-scale pilot studies of various measures: physical functioning, health perceptions, energy/fatigue, sleep, role functioning, pain, physical/psychophysiologic symptoms, family functioning, and sexual functioning. The purpose of the pilot studies varied according to the particular set of measures; however, they generally addressed administrative issues and tested a large item pool so the best items could be selected empirically. From a sample size of 50–100 patients, the MOS identified items with poor variability or a high percentage of missing responses as bad items and revised or eliminated them. Unclear instructions were clarified. By examining correlations among items, we identified items that did not converge (i.e., were not strongly related) with items intended to assess the same concept or that were too strongly correlated with items intended to measure distinct concepts. The importance of these pilot studies is exemplified by the expenditure of more than one year on this phase of the MOS. The results were documented in project memoranda and are summarized in corresponding chapters.

Techniques for Combining Items into Scales

Groups of items that could possibly be combined into a single score were first hypothesized. Hypotheses were based on logical combinations of items appearing from their content to measure the same construct. For many of the MOS measures, hypotheses were well grounded in prior work on the measures.

Multitrait scaling was used as the method for evaluating the hypothesized item groupings. The most commonly used method for evaluating the underlying structure of a set of related concepts in order to develop a set of measures of those concepts is exploratory factor analysis (Ford, MacCallum, and Tait, 1986; Montgomery, Shadish, Orwin, et al.,

1987). This method is appropriate for exploring the relationships among a universe of items in the beginning phases of developing an understanding of the underlying dimensions of the items and was occasionally used during the pilot testing of some of the measures. Exploratory factor analysis, however, has a number of limitations. The resulting item structure depends on the choices regarding the factor model (principal components or common factor analysis), the number of factors that are appropriate, the rotation method selected, and the other items that are included in the analysis. "The decisions made at each choice point can have a substantial impact on the results of the factor analysis and on subsequent interpretation of these results" (Ford, MacCallum, and Tait, 1986). In addition, the interrelationship of variables is left unspecified, and it is impossible to test directly alternative theoretical structures underlying the data.

When theoretical progress on a concept has advanced beyond exploratory development and the hypotheses about its underlying structure are fairly good, confirmatory analysis is more informative than exploratory analysis. Multitrait scaling was selected as the primary scaling method for use in the MOS because it is a confirmatory approach that allows a direct test of a priori structures.

Multitrait Scaling

Multitrait scaling is based on the traditional Likert (1932) method of summated ratings. When responses to several questionnaire items are summed into a single scale score, it is generally termed a summated or a "Likert-type" scale. Summated scales are constructed by summing the items in each hypothesized scale, assigning equal weights to the items. A simple example of a summated ratings scale illustrates this method. Suppose you have two items—"How often during the last four weeks did you have a lot of energy?" and "How often during the last four weeks did you feel tired?"—each with the following response choices:

(1) none of the time
(2) a little of the time
(3) some of the time
(4) most of the time
(5) all of the time.

A summated rating (Likert) scale of these two items involves first reversing the scores on the second item (i.e., 1 = all of the time, 5 =

none of the time) to make a high score on both items refer to energy, and then adding the item scores. The lowest possible score on this summated scale is 2, obtained from two minimum item scores of 1 each, and the highest possible score is 10, obtained from two maximum item scores of 5 each.

A number of analyses must be performed to determine whether a set of items can be appropriately combined into a summated rating scale. In multitrait scaling several scaling criteria are added to those usually associated with Likert scaling. Multitrait scaling follows five steps to determine whether:

(1) each item in a hypothesized grouping is substantially linearly related to the total score computed from other items in that group (a traditional criterion of convergence usually expressed in terms of internal consistency);

(2) each item correlates significantly higher with the construct it is hypothesized to measure than with other constructs (item discrimination criterion);

(3) item groups not hypothesized a priori are not identifiable from the data (factor analytic test);

(4) items in the same scale contain the same proportion of information about the construct (test for approximately equal item-total correlations); and

(5) items measuring the same construct have equal variances and therefore do not need to be standardized before combining them in the same scale (equal variances criterion).

If items in each hypothesized grouping satisfy these criteria, simple summation (or averaging) of items to derive a scale score is appropriate. If the first two scaling criteria are not satisfied in a priori hypothesized groupings, item groupings should be revised. If unhypothesized groupings are identified using factor analysis, these should be evaluated according to the other four scaling criteria. The fourth criterion is often relaxed as long as each item contributes substantially to the total. However, if more stringent criteria are being applied and the fourth scaling criterion is not satisfied, unequal weights can be used for different items. Items should be standardized prior to combining whenever their variances differ significantly (fifth scaling criterion). Equality of variances can be assessed using multiple range tests (Levy, 1975).

Multitrait scaling involves examining item frequencies, means, standard deviations, item-scale correlations (corrected for overlap), scale internal-consistency reliability estimates, and correlations among scales. Multitrait scaling goes beyond traditional tests of internal consistency primarily because it tests item discrimination across scales, as shown in step 2 of the 5-step scaling process. Thus, items are evaluated with respect to how well they represent a particular construct relative to other constructs.

All computations were performed using the Multitrait Analysis Program (MAP), which was derived from ANLITH (Analysis of Item-Test Homogeneity program), written by Thomas Gronek at IBM and Thomas Tyler at the Academic Computing Center at Southern Illinois University. The ANLITH program was first modified for use with SAS on the IBM at The RAND Corporation by William H. Rogers, Patti Camp, and John E. Ware, Jr. The MAP program represents a modification of ANLITH for use with SAS on the IBM PC and the VAX-780 at The RAND Corporation (Hays and Hayashi, 1990; Hays, Hayashi, Carson, and Ware, 1988).

Prior to the multitrait scaling analyses, it is necessary to examine item variability. We look for comparable item variances, roughly symmetrical item response distributions, and a standard deviation near 1.0 (for 5-point scales). If all of these conditions are met, then items can be combined into scales without weighting. There are exceptions to these criteria, however. In cases where an item reflects an uncommon but serious state, it might be preferable to retain a poorly distributed item in order to represent fully a range of health states. Because most of the items in the MOS measures are based on items from prior measures or from measures developed during pilot studies, the tendency was not to eliminate final items during scale construction because of poor variability. Poor item variability was a basis for eliminating items during pilot study analyses.

When items differed substantially in the number of response options, the items were standardized prior to combining in order to weight them equally. If the number of options was the same or differed only by one, the items were combined without standardizing unless their variances differed dramatically.

Item-scale correlations are the fundamental elements of multitrait scaling (Ware, Snyder, Wright, et al., 1983). The first two steps in multitrait scaling analysis involve examining a matrix in which items are rows and scales are columns. Each row contains correlations between one item and all scales, including the one it is hypothesized to be part of. Each column contains correlations between one scale and all items in the analysis, including those hypothesized to be part of that scale and those hypothesized to be part of other scales. Correlations between items and the scale they are a part of are corrected for overlap (Howard and Forehand, 1962) so that estimates of the item-scale correlation are not spuriously inflated.

Item convergence is supported if an item correlates substantially (a corrected correlation of 0.30 or above was used as our standard) with the scale it is hypothesized to represent. Any item not meeting this criterion is eliminated from that scale. For MOS scales that had a previous history of development and for which analyses were intended to refine rather than develop anew, a more stringent criterion of 0.40 was used.

Satisfaction of the second multitrait scaling criterion is obtained if the correlation between the item and the scale it is hypothesized to measure is significantly higher than the correlation of that item with any other scale. This test of item discrimination (Campbell and Fiske, 1959; Jackson, 1970; Thorndike, 1967a) is satisfied and a scaling "success" counted whenever the correlation between an item and its hypothesized scale is substantially higher than other correlations in the same row. A "definite" scaling success is defined by a correlation between an item and its hypothesized scale that is more than two standard errors larger than another correlation in the same row. When a correlation between an item and its hypothesized scale is significantly lower than another correlation in the same row, a "definite" scaling error is counted. When the correlation between the item and other scales in the same row is within two standard errors of its correlation with its hypothesized scale, a "probable" scaling error is counted.

Items that consistently accounted for definite scaling errors were excluded from the scale in question. Inclusion or exclusion of items associated with probable scaling errors depends on several factors, including the number of subjects in the analysis, the number of items in the scale, the internal-consistency reliability, and the strength of associations between the constructs involved. If measures are being constructed that are known to be related theoretically (e.g., depression and anxiety), probable errors associated with items in the two scale groupings are more likely to be tolerated, at least early in the process of scale development. When scale development is in more advanced stages of refinement, like the MOS measures, we were less tolerant of probable errors.

Item-scale correlations uncorrected for overlapping items are calculated using the following formula (Tyler and Fiske, 1968):

$$r_1 = \frac{n * X_J X_W - (\Sigma X_J)(\Sigma X_W)}{n^2 S_W S_J} \quad \text{Where } J = \text{item}$$
$$W = \text{scale with } J \text{ in it.}$$

Corrected item-scale correlations are calculated using the following formula (Howard and Forehand, 1962):

$$r_2 = \frac{r_1 S_W - S_J}{[S_W^2 + S_J^2 - 2(r_1)(S_W)(S_J)]^{1/2}} \quad .$$

Missing Data in Multitrait Scaling When summated ratings scales are scored, substitutions might need to be made for missing item responses. Four options are possible: (1) midpoint of the possible scale range, (2) sample central tendency statistics (mean, median, or modal score for the item in question), (3) regression estimate, and (4) respondent central tendency statistic (mean, median, or modal score for that respondent across either all items in the battery or other items in the same scale). When the range of response values differs for items used (e.g., one item with four possible responses and another with five), responses can be prorated to estimate the missing response.

In the multitrait analyses, the MAP program estimates missing values using option (4) above with the mean as the central tendency statistic. The MOS estimated missing values for respondents with data for at least half of the items in a scale. Because of this, sample sizes in each multitrait analysis varied. The MAP program provides two additional missing value options: (1) respondents can be excluded if they have missing data on any item in any item grouping, and (2) scores can be estimated if respondents answer at least one item for all scales.

Factor Analysis Exploratory factor analysis was sometimes used to test for unhypothesized item groupings, especially in the pilot studies. In exploratory factor analysis, the factors identified represent underlying dimensions that define the measured items. Factor analysis was also used to guide in the development of overall indexes (i.e., combining items across constructs). For this purpose, the size of the first factor was evaluated in terms of the variance accounted for and items were identified that correlated at least 0.30 with the first unrotated principal component or factor.

Both principal components analysis and common factor analysis were performed, depending on the situation. Factors were extracted from a matrix of product-moment correlations among item scores with unities (principal components) or communality estimates (principal axes) in the matrix diagonal. When unities are used as communality estimates, all of the variance and covariance among items is explained by the components. In contrast, when communalities are inserted in the matrix diagonal, only the covariance among items and the portion of the total variance due to common factors are explained. In principal components analysis, no distinction is made among common, specific, and error variance. Common factor analysis provides a solution based on common variance among the items, excluding unique variance (Ford, MacCallum, and Tait, 1986).

In order to achieve simple structure, factor rotation was conducted. The decision regarding the number of factors to rotate is a central issue in exploratory factor analysis (Rummel, 1970). The initial unrotated solution was evaluated using various criteria for determining the number of factors to rotate:

(1) Guttman's (1954) weakest lower bound, in which the number of factors to rotate is indicated by the number of eigenvalues exceeding 1.0 when unities are inserted in the matrix diagonal (this is the most commonly used criterion);

(2) Cattell's (1966) scree test, which involves interpreting the eigenvalue plot across factors and identifying the point at which the negative slope of the curve levels off and begins the "scree";

(3) parallel analysis (Humphreys and Ilgen, 1969), in which actual data eigenvalues derived using unities (Allen, 1986; Holden, Longman, Cota, and Fekken, 1989) or squared multiple correlation (Montanelli and Humphreys, 1976) communality estimates are compared with random data eigenvalues derived from a correlation matrix produced from normally distributed random numbers. Parallel analysis sets an upper bound for the number of factors to rotate based on the number of actual data eigenvalues that exceed the corresponding random data eigenvalues (Hays, 1985, 1987; Montanelli and Humphreys, 1976; Silverstein, 1987); and

(4) use of trial rotations when the decision as to the best number of factors for final rotation is ambiguous according to the preceding criteria. Trial rotations are evaluated in terms of interpretability and the meaningfulness and desirability of alterations in major factors when additional factors are rotated.

Both orthogonal and oblique rotations were performed. Oblique rotations are generally preferred because "it is more sensible to rotate the factors obliquely and then determine the tenability of the orthogonality assumption" (Ford, MacCallum, and Tait, 1986). Oblique rotations generally produce a more realistic representation of the factors (Rummel, 1970).

Guttman Scalogram Analysis Scalogram Analysis (Guttman, 1944) or Guttman scaling is sometimes used to construct multi-item measures. Guttman scales were avoided for the final M O S measures for several reasons. Guttman scales require a dichotomous response format, limiting responses to two choices (e.g., yes or no), which considerably restricts the amount of information that can be obtained with any one item. Guttman scales also tend to be limited to a few items, because as the number of items exceeds five or six, it is hard to achieve a realistic ordering of difficulty. Thus the "richness" of a construct is hard to represent adequately and precision is limited. When Guttman scale levels are slightly ambiguous and variability in a certain item is skewed, a different ordering of items might be obtained in different samples of people. Guttman scaling ignores measurement error and is deterministic in the sense that all individuals are assumed to adhere to the same basic response model. The experience in the H I E with Guttman scales was that scoring people who do not fall into one of the perfect scale type categories is cumbersome and time-consuming.

Calculation of Scale Scores Scale scores were calculated by averaging item scores for all respondents that had nonmissing data for half or more of the items in the scale. Missing values were assigned for the scale to those who had missing data for more than half the items in the scale. Because of the distribution of missing values for items in the scales, the number of missing values for scales was similar to that obtained if we had used a more stringent criterion of 90% nonmissing items before allowing scale scores. Most respondents either answered half or more of the scale items or answered none of the items. Most scales were transformed so that the lowest possible score was 0 and the highest possible score 100, using the following formula:

$$100 \times \frac{(\text{observed score} - \text{minimum possible score})}{(\text{maximum possible score} - \text{minimum possible score})}$$

For many of the single items, however, the raw scale scores were retained.

Variability of Scales After multitrait scaling studies were completed, the variability of resulting score distributions was studied. Good variability means that the scores are spread over the full range of the measure and that the distributions are roughly normal. The distributions of each final measure, including single-item measures, were evaluated in a number of ways: by seeing whether the full range of scores is observed and, if not, what the range is; by analyzing the percentage who receive a perfect score (or the percentage with some limitations); and by looking at the shape of the frequency distribution. The shape of distributions was inspected to identify measures yielding nonnormal (i.e., skewed or kurtotic) score distributions. Skewed distributions are those that are bunched up at one end of the distribution. Positive skew means that the tail is to the right and the hump is to the left. Negative skew means that the tail is to the left and the hump is to the right. The skewness statistic ranges from negative to positive infinity. The closer the skewness statistic is to zero, the more normal the distribution. The highest skewness observed in the MOS was 3.3 for the mobility measure. Kurtosis refers to whether the distribution is more peaked (leptokurtic) or more flat (platykurtic) than normal. The kurtosis statistic ranges from -2 to positive infinity. A high positive statistic indicates a more peaked distribution, a high negative statistic a flatter one. Thus, the closer the score is to zero, the more normal the distribution.

Both skewness and kurtosis are interpreted in terms of whether they are statistically different from zero, using a t-test. This test uses a standard error based on the sample size. The standard error for skewness is the square root of $6/N$, and the standard error for kurtosis is the square root of $24/N$. In the large MOS sample, these standard errors are small and a significant statistic is easy to obtain. Thus, more weight was given to the more qualitative approaches evaluation of the score distributions.

Variability of scores on health status measures might be insufficient for many reasons. Assuming there is actual variability in the construct being measured, insufficient variability might indicate that the items do not adequately assess the particular health construct of interest; do not adequately detect differences in some range of values between the extremes (e.g., distances between the levels represented by the items might be too large, and scores might not reflect important differences between the health states of respondents); and do not assess important differences in health states at one or the other end of the continuum (e.g., items assessing severe limitations only). Addition of items that more precisely assess clinically significant differences between scale levels or that increase the range of measurement should increase the variability of resulting score distributions and the usefulness of the scale in detecting actual differences in health status.

Reliability and Stability Reliability refers to the consistency of the score or to the extent to which a score is free of random error. Reliability of measurement refers to the extent to which measured variance reflects true score rather than random error. To the extent a score is unreliable, it becomes more difficult to observe or to measure the true situation. A reliability coefficient is an estimate of the proportion of total variance that is true score variance, as expressed in the following formula (Kerlinger and Pedhazur, 1973): reliability $= 1 - (V_e / V_t)$, where V_e equals the error variance and V_t is the total measured variance.

For multi-item scales constructed using multitrait scaling techniques, the internal consistency of the scale is the appropriate indicator of reliability. For single-item measures and multi-item measures constructed according to other techniques, test-retest reliability must be used. When reliability estimates are unavailable, an inference about reliability can be made based on studies of correlations between the measure and other variables.

Adequate reliability is a prerequisite for using a score for any purpose (Thorndike, 1967b). The criterion for "adequate" depends on the purpose of the measure. For purposes of group comparisons, including correlational studies, reliability need not be as high as it would have to be to make individual comparisons. Reliability of 0.50 or above is considered acceptable for group comparisons (Helmstadter, 1964). Coefficients of 0.90 or greater are acceptable for individual comparisons, including evaluation of changes in an individual over time (Helmstadter, 1964). Nunnally (1978) suggests that in the early stages of research, reliabilities of 0.50 or 0.60 suffice. As the theory and methods become more refined, additional resources can be allocated to improving the reliabilities of the more important concepts (e.g., by adding more items). Even then, in basic research, the burden imposed by the number of items necessary to obtain reliabilities of 0.80 might exceed the value of the increased reliability.

Internal-Consistency Reliability The internal-consistency approach was used to estimate reliability for all multi-item scales. This approach considers common variance (shared by all items in a scale) to be true score (reliable variance) and unique item variance to be error. The reliability coefficient it yields, coefficient alpha (Cronbach, 1951), is a function of two properties of scale items: item homogeneity or the extent to which the items covary or have something in common and the number of items in the scale. Reliability is increased when either of these properties increases. The relationships among internal-consistency reliability, homogeneity, and scale length are shown in the following formula (Nunnally, 1978): $r_{tt} = k r_{ii}/(1 + (k - 1)r_{ii}$ where r_{tt} is the internal-consistency reliability of a score, k is the number of items used to compute the scale score, and r_{ii} is the estimated reliability for a single item and can be interpreted as the average inter-item correlation (Fiske, 1966; Tyler and Fiske, 1968).

Internal consistency estimates were made using the analysis-of-variance approach to reliability (Guilford, 1954). The analysis of variance is a one-way repeated measures design with items functioning as the repeated measures. R_{tt} (alpha) is calculated by using the Hoyt (1941) formula for reliability:

$$R_{tt} = 1 - \frac{MS_{within}}{MS_{respondents}} - \frac{MS_{respondents} - MS_{within}}{MS_{respondents}}$$

Calculation formulas for R_{ii} (intra-class correlation for items, average correlation between items), R_{gg} (coefficient of homogeneity of persons), and R_{pp} (intra-class correlation for persons, average correlation between persons) are provided below:

$$R_{ii} = R_{tt}/(k + R_{tt} - (k*R_{tt}))$$
$$R_{gg} = 1 - (MS_{within}/MS_{items})$$
$$R_{pp} = R_{gg}/(N + R_{gg} - (N*R_{gg}))$$

where k is the number of items in the scale, and N is the number of respondents.

Because the reliability coefficient is a function of differences between individuals, it will tend to be larger for samples that vary more on the trait being studied (Aiken, 1982; Nunnally, 1978). Indeed, for some measures the reliability increased in this patient sample over that observed in a general population. This is consistent with the fact that scores on these health measures tend to be more skewed in general populations than in patient samples.

For most purposes of the MOS, the aim was to achieve an internal-consistency reliability of between 0.70 and 0.80, using a minimum of from two to four items per measure. However, for the short-form measures that might be used to assess patients routinely in office practice, the MOS attempted to achieve reliabilities approaching 0.90 in order to increase their usefulness in assessing individual patients over time. Measures that approach the 0.90 standard are potentially useful for individual assessment. Measures to be used for individual assessment can be supplemented by additional items to increase their reliability or used as they are with the knowledge that standard errors of measurement are somewhat larger than ideal.

Estimating Reliability For Single-Item Measures Test-retest reliability can be used for single items as well as for multi-item scales. In test-retest reliability, questions are administered to the same group of people at two points in time, and a correlation between the two times is computed. The time difference between the two administrations must be short enough so that substantial change in the attribute being measured is unlikely but long enough so respondents will not remember their previous responses. If change has occurred the true reliability will be underestimated. If respondents remember their previous responses, the true reliability will be overestimated (Anastasi, 1976; Nachmias and Nachmias, 1981).

As the time difference between the two measures increases, the coefficient can become an indicator of stability rather than reliability. This shift is more true for constructs that tend to change over time (e.g., health) than for those that tend to be relatively stable (e.g., attitudes, beliefs) (Nunnally, 1978) and for younger versus older adults (Finn, 1986). The degree to which stability and reliability are represented in a test-retest coefficient depends on the time interval, the nature of the measure, and the characteristics of the respondents. The relative amount of reliability and stability of measures can be estimated using sophisticated panel models (Werts, Linn, and Jöreskog, 1978; Wheaton, Muthen, Alwin, and Summers, 1977; Wiley and Wiley, 1970).

The MOS was able to evaluate the correlation of some single-item measures administered on an average of four months apart. Because this time difference is substantial enough to expect a real change in health, it provides a lower-bound estimate of reliability.

In addition to test-retest reliability, we were able to glean something about the reliability of the single-item measures based on their correlations with other health measures. The reliability of a measure limits the degree of validity that is possible. This means that the correlation between one measure and another can never exceed the square root of the product of the reliabilities of these measures (Nunnally, 1978). Thus, if both measures have reliabilities of 0.70, their intercorrelation, in theory, will not be any larger than 0.70. This principle allows us to evaluate the reliability of single-item measures. For example, if a single-item measure of health correlates 0.70 with another measure of health whose reliability is about 0.70, it can be inferred that the single-item measure is adequate for group comparison. This is referred to as alternate-forms reliability. Because of the noncomparability of the alternate forms, it is considered a lower-bound estimate of reliability.

Evaluating Reliability in Disadvantaged Groups Reliability tends to be poorer in more disadvantaged groups such as those with low education (Andrews, 1984; Ware, Brook, Davies-Avery, et al., 1980). The suggested cause of this is that less educated people have difficulty reading and understanding the questions or are less familiar with questionnaire procedures. Of direct relevance to the MOS were three additional groups of patients for whom reliability might be poor: the more severely ill, the very old, and the depressed. For comparisons to be made on outcome measures across groups diverse in these characteristics, it is important to test the reliability separately to assure that minimum standards are met for each of them.

The MOS tested the internal-consistency reliability of selected health scales constructed according to multitrait scaling techniques separately for four groups: (1) those with low education (less than a high school education); (2) the very old (over age 70); (3) those with a serious chronic condition; and (4) the depressed (those having depressive symptoms using an 8-item screener for depression [Burnam, Wells, Leake, et al., 1987]).

The reliability of the measures of psychological distress and well-being (chapter 7) and of the short-form measures (Stewart, Hays, and Ware, 1988) was evaluated for one or more of these subgroups. In all cases, reliabilities were comparable. Time constraints precluded the evaluation of all measures in these subgroups; however, we expect that similar findings would be observed for other measures.

Assigning Labels to Measures The importance of the process of labeling measures is often overlooked. When a measure is used later in various clinical studies, often the detailed content of the measure is abbreviated, and readers interpret the results based on the label. Because labels are often vague (e.g., functional status, emotional functioning; subjective well-being), more attention should be given to making this process more precise. Extended labels should be assigned that clearly indicate the nature of the measure, in order to avoid confusion and misinterpretation. The MOS provides a table of definitions of each of the MOS measures (chapter 20). These extended labels include information on the time frame of the questions and summarize the item content of multi-item measures. Information is also provided on the direction of scoring in the label of each variable. The sign (+) indicates that a high score represents better health (or is more positive), and the sign (−) indicates that a high score represents poorer health. This sign facilitates interpretation of tabulated results without having to refer to scoring information.

6. Physical Functioning Measures

Anita L. Stewart and Caren J. Kamberg

Definition and Issues

Physical functioning refers to the performance of or the capacity to perform a variety of physical activities normal for people in good health. Such physical activities include bathing, dressing, walking, bending, climbing stairs, and running. Limitations in physical activities are frequently due to physical health problems such as shortness of breath, joint problems, overweight, and back problems (Stewart, Ware, and Brook, 1982).

At the time measures of physical functioning were selected for the MOS, a number of conceptual and methodological issues remained unresolved. One was the identification of appropriate content. Since most activities of daily life are physical in some sense, theoretically all activities could be included. For example, shopping, housecleaning, and using tools are daily physical activities but can also be classified as role activities. Therefore, many measures combine questions about physical and other activities into one measure, labeled "functional status" or "activities of daily living" (Canadian Sickness Survey, 1960; Patrick, Bush, and Chen, 1973a, 1973b; Reynolds, Rushing, and Miles, 1974; Berdit and Williamson, 1973; Deniston and Jette, 1980; Parkerson, Gehlbach, Wagner, et al., 1981). The problem with including all daily activities in a physical functioning measure is that many factors other than physical health determine whether people can perform daily activities. For example, the ability to work depends on the physical difficulty of the work. Whether or not health interferes with walking is more likely to reflect physical capacity. A review of empirical studies of the relationships between role activities and physical activities shows that physical limitations only partially explain limitations in role activities (Stewart, Ware, and Brook, 1978). For this reason, social and role activities were treated as separate content areas in the MOS. The content of MOS physical functioning measures was thus limited to those physical activities most likely to be the same for all people regardless of their life situation such as dressing, walking, bending, climbing stairs, and lifting heavy objects. Three categories of physical activities were included: self-care activities (bathing, dressing); activities related to mobility (getting around indoors and outdoors and in the community); and other physical activities (running, walking, using stairs, lifting, bending).

A second issue was coarseness. Available physical functioning measures define relatively few scale levels. For example, the twenty-two items in the Personal Functioning Index define only six scale levels (Stewart, Ware, and Brook, 1982). To detect small differences in physical functioning, more scale levels need to be developed. This can be achieved by asking about a broader range of physical activities, asking about the degree of limitation and not merely whether or not people can perform the activity, and using a scaling method that avoids aggregation at a particular scale level. It is also important that added scale levels be well represented in the samples being studied. For this reason, additional scale levels in the MOS physical functioning measure were concentrated in the middle and upper range of the scale, where most patients function.

A third issue focused on the range of physical activities. Most available scales emphasize basic physical activities which are performed without limitations for most people in general populations. Activities such as bathing, dressing, and feeding are the entire focus of some measures because they were developed for older populations (Katz, Ford, Moskowitz, et al., 1963). The most strenuous activities assessed by Jette and Deniston (1978) are climbing stairs and walking outside. The implications are twofold: (1) score distributions tend to be skewed, with most people receiving a perfect score, and (2) a perfect score is simply the absence of serious physical limitations rather than a state of positive physical functioning. By extending the range of assessment into more strenuous physical activities, the precision of these measures can be improved. Examples of measures that attempt to tap the positive end of the physical functioning continuum have been published (Stewart, Ware, and Brook, 1981, 1982). Nevertheless, because many people with chronic conditions are older, it is also important to retain the ability to identify limitations in basic physical activities such as dressing, bathing, or walking a block.

A fourth issue relates to whether the extent of difficulty or the need for help should be assessed as opposed to whether people can perform each activity. A way to enhance the sensitivity of measures is to assess the extent of difficulty or the need for help in performing each activity rather than to assess mere performance. Several available measures assess degree of difficulty or pain associated with various physical activities (Nagi, 1969; Stewart, Ware, and Brook, 1978; Jette and Deniston, 1978; Deniston and Jette, 1980; Fries, Spitz, and Kraines, 1980; Meenan, 1986; Parkerson, Gehlbach, Wagner, et al., 1981). Jette and Deniston measured both pain and difficulty. The usefulness of these approaches to increase the precision of measurement was evaluated in the physical functioning pilot studies.

A fifth issue asks whether the degree of difficulty and the need for help should be assessed separately. It has been suggested that an increase in dependence—obtaining help from another person—might decrease functional pain and difficulty (Jette and Deniston, 1978). The literature reveals no tests of the incremental validity of these separate measures. Separate measures of pain, difficulty, and dependence were constructed by Deniston and Jette (1980). Based on their correlations with other measures, it appears that dependence is less related to other health measures than pain and difficulty. This concept is tested in the pilot studies.

A sixth issue relates to aggregating categories of physical functioning. Although many available measures assess limitations in three categories of physical activities—self-care, mobility, and other physical activities—there is no consensus on whether separate scales should be constructed for each or whether the information the scales contain is just as well summarized in an aggregate physical functioning measure. Three available measures combine items measuring self-care activities, mobility, and other physical activities into a single measure (Haber, 1970; Nagi, 1976; Stewart, Ware, and Brook, 1982). Haber and Nagi considered limitations in self-care and mobility more severe than those in other physical activities but did not empirically test their assumption. Stewart, Ware, and Brook scored limitations in self-care as the most extreme and limitations in mobility as the next most extreme, based on empirical tests. Others developed separate scales of each (Gilson, Gilson, Bergner, et al., 1975; Bergner, Bobbitt, Carter, and Gilson, 1981), but no empirical evidence of their independence was presented.

Because mobility is conceptually distinct from self-care and other physical activities, whether it could be scored as a separate measure of physical functioning was tested empirically. The ability to go where one wants, when one wants, without help might be more strongly related to peoples' well-being than to their actual functioning in other physical activities. Having a separate measure of mobility would facilitate such studies.

A seventh issue in the assessment of physical functioning has been the lack of consideration of people's values for different levels of functioning. This is of special importance in measures of physical functioning, especially as we attempt to incorporate into these measures activities that many people do not care to perform, such as running. By incorporating a measure of satisfaction with functioning into a physical functioning battery, patients' preferences for different levels of functioning are taken into account. Such a measure would be somewhat independent of a measure of physical functioning. We can imagine people who are satisfied with less than perfect physical functioning scores because of the minimal physical demands their daily life makes upon them. We can also imagine people who are unsatisfied despite the fact that they receive high physical functioning scores because they desire an extremely physically active life.

With few exceptions, evaluations of physical functioning in terms of satisfaction have rarely been assessed. A modification of the Health Assessment Questionnaire assessed whether people were or were not satisfied with various physical activities (Pincus, Summey, Soraci, et al., 1983). Berki and Ashcraft (1979) asked about the degree of satisfaction on a 5-point scale from extremely satisfied to extremely dissatisfied with six aspects of physical functioning (e.g., satisfaction with your physical ability to do things you want to do, your physical fitness, your ability to get around outdoors).

A final issue pertains to the method of scoring of the measures. Our prior work involved Guttman scaling with its complicated scoring algorithms (Stewart, Ware, and Brook, 1981). Simpler methods of scoring need to be used.

Content and Measurement Strategy

Pilot Study Five goals guided the development of the physical functioning measures. Comprehensiveness was assured by assessing

three categories of activities—self-care, mobility, physical activities—
and a range of physical activities from very basic to fairly difficult. We
attempted to capture more than merely whether people could or could
not do various activities by assessing the amount of help needed in
performing these activities (independence) and the discomfort, effort,
or difficulty experienced in attempting their performance. We also
assessed only limitations in physical functioning due to poor health and
people's evaluation of their physical functioning (i.e., satisfaction with
functioning). The use of cumulative (Guttman) scales was discontinued
in favor of summated ratings scales to enable more sensitive scales and
to make scale scoring easier.

To develop the MOS battery, two pilot studies were conducted in
which these issues were addressed. The pilot study samples were
obtained from a medicine outpatient clinic in an urban setting and from
a rural health clinic.

To meet the goal of assessing a range of physical activities, a
representative set of twenty-three activities was selected from nine
existing measures of physical functioning. Four potential measures
were tested: (1) short-form physical functioning, (2) long-form physical
functioning (degree of pain or difficulty), (3) independence (need for
help) in basic activities, and (4) mobility. The strategy was to select a
short-form measure (the 6-item physical functioning measure from the
MOS Short-Form General Health Survey) and determine whether the
long-form measure contributed more information. We then tested
whether measures of independence in basic physical activities and
mobility were redundant in relation to the long-form physical functioning measure.

For the evaluation of the long-form measure, the MOS assessed the
degree of pain and difficulty associated with each of twenty-three
activities, using published response scales (Pincus, Summey, Soraci, et
al., 1983; Jette and Deniston, 1978). The 6-item short-form measure
correlated at least as high as the 23-item long-form measure with a set of
health measures and age. Further tests of the incremental validity of the
long-form measure showed that it did not contribute over and above the
short-form measure in any of four tests. However, the number who
reported one or more limitations was only 56% for the short-form
measure and 75% for the long-form measure, indicating substantially
greater sensitivity with the use of the long-form measure. We thus
decided to further develop the long-form measure by building on the six
items that performed well in the short-form measure. Eight items from

the item pool were added to the six existing short-form items. Based on item response distributions from the first pilot study, the item response choices were revised to ask about degree of limitations (limited a lot, limited a little, not limited) to more easily assess the degree of pain and difficulty. Ten of the fourteen pilot physical functioning items were retained based on item-scale correlations in the second pilot study. Two self-care items were eliminated because of low prevalence and low item-total correlations; "walking uphill" was eliminated because of its conceptual overlap with climbing stairs, and "standing for long periods" was eliminated because it was less physical than other items.

A set of fifteen items measuring independence in the most basic or elementary activities (e.g., shopping, preparing foods) was tested. For all items, the MOS asked about the extent of need for help (four levels). Most people did not require help with these fifteen basic activities (the range was 99% [eating] to 75% [climbing several flights of stairs]). Cross-tabulations of comparable items, those for which we asked both whether they needed help and extent of pain or difficulty, revealed very high agreement. Of those who said they had no pain or difficulty, 97–100% said they needed no help. The converse was also true. Correlations of comparable items with validity variables were either the same or the independence items correlated lower than the items from the long form. In regression analyses predicting a variety of health measures, the independence measure did not predict any additional variance over and above the long-form measure. From these results, we concluded that the independence in basic physical activities measure added little information over and above the long-form physical functioning measure, and the "need for help" measure was eliminated.

Four mobility items were developed: (1) the need for help in traveling around the community; (2) the amount of the time, if at all, a person was in bed or in a chair all or most of the day; (3) limitations in ability to use public transportation; and (4) limitations in ability to drive a car due to health. These items were adapted from those used in the HIE (Stewart, Ware, and Brook, 1978) and from the Rheumatology Rehabilitation Questionnaire (Spiegel, personal communication). The mobility measure predicted a significant amount of additional variance in a current health criterion variable over and above the long-form physical functioning measure. Thus, the mobility measure is an essential component of the set of physical functioning measures.

Six items pertaining to satisfaction with physical functioning adapted from Berki and Ashcraft (1979) were included in the first pilot study. These items were highly intercorrelated (from 0.82 to 0.92), indicating that satisfactory reliability could be achieved with fewer items. The MOS eliminated three items and added one item based on written comments to an open-ended question. These four items were administered in the second pilot study with very high reliability (0.93), suggesting that a single item might suffice.

Final Items Based on pilot study results, items assessing the following aspects of physical functioning were included in the final battery: physical functioning (ten items), satisfaction with physical ability (one item), and mobility (three items) (see pages 375–376 in the appendix). The ten physical functioning items assess the extent of health-related limitations in various activities, ranging from basic (bathing or dressing) to strenuous (running). Respondents were asked if their health limited them in these activities. Three response choices were offered: limited a lot, limited a little, not limited at all. Three mobility items refer to independence in traveling around the community, being in bed or a chair most or all of the day because of health, and problems using public transportation due to health. The response choices for the three mobility items were unique to each item. Two of the mobility items had five response choices, indicating increasing proportions of time the person had the limitation. The item responses to the ability to use public transportation were: (1) no, because of my health; (2) no, for some other reason; (3) yes, able to use public transportation.

Construction and Evaluation of Measures

Analysis Plan The general goals of the analysis plan were to confirm that the multi-item scales for physical functioning and mobility would satisfy scaling assumptions, including tests of internal consistency and item discriminant validity. Items were first evaluated to assure adequate variability. Multitrait scaling techniques were used to evaluate the convergent and discriminant validity of the items in the hypothesized scales. The variability and interval properties of the satisfaction with physical ability item was evaluated. Because each mobility item had a different response choice, it was necessary to pursue several alternative possibilities for constructing a scale. For all analyses, the mobility item pertaining to ability to use public transportation was dichotomized such that 0 = unable to use public transportation because of health and

1 = other responses (able to use public transportation or unable to use it for a reason other than health).

The following configurations of the three mobility items were evaluated: (1) only the two mobility items that had five response choices, without recoding the responses; (2) same as number one but adding the public transportation item scored dichotomously; (3) collapsing the two items with five response choices into three response choices and including the dichotomous public transportation item; (4) dichotomizing all three items; and (5) standardizing all three items.

Validity variables in the multitrait analysis included those conceptually related to physical functioning, including other measures of functioning and measures of general health. The measure of role limitations due to physical health was expected to provide the most stringent test because its items attributed limitations to physical health problems. Other measures included current health, physical/psychophysiologic symptoms, energy/fatigue, and social activity limitations due to health.

Item Variability A summary of physical functioning items and their frequencies are shown in Table 6–1. Item means and standard deviations are presented in the multitrait scaling analysis table for those items contained in multi-item scales. The percentage that reported being limited at all ranged from 10% for the bathing and dressing item to 76% for the vigorous activities item. These results are in contrast to those for a general nonaged population in which the percentages limited on comparable items ranged from 1% to 16% (Stewart, Ware, and Brook, 1982). For those with limitations, responses were fairly evenly divided between the "limited a lot" and "limited a little" categories, indicating that those who report being limited in their performance of these activities differ in the degree of their limitations. This distinction appears to improve the amount of information obtained, in contrast to a dichotomous measure.

A fairly small percentage of patients in this sample was identified as limited on any of the mobility items (see Table 6–2). Only about 10% of patients needed any help in getting around the community. However, 22% reported at least occasionally being in bed or in a chair most or all of the day because of health, although some of these (14%) reported doing so only occasionally. Only 4% reported being unable to use public transportation because of health. Because we scored the public transportation item dichotomously, this distribution is quite poor for

Table 6–1 Frequency and Percentage Distribution of Physical Functioning Items: PAQ Baseline Sample (N = 3,053)

Abbreviated Item Content	Item Variable Name	ITEM RESPONSE[a]					
		Limited a Lot (1)		Limited a Little (2)		Not Limited (3)	
		f	%	f	%	f	%
Vigorous activities	PF 1	1,224	42.5	975	33.9	679	23.6
Moderate activities	PF 2	370	12.7	798	27.3	1,749	59.9
Lifting, carrying groceries	PF 3	278	9.5	730	24.9	1,925	65.6
Climbing several flights of stairs	PF 4	607	20.8	995	34.2	1,310	45.0
Climbing one flight of stairs	PF 5	195	6.7	606	20.8	2,109	72.5
Bending, kneeling, stooping	PF 6	346	11.8	951	32.6	1,621	55.5
Walking more than one mile	PF 7	658	22.6	778	26.8	1,471	50.6
Walking several blocks	PF 8	431	14.8	533	18.3	1,952	66.9
Walking one block	PF 9	173	5.9	368	12.6	2,383	81.5
Bathing or dressing	PF 10	63	2.1	239	8.1	2,631	89.6

[a] Percentage of those who responded to each item. Percentage missing ranged from 3.9% to 5.7% across items.

purposes of multitrait analysis. The remaining items had sufficient variability to warrant their inclusion in the multitrait scaling analyses.

Scale Construction Five multitrait scaling analyses were performed, one for each way of scoring the mobility items outlined in the analysis plan. In the first analysis—scoring mobility in terms of only the two items with five response choices—all items met the criterion of convergent validity and eleven of the twelve items met the criterion of discriminant validity (Table 6–3). Item-scale correlations ranged from 0.48 to 0.80 for physical functioning and were 0.56 for each of the two mobility items. The correlation of the mobility item pertaining to being in a bed or chair most or all of the day (MOB2) with the physical functioning scale was within two standard deviations of its correlation with the mobility scale. In all additional analyses, which varied in terms of how mobility was scored, one or more items in the mobility scale also failed tests of discriminant validity. Because results using the first method of scoring mobility were preferable, we scored mobility in

Table 6–2 Frequency and Percentage Distribution of Mobility Items: PAQ Baseline Sample (N = 3,053)

Item Content	Item Variable Name	Item Response Choices	f	%
When you travel around your community, does someone have to assist you because of your health?	MOB1	1–Yes, all of the time	49	1.6
		2–Yes, most of the time	35	1.2
		3–Yes, some of the time	88	3.0
		4–Yes, a little of the time	138	4.6
		5–No, none of the time	2,662	89.5
		Total		99.9
		% of total missing		2.6
Are you in bed or in a chair most or all of the day because of your health?	MOB2	1–Yes, every day	50	1.7
		2–Yes, most days	48	1.6
		3–Yes, some days	110	3.7
		4–Yes, occasionally	431	14.5
		5–No, never	2,332	78.5
		Total		100.0
		% of total missing		2.7
Are you able to use public transportation?	MOB3	1–No, because of my health	130	4.4
		2–No, for some other reason	205	6.9
		3–Yes, able to use public transportation	2,617	88.6
		Total		99.9
		% of total missing		3.3

terms of the two items. However, this scale is, therefore, not as unique as we would like.

For the satisfaction with physical ability measure, the frequency and percentage distribution and the mean physical functioning scores (for purposes of evaluating the intervals between levels) are shown in Table 6–4. Although most people fell in the "satisfied" half of the scale (68%), responses were well distributed across the first three "satisfied" categories. Only 13% reported being completely satisfied. However, inspection of the mean physical functioning scores suggests that the "very satisfied" category is nearly the same as the "completely satisfied" category. The intervals between the five other categories are fairly

Table 6–3 Item-Scale Correlation Matrix, Physical Functioning: P A Q Baseline Sample (N = 2,568)

Item	Mean	S D	P H Y S	M O B	P F S A T
PF1	1.84	.80	.62[a]	.31	.56
PF2	2.49	.70	.77[a]	.49	.54
PF3	2.58	.65	.75[a]	.52	.49
PF4	2.26	.77	.77[a]	.40	.55
PF5	2.67	.58	.77[a]	.51	.46
PF6	2.45	.68	.70[a]	.42	.48
PF7	2.30	.80	.78[a]	.43	.55
PF8	2.54	.72	.80[a]	.49	.50
PF9	2.77	.53	.72[a]	.55	.42
PF10	2.88	.38	.48[a]	.44	.31
MOB1	4.82	.64	.46	.56[a]	.31
MOB2	4.68	.75	.55	.56[a]	.42

Note: Standard Error of Correlation = .02. P H Y S = Physical functioning; M O B = Mobility; P F S A T = Satisfaction with physical abilities; R O L P H Y = Role limitations due to physical health; C U R R = Current health; S Y M P = Physical/psychophysiologic symptoms; E N E R G Y = Energy/fatigue; S O C = Social activity limitations due to health.
[a] Denotes hypothesized item groupings and item-scale correlation corrected for overlap (chapter 5).

equivalent, ranging from about 13 to 18 points on the physical functioning scale.

Scoring Rules The 10-item physical functioning scale was scored by averaging the item responses across all nonmissing items. No recoding was necessary because a high item score indicated better functioning. Persons missing more than five of the ten items were assigned a missing score on the scale. In addition, if persons who received a missing score based on this algorithm had responded "not limited" to the vigorous activities item, they were instead assigned a perfect score. The logic was that if we knew these persons were not limited in vigorous activities, we could assume they were not limited on any remaining missing items. The score was then transformed to a 0–100 scale. A high score means better functioning.

The item pertaining to vigorous activities had the largest percentage missing (5.7%). The percentage missing on the remaining nine items ranged from 3.9% to 4.4%. Eleven percent of the sample missed one or more items. Three percent were missing all ten items; thus, scores could not be estimated for them based on other items. Most of those who were

ROLPHY	CURR	SYMP	ENERGY	SOC
.50	.49	−.37	.42	.26
.57	.51	−.41	.48	.41
.55	.47	−.41	.44	.39
.51	.49	−.41	.45	.33
.48	.44	−.36	.41	.34
.51	.44	−.41	.39	.32
.53	.50	−.41	.47	.36
.53	.48	−.38	.45	.38
.46	.41	−.32	.39	.36
.35	.31	−.26	.28	.32
.36	.32	−.25	.31	.35
.50	.45	−.40	.44	.49

Table 6–4 Frequency, Percentage, and Mean Physical Functioning Scale Scores for Respondents in Six Satisfaction Categories

Category	Transformed Score	f	%	Mean
1–Completely satisfied	100	387	13.1	90.8
2–Very satisfied	80	822	27.8	88.8
3–Somewhat satisfied	60	792	26.7	73.7
4–Somewhat dissatisfied	40	577	19.5	60.6
5–Very dissatisfied	20	292	9.9	42.2
6–Completely dissatisfied	0	92	3.1	29.1

missing any items were missing only one (6%). Thus, our estimates of scores for those with missing items are probably fairly accurate.

The satisfaction with physical ability measure was created simply using the raw item, which was reversed so that a high score means greater satisfaction, and transformed to a 0–100 scale.

The mobility measure was scored by summing responses to the two items. No recoding of the items is required, and a high score indicates greater mobility. A missing score was assigned if either item was missing. The score was transformed to a 0–100 scale.

Characteristics of Measures

Descriptive Statistics Descriptive statistics for the physical functioning measures are shown in Table 6–5. Indicated in the table are the number of items in each measure (k), the mean and standard deviation, the percentage who were limited, the observed range, the percentage missing, and the internal-consistency reliability. The percentage identified as having any limitations ranged from 24 for mobility to 87 for satisfaction with physical ability, using the most stringent definition of any limitations.

Variability All possible scale levels were observed for all measures. Physical functioning was skewed, with people tending to receive positive scores; 81% were identified as having limitations and 79 was the median score. Mobility was skewed, with most people having no limitations (76%). Twelve percent of this sample received the next highest score. Thus, 88% of the sample received one of the two highest possible scores of a possible nine scale levels, even though there were people scoring at all possible scale levels.

Reliability The internal-consistency reliability of the 10-item physical functioning scale was 0.92 and that of the 2-item mobility scale was 0.71, both of which are more than adequate for group comparisons.

Table 6–5 Descriptive Statistics and Reliability Coefficients for Physical Functioning and Mobility Scales: PAQ Baseline Sample $(N = 3,053)$

Scale[a]	k	Mean	SD	% Limited	Observed Range	% Missing	Reliability
Physical functioning (+)	10	73.2	26.4	81	0–100	3.4	.92
Mobility (+)	2	93.3	16.1	24	0–100	2.4	.71
Satisfaction with physical ability (+)	1	61.0	25.8	87[b]	0–100	3.0	.63[c]

[a] A (+) high score indicates better health.
[b] 87% less than completely satisfied; 59% less than completely or very satisfied.
[c] Alternate forms reliability.

Table 6–6 Correlations among Physical Functioning Measures: PAQ
Baseline Sample

Measure[a]	PHYS	MOB	PFSAT
Physical Functioning (PHYS)(+)	(.92)		
Mobility (MOB)(+)	.58	(.71)	
Satisfaction with Physical Ability (PFSAT)(+)	.63	.42	—

Note: Internal consistency reliability on the diagonal (where available). *N* ranges from 2,993 to 3,036.
All coefficients are significant ($p < .001$).
[a] A (+) high score indicates better health.

The internal-consistency reliability of the 10-item scale is above the criterion for individual comparisons.

Validity The correlations among the three physical functioning measures included in the baseline sample are shown in Table 6–6. These correlations are moderate and indicate that all the measures assess a similar construct. However, the correlations are low enough to suggest that they are independent.

In a factor analysis of the three measures, a single factor was identified that explained 70% of the common variance. Factor loadings ranged from 0.79 for mobility to 0.89 for physical functioning.

The correlation of physical functioning with satisfaction with physical abilities was 0.63. Of patients who received perfect physical functioning scores, 15% were not completely or very satisfied with their physical abilities. Of those who did not receive perfect physical functioning scores, 31% were completely or very satisfied with their physical abilities. Of patients who were not completely or very satisfied, the full range of physical functioning scores was observed. These two concepts thus appear to be quite distinct.

Resolution of Issues and Future Directions

The measurement of physical functioning focused specifically on physical activities, leaving the assessment of functioning in other daily activities to other measures and thereby assuring that MOS measures of physical functioning are distinct from measures of social and role functioning. This allows the possibility that measures of each can be interpreted separately in relation to other variables and that further studies can evaluate the relationships among measures of different types of function. The MOS measures of physical functioning focus specifi-cally on health-related limitations in physical activities, including self-care activities, mobility, and satisfaction with physical abilities.

The coarseness of most existing scales was improved by developing a physical functioning scale that potentially has twenty-one scale levels, all of which were represented. This is a great increase over the number of scale levels typically available, such as the 6-level scale constructed from twenty-two items for the HIE and the seven levels available in the MOS 6-item short-form measure. This 10-item measure contains infor-mation on extent of limitation in a wide variety of basic and strenuous activities. To our knowledge, no other measure reflects both of these features. The measure should therefore be more sensitive to small differences in physical functioning than previous measures. Although the scale was skewed with people tending to report positive functioning, it was not nearly as skewed as in general populations. This suggests that in patient populations, the distribution of physical functioning mea-sures is more normal, thus making the measures more useful analyt-ically.

The pilot studies indicated that it is unnecessary to ask separately about the need for help with basic activities as long as one asks about the extent of limitations in performing these activities. That is, the need for help is typically incorporated when people report being limited. However, the need for help in getting around the community may be a different type of problem that warrants separate assessment, as indi-cated by our pilot study results that mobility contains information over and above physical activities limitations. For this reason, one of the items in the mobility scale pertains to independence in getting around. These findings and conclusions are based on the MOS patient popula-tion that includes some elderly. Because the need for help is more salient in older populations, this issue may need to be reevaluated in studies that focus entirely on the elderly.

Information on self-care activities was successfully combined with other physical activities. The concept of mobility appears to be distinct. Because mobility concerns something more than simply being limited in a specified set of physical activities, it is scored and interpreted sep-arately. Because of the severe restriction on people's lives caused by limitations in mobility, this concept warrants considerable attention. Although being able to get around without help is probably the most important aspect of mobility, subsequent work on this measure should incorporate information on the extent of difficulty in getting around and whether people are satisfied with their ability to get around.

Although the measure of satisfaction with physical abilities was originally developed based on the idea that many people who receive a perfect physical functioning score might nonetheless be dissatisfied, the converse may be even more important. Thus, information on physical functioning levels is incomplete if the question of whether or not the person is satisfied with that level is not taken into account. The finding that 31% of those with nonperfect physical functioning scores are completely or very satisfied suggests that it is important to understand patients' values with respect to specific types of functioning. Apparently, for many patients with less than perfect physical functioning, that level appears to allow them to do what they want to do. This issue requires further research.

The finding that 15% of patients with perfect physical functioning scores are not completely or very satisfied with their physical functioning suggests that there are other components of physical abilities that have not been tapped. Although these components may not be necessary in evaluating medical care, it does indicate that the satisfaction measure detects some problems that the physical functioning measure does not. This conclusion is also supported by the observation of a full range of physical functioning scores for those patients who were not completely or very satisfied.

Despite the promise of the 6-item short-form measure, the 10-item long-form measure is so similar in length that we recommend using the long-form measure whenever possible. The long-form measure has several advantages over the short-form measure, the most important of which is its potential for added sensitivity to small differences in physical functioning. Although the response format of the 6-item version can be modified to detect differences in extent of limitations, thus increasing its sensitivity to some extent, the 10-item version will do so even better.

The set of three physical functioning measures provides an adequately comprehensive approach to the assessment of physical functioning. We recommend using all three together.

7. Psychological Distress/Well-Being and Cognitive Functioning Measures

Anita L. Stewart, John E. Ware, Jr., Cathy D. Sherbourne, and Kenneth B. Wells

Definition and Issues: Psychological Distress and Well-Being

Psychological distress and well-being pertain to positive and negative affective states such as feeling happy, peaceful, anxious, depressed, or blue. The focus is on the quality of the feelings themselves and not on making a diagnostic classification of an affective disorder.

In the assessment of psychological distress and well-being, long considered a primary indicator of mental health, two historic issues, affective vs. somatic symptoms and negative vs. positive emotions, have already been resolved. Early conceptualizations of mental health included physical or somatic symptoms as well as negative affect, functional status, energy, general health, and other health problems (Ware, Johnston, Davies-Avery, et al., 1979). In diagnosing mental disorders, the entire syndrome of distress is important, including the somatic aspects. In assessing general distress and well-being, however, to include somatic problems dilutes its validity. Newer instruments thus focus less on the somatic and more on the affective components of mental health to be appropriate for patient groups as well as general populations.

Measures have historically focused on negative states such as depression and anxiety. Using such definitions, the best status that can be defined is the absence of distress. However, positive states such as feeling happy, cheerful, interested in life, and peaceful are increasingly being included (Bradburn, 1969; Dupuy, 1973, 1984; Goldberg, 1978; Goldberg and Hillier, 1978; Veit and Ware, 1983). Including these positive feelings is important because a substantial proportion of people rarely report symptoms of distress (Veit and Ware, 1983). Additionally, some clinically and socially relevant changes are not tapped by measures of distress (Ware, 1986). And disease, treatment, and other stressful life events might not increase distress but simply take the joy out of life (Ware, 1986).

The MOS considers psychological distress and well-being not as mental health per se but rather as indicators of mental health. There are good reasons for questioning the practice of interpreting more positive and fewer negative feelings to mean better mental health. Because psychological distress and well-being often depend on the social and environmental circumstances of the individual, only part of these feelings reflect mental health (Jahoda, 1958). If a person feels distressed by a particular situation, it should not be concluded that the person is not mentally healthy. The mentally healthy are not immune to anxiety and depression, because healthy adaptation requires an accurate perception of the world, which often evokes pain (Vaillant, 1977). Since one of the goals of medical and mental health care is to relieve distress, if not to promote positive affect, and the existence of such distress is often the reason people seek care, these feelings are important in their own right, regardless of whether the absence of negative feelings is healthy.

Definition and Issues: Cognitive Functioning

The highly abstract cognitive or intellectual functioning concept has been defined in multiple terms: memory, perception, ability to reason abstractly, psychomotor ability, attention span and concentration, confusion, comprehension, problem solving and judgment, learning ability, intelligence, mental alertness, and orientation in time and space (Kane and Kane, 1981; Gilson, Bergner, Bobbitt, and Carter, 1978). Although cognitive functioning can theoretically be defined in both negative and positive ways, for purposes of defining health, it is usually defined negatively or in terms of impairment, ranging from somewhat minor impairment, such as forgetfulness and limited attention span, to more severe impairment, such as disorientation in time and space.

Cognitive impairment can have an impact on people's ability to function in other areas of their lives (Kane and Kane, 1981). Cognitive impairment can also interfere with successful participation in the treatment process, but clinicians often have difficulty recognizing cognitive impairment in their patients (Anthony, LeResche, Niaz, et al., 1982; Williamson, Stokoe, Gray, et al., 1964; Knights and Folstein, 1977; DePaulo and Folstein, 1978). Pain, fatigue, and psychological distress can adversely affect cognitive functioning.

Measurement of cognitive functioning from several viewpoints— those of the person assessed, the family, and a trained clinician—is perhaps essential because no one measure captures all aspects of cognitive functioning. Severe and moderately severe cognitive problems can be observed by family, friends, and others. Milder forms of impairment (e.g., forgetfulness, difficulty concentrating) can be perceived by the individual.

In the MOS, for purposes of inclusion in the profile of functioning and well-being, we were interested in assessing day-to-day problems in cognitive functioning that the patient would be aware of. Cognitive functioning was also assessed in the MOS by a trained clinician, but that measure was for the purpose of identifying those with severe impairments and is not described here. A self-administered measure presents two problems: patients might be unaware of cognitive impairment, and, even if they are aware of it, they might hesitate to report it. The question was whether a self-administered, reliable, and valid measure could be developed that was independent of the measures of psychological distress and well-being.

Measures: Psychological Distress and Well-Being

The basis for the MOS measures was the Mental Health Inventory (MHI), which was developed for the Health Insurance Experiment (HIE). The MHI was based upon the General Well-Being Schedule (GWB) administered in the 1971 Health and Nutrition Examination Survey (Dupuy, 1973) and on items described by Costello and Comrey (1967), the Social Psychiatry Research Unit (1977), Dohrenwend, Shrout, Egri, et al. (1980), Beck (1967a, 1967b), and Zung (1965). The reasons for the selection of the MHI were its emphasis on the most commonly researched dimensions, including positive affect; the variability of its scores throughout the range of affective states; its reliability and validity in different settings, including primary care; and previous successful use.

The MHI, a general population mental health survey, is a 38-item self-administered questionnaire, designed specifically to measure mental health in terms of psychological distress and well-being. Unlike earlier surveys that assessed a variety of general health constructs (e.g., health habits, general symptoms, health perceptions) (Ware, Johnston, Davies-Avery, et al., 1979), the MHI focused primarily on affective states. The MHI defines a hierarchy of concepts which have been empirically confirmed (Veit and Ware, 1983). In addition to a total MHI score, scores are available for psychological distress and psychological well-being. Three subscales represent the dimensions within psychological distress: anxiety, depression, and loss of behavioral-emotional control. Two subscales represent the dimensions within psychological well-being: general positive affect and emotional ties.

The total MHI score had a high reliability in all HIE sites. Its internal-consistency reliability was 0.96 in the total HIE sample. The internal-consistency reliabilities of the subscales scored from the MHI ranged from 0.81 for the emotional ties scale to 0.92 for the general positive affect scale (Veit and Ware, 1983). The validity of the MHI has been evaluated in terms of a construct validity model. Specifically, hypothesized correlations have been confirmed with other health status measures (Ware, Davies-Avery, and Brook, 1980); measures of social contacts and social supports (Donald and Ware, 1982; Williams, Ware, and Donald, 1981); stressful life events (Ware, Johnston, and Davies-Avery, 1979; Williams, Ware, and Donald, 1981); and clinically diagnosed depression (Cassileth, Lusk, Strouse, et al., 1984).

The positive well-being and anxiety subscales of the MHI were sensitive to treatment differences in a study of antihypertensive drugs (Croog, Levine, Testa, et al., 1986; Levine, Croog, Sudilovsky, et al., 1987). The subscales predict significantly subsequent medical expenditures and use of mental health services (Manning, Newhouse, and Ware, 1982). The total MHI score is a good predictor of the use of outpatient mental health services and of the use of prescribed psychotropic drugs (Wells, Manning, Duan, et al., 1982; Ware, Manning, Duan, et al., 1984).

For the chronically ill, three issues remain to be resolved in using the MHI; (1) the dimensionality needs further evaluation; (2) the concept of emotional ties needs to include loneliness; and (3) more practical and shorter measures need to be developed.

One issue is to assure that the MHI subscales are independent enough to warrant scoring separately. The MHI subscales were developed in the HIE to be as independent as possible. However, the HIE consisted of a general population with relatively little distress. The issue is thus whether the subscales would be independent of one another in a sample such as the MOS, which includes the chronically ill and clinically depressed. To describe this issue, we will first define the concepts represented by the MHI subscales. The MOS focused on the dimensions most commonly assessed, which include depression, anxiety, loneliness and feelings of belonging, positive affect, and behavioral-emotional control.

General depression, as opposed to clinical depression, has been defined as a syndrome or collection of various feelings or perceptions, somatic or bodily manifestations, and behaviors (Beck, 1967a, 1967b; Brown and Harris, 1978; Ware, Johnston, Davies-Avery, et al., 1979). The emotions or feelings usually associated with general depression include feelings of worthlessness, meaninglessness, hopelessness or pessimism, loneliness, sadness, restlessness; and feeling blue, down-hearted, or discouraged. Somatic symptoms of depressed mood include: insomnia, low energy or fatigue, and loss of appetite, with resulting weight loss. Behavioral manifestations of depressed mood include social withdrawal, loss of interest in people and things, loss of sexual interest or pleasure, and impaired functioning.

Anxiety is defined by both affective and somatic symptoms. The affective symptoms include nervousness, restlessness, tension, and jumpiness. The somatic symptoms include increased sweating and upset stomach.

Loneliness, a feeling of being cut off or separated from others, has been defined as "a subjective state of reflecting the person's assessment of the quality and quantity of relationships" (Jones, Hansson, and Cutrona, 1984) or the unpleasant feeling resulting from a discrepancy between actual and desired social contact. At the opposite pole are feelings of belonging, such as feeling loved and wanted. The concept of feelings of belonging/loneliness, which derives from the assumption that intimate and social relationships are essential to psychological well-being, emphasizes the person's subjective impressions or inner experience rather than the existence of such relationships (Jones, 1985).

Positive affect, sometimes referred to as psychological well-being, has been defined in terms of cheerfulness, happiness, lightheartedness, optimism, satisfaction, and enjoyment of people and activities. It can also include feelings of belonging, which defines the positive end of the loneliness/belonging continuum.

Other aspects of mental health related to psychological distress/well-being include control of behavior, thoughts, emotions, and feelings;

fear of going crazy or losing one's mind; and emotional stability (Brown and Harris, 1978; Dupuy, 1973; Social Psychiatry Research Unit, 1977; Ware, Johnston, Davies-Avery, et al., 1979; Veit and Ware, 1983). These components have collectively been defined as behavioral-emotional control (Ware, Johnston, Davies-Avery, et al., 1979).

The distinction between depression and loss of behavioral-emotional control needed special attention. In the original HANES version of the GWB, this concept was labeled self-control and included three items pertaining to control of behavior, thoughts, feelings; losing one's mind or control over the way one acts, talks, feels, or remembers; and feelings of emotional stability and being sure. These three items were adopted for the HIE version of the MHI. The HIE measure of this concept also included crying, feeling so down in the dumps that nothing could cheer you up, having nothing to look forward to, and suicidal thoughts. All reflect severe depression and hopelessness. In fact, in the factor analyses and multitrait scaling analyses reported for these items (Ware, Johnston, Davies-Avery, et al., 1979; Ware, Veit, and Sherbourne, 1985), the behavioral-emotional control items did not always discriminate from the measure of depression. Because the MHI had been developed in a general nonaged population, we felt that the MOS could make a major contribution by testing the uniqueness of these concepts in a patient population consisting of a large number of patients with depression.

The second issue for the MOS was that the MHI underrepresented the concept of loneliness and feelings of belonging. Only two items were included to tap this concept, both worded positively and labeled "emotional ties." Although the emotional ties scale had a high internal-consistency reliability (0.81), a more comprehensive measure that incorporated feelings of loneliness was needed to evaluate patients with depression and chronic disease.

One of the most widely used loneliness measures is the revised UCLA Loneliness Scale developed by Russell and colleagues (Russell, Peplau, and Cutrona, 1980; Russell, Peplau, and Ferguson, 1978). This measure contains items that reflect feelings of belonging (e.g., "there are people I feel close to"; "I feel part of a group of friends"). The 20-item scale contains a balance of ten positively and ten negatively worded items, some focusing on affect (e.g., feelings of loneliness) and others on behaviors (e.g., lack of companionship). The scale has a coefficient alpha of 0.94 and a test-retest reliability of 0.73 over a two-month period (Peplau, 1985). Its validity has been demonstrated, and some

evidence suggests that it is distinct from depression and anxiety measures (Russell, 1982).

The third issue was the need for more practical measures. Although a
5-item version of the MHI was available, more information on its
reliability and validity was needed. Additionally, because the reliabilities of the MHI subscales and index are high, respondent burden
could be reduced without compromising the quality of the measures.
An intermediate-length measure somewhere between the 5-item short
form and the full-length MHI would be useful.

Measures: Cognitive Functioning

Two measures that were either self-administered or could easily be
adapted into a self-administered form were found. The Sickness Impact
Profile (SIP) assesses cognitive impairment in a subscale labeled "alert-
ness behavior" (Bergner, Bobbitt, Carter, and Gilson, 1981; Gilson,
Bergner, Bobbitt, and Carter, 1978). The Psychiatric Epidemiology
Research Interview (PERI) has a subscale labeled "confused thinking"
(Dohrenwend, Shrout, Egri, and Mendelsohn, 1980; Dohrenwend,
Levav, and Shrout, 1983; Social Psychiatry Research Unit, 1977,
1984). The entire PERI was developed for investigating dimensions of
psychopathology and for psychiatric screening in a general population
(Dohrenwend, Levav, and Shrout, 1983).

Seven categories or aspects of cognitive functioning were identified
and tapped by one or both measures: confusion, thinking, concentration, attention, memory, reasoning, and psychomotor (Table 7–1). SIP
items are phrased in terms of whether or not a statement is true for
respondents "today." The time frame for the PERI items is over the past
year.

Content and Measurement Strategy

Pilot Study A pilot study was conducted to try to improve the MHI
measure of emotional ties which contained two positively worded items
by adding items asking about the negative emotion of loneliness. In the
pilot study, the MOS fielded eight items, including the two MHI items
and six items adapted from the UCLA Loneliness Scale that focused on
feelings of loneliness. The pilot study included patients from a rural

Table 7–1 Cognitive Functioning Categories Measured by PERI[a] and SIP[b]

Category/Item Content	PERI	SIP
Confusion		
Confused, start several actions at a time		x
Confused and had trouble thinking[c]	x	
Behave as if confused or disoriented in place or time		x
Thinking		
Not able to think straight	x	
Confused and had trouble thinking[c]	x	
Difficulty doing activities involving concentration and thinking[c]		x
Concentration		
Losing your train of thought	x	
Difficulty doing activities involving concentration and thinking[c]		x
Trouble concentrating or keeping mind on what you were doing[c]	x	
Attention		
Do not finish things I start		x
Do not keep attention on any activity for long		x
Memory		
Forget a lot		x
Trouble remembering	x	
Reasoning		
Difficulty reasoning and solving problems		x
Psychomotor		
More minor accidents		x
React slowly to things said or done		x
Make more mistakes than usual		x

[a] Psychiatric Epidemiology Rating Index (Dohrenwend, Shrout, Egri, and Mendelsohn, 1980; Dohrenwend, Levav, and Shrout, 1983; Social Psychiatry Research Unit, 1977, 1984).
[b] Sickness Impact Profile (Bergner, Bobbitt, Carter, and Gilson, 1981; Gilson, Bergner, Bobbitt, and Carter, 1978).
[c] Confounded item, including two aspects of cognitive impairment.

health clinic. Based on the pilot, five items were selected: the two original MHI items and three of the UCLA items, one positively and two negatively worded. The internal-consistency reliability of this 5-item scale was 0.88.

Psychological Distress/Well-Being Final Items To provide a slightly shorter battery, a subset of items was selected from the 38-item MHI. Before the MOS items were chosen, a set of eighteen items from the MHI were selected by John Ware and Kenneth Wells for a study to validate a telephone diagnostic interview for depressive disorder. That study needed a shorter version of the MHI that could be telephone administered. The eighteen items were chosen to include: (1) all items from the short-form MHI-5; (2) at least four items each from the anxiety, depression, behavioral-emotional control, and positive affect subscales, representing the range of content of the MHI; (3) one of the two emotional ties items, referred to in the MOS as feelings of belonging; (4) items that best discriminated between each MHI subscale; and (5) items with a common response choice to facilitate telephone administration and minimize the number of items that had to be revised. To telephone administer these items, the same response format was needed for each item. The response format referring to frequency was selected, which necessitated some item revisions. The 18-item version was subsequently tested by Weinstein, Berwick, Goldman, et al. (1989) as a screening measure for depression and anxiety disorders.

Items for the MOS were selected in a hierarchical manner in this order: seventeen of the eighteen items developed for the depression interview validation study (which included the five items in the MHI-5), the five belonging/loneliness items from the pilot study, and twelve of the remaining twenty-two HIE items. One of the eighteen items (able to relax without difficulty) was not included in the MOS battery because of questionable content validity as a positive affect item (Veit and Ware, 1983). The selection goals for the twelve last items were: (1) to include items from all four constructs for which items remained (anxiety, depression, behavioral-emotional control, positive affect); (2) to retain items that best represented a range of severity of each construct; (3) to retain items that best discriminated within each subscale; and (4) to retain items that did not overlap with other concepts being developed in the MOS such as energy/fatigue or sleep.

A summary of the psychological distress and well-being items included in the MOS and their relationship to earlier versions of the MHI is presented in Table 7–2. Items are ordered by hypothesized construct, and the presence of items in the various batteries is indicated. The earliest versions of these concepts also included items pertaining to general health and vitality, as shown in the table. For purposes of the MOS, we sometimes revised the response choices from the HIE version to simplify them.

The final MOS psychological distress/well-being battery consists of seven anxiety items, six depression items, eight behavioral-emotional control items, seven positive affect items, and five loneliness/belonging items, for a total of thirty-three items (which include the 5-item and the 17-item versions).

Cognitive Functioning Final Items In the MOS self-administered measure, all categories of cognitive functioning identified in our review of measures are represented. All items were selected from one instrument to avoid mixing items across instruments. The SIP items were more comprehensive; therefore, one SIP item from each category was selected. This resulted in six items, because concentration and thinking were combined in one category in the SIP.

The SIP asked whether each statement was currently true for respondents and then weighted the scores. To be consistent with the MOS psychological distress/well-being items and to provide a more sensitive scale, the MOS asked how often each problem had occurred during the past month and provided six response choices ranging from "none of the time" to "all of the time."

Summary of Final Items Six items assessing cognitive functioning and thirty-three items assessing psychological distress and well-being were included, organized according to the *hypothesized* categories in Table 7–3. Actual items are shown in the Appendix, pages 381–394.

Construction and Evaluation of Measures

Analysis Plan In addition to the PAQ baseline sample, the 17-item psychological distress and well-being battery, which includes the 5-item measure, was also administered to a subsample of participants in the Los Angeles site of the National Institute of Mental Health Epidemiologic Catchment Area (ECA) sample. All analyses were performed on the PAQ baseline sample, and selected analyses were performed on the ECA sample as well.

Although the ECA sample, consisting of 230 English-speaking adults, was a community-based sample, depressed people were oversampled. Sample ages ranged from eighteen to eighty-one (mean age thirty-nine), with 54% male, 60% non-Hispanic white, and 26% Hispanic. The ECA sample design is presented elsewhere (Wells, Burnam, Leake, et al., 1988).

Multitrait scaling techniques were used to evaluate the scales. More

Table 7–2 Summary of Psychological Distress/Well-Being Items across Studies

Hypothesized Construct/ Abbreviated Item Content	Type of Response[b]	HANES GWB
Number of items		18
Anxiety		
Very nervous person	AT	
Bothered by nervousness	U	x
Bothered by nervousness	AT	
Felt tense, high strung	AT	
Difficulty trying to calm down	AL	
Anxious, worried	U	x
Anxious, worried	AT	
Rattles, upset, flustered	AL	
Restless, fidgety, impatient	AT	
Hands shake when doing things	AL	
Nervous or jumpy	AL	
Under strain, stress, pressure	U	x
Relaxed vs. high strung	U	
Generally tense, feel tension	U	x
Generally tense, feel tension	U	
Depression		
In low or very low spirits	AT	
Downhearted and blue	AT	x
How depressed at worst	U	
Time feel depressed	AT	
Moody, brooded about things	AT	
Depression interfered	AL	
Feel depressed	U	x
Feel depressed	U	
Sad, discouraged, hopeless	U	
Behavioral/emotional control		
Down in the dumps	AT	
Nothing to look forward to	AT	
Firm control of behavior	U	x
Firm control of behavior	AT	
Felt like crying	AL	
Others better off if dead	AL	
Losing mind, losing control	U	x

BATTERY/STUDY[a]					
HIE GWB	HIE MHI15	HIE MHI38	MOS MHI17	MOS MHI5	MOS Total
22	15	38	17	5	33
		x	x	x	x
x		x			
					x
		x	x		x
		x			x
x	x	x			
			x		x
		x			x
		x	x		x
		x			
		x			
x	x	x[c]			
x	x				
x	x				
		x	x		x
x	x	x	x	x	x
					x
			x		x
		x	x		x
					x
x	x	x			
x	x				
		x	x	x	x
		x	x		x
x	x	x			
			x		x
		x			x
		x			x
x	x	x			x

Table 7–2 (*Cont.*)

Hypothesized Construct/ Abbreviated Item Content	Type of Response[b]	HANES GWB
Emotionally stable, sure	AT	x
Emotionally stable	AT	
Think about taking own life	U	
Nothing turned out as wanted	AL	
General positive affect		
Happy person	AT	
Generally enjoyed things	AT	
Calm and peaceful	AT	
Happy, satisfied, pleased	U·	x
Happy, satisfied, pleased	U	
Living a wonderful adventure	AT	
Cheerful, lighthearted	U	x
Cheerful, lighthearted	AT	
Daily life interesting	AT	x
Relaxed, free of tension	AT	
Expect an interesting day	AL	
Future hopeful, promising	AT	
Relax without difficulty	AT	
Waking up fresh, rested[c]	U	
Emotional ties/loneliness		
Felt loved and wanted	AT	
Love relationships full	AT	
Time felt lonely	AT	
Felt isolated	AT	
Felt left out	AT	
People felt close to	AT	
General health		
Feeling in general	U	x
Feeling in general	U	
Healthy enough to do things	U	
Bothered by illness	U	
Concerned, worried, fears	U	x
Concerned, worried, fears	U	
Vitality		
Energy, pep, vitality	U	x
Energy, pep, vitality	U	
Active, vigorous vs. dull	U	

| BATTERY/STUDY[a] | | | | | |
HIE GWB	HIE MHI15	HIE MHI38	MOS MHI17	MOS MHI5	MOS Total
x	x				
		x	x		x
		x			x
		x			
		x	x	x	x
		x			x
		x	x	x	x
x	x	x[c]			x
		x			x
x	x	x	x		x
x	x	x	x		x
		x			
		x			
		x			
		x[c]	d		
		x			
		x	x		x
		x			x
		x[c]			
					x
					x
					x
x	x				
x					
x					
x					
x					
x					

Table 7–2 (*cont.*)

Hypothesized Construct/ Abbreviated Item Content	Type of Response[b]	HANES GWB
Tired, wornout, used up	AT	x
Waking up fresh, rested[c]	U	x
Waking up fresh, rested[c]	AT	

[a]HANES GWB = GWB included in the Health and Nutrition Examination Survey, 1971; HIE-GWB = HIS-GWB, preliminary general well-being measure for the Health Insurance Experiment fielded only at enrollment in first site; HIE-MHI15 = Preliminary mental health measure scored from HIS GWB, excluding concepts of general health and vitality; HIE-MHI38 = final mental health battery included in the Health Insurance Experiment; MOS-MHI17 = short-form mental health battery developed for telephone administration (subset of MOS battery); MOS-MHI5 = short-form mental health battery (subset of MOS battery); MOS-Total = mental health battery included in the Medical Outcomes Study.

stringent criteria than those typically used were applied, deleting items from scales if a probable scaling error was observed, because the scales had been evaluated so extensively prior to the MOS work.

Consistent with earlier work on the MHI (Veit and Ware, 1983; Ware, Veit, and Sherbourne, 1985), the MOS began by testing a 6-scale and 5-scale model corresponding to the hypothesized subscale item groupings described above for the full battery.

Six-scale model:
Anxiety (7 items)
Depression (7 items)
Behavioral-emotional control (8 items)
Belonging/loneliness (5 items)
Positive affect (7 items)
Cognitive functioning (6 items)

Five-scale model:
Anxiety (7 items)
Depression/behavioral-emotional control (14 items)
Belonging/loneliness (5 items)
Positive affect (7 items)
Cognitive functioning (7 items)

The test of these components as separate entities does not imply that they will be completely independent. From a clinical point of view, we expect them to overlap considerably. However, to the extent that the separate concepts discriminate from one another, we are better able to evaluate the importance of each separate component. These models differ slightly from previous work because a broader belonging/loneliness dimension is hypothesized. To test the discriminant validity

BATTERY/STUDY[a]					
HIE GWB	HIE MHI15	HIE MHI38	MOS MHI17	MOS MHI5	MOS Total
x					
x					

[b]AT = all ot the time–none of the time; AL = always–never; U = unique.
[c]This item was included in the MHI38 total score only; it was not included in the hypothesized subscale.
[d]This item was included in the MHI18 but excluded from the MOS battery (see text).
[e]This item was included in the Vitality measure in the HIS GWB and in the General Positive Affect measure in the MHI38.

Table 7–3 Summary of the Number of Items Assessing Hypothesized Subscales of Psychological Distress/Well-being and Cognitive Functioning

	NUMBER OF ITEMS		
	Full Battery	17-item Version	5-item Version
Cognitive functioning	6	0	0
Psychological distress and well-being			
Anxiety	7	4	1
Depression	6	4	1
Behavioral-emotional control	8	4	1
Belonging/loneliness	5	1	0
Positive affect	7	4	2

of items in these subscales, the following validity measures were included in the multitrait scaling matrix: health distress, role limitations due to emotional problems, energy/fatigue, social activity limitations due to health, and current health. Because each validity measure has some conceptual similarity to one or more of the mental health concepts, it was important to assure that the measures were independent of each concept.

The 17-item battery also included items in the originally hypothesized item groupings. We were certain that an overall index could be scored from the 17-item battery, but we wanted to test whether the same subscales would discriminate from each other as in the 33-item battery. Even if the subscales would discriminate using the full battery, it was possible that the reduced number of items per concept would compromise this. Rather than test all models as outlined for the full battery, we decided to try to replicate the final structure determined in the analysis of the full battery. Although the 17-item battery was administered to two samples, the sample size in the ECA sample was too small to draw firm conclusions regarding discriminant validity. Thus, the structure of the 17-item version was tested only in the MOS baseline sample. The reliability of the resulting measures is reported for the ECA sample.

Three overall indexes of the psychological distress and well-being items were tested: (1) all thirty-three items from the full battery, (2) the 17-items, and (3) the 5-item short form. These indexes were intended to reflect the combination of positive and negative states for use as summary scores. We were able to test the full 33-item index only in the MOS PAQ baseline sample. The 17-item and 5-item indexes were also tested in the ECA sample.

Item Variability The abbreviated item content and variable names for each of the items are presented in Table 7–4 for the MOS PAQ baseline sample, along with the percentage distributions for the items. The means and standard deviations for the thirty-nine items are shown in the multitrait analysis tables (Tables 7–5 and 7–6).

All psychological distress and well-being items exhibited a reasonable spread of responses, with few exceptions. Although the skew was less pronounced for the positive affect items, items tended to reflect more positive affect and less negative affect. Two items were extremely skewed: thinking about taking own life and thinking others would be better off if you were dead. Standard deviations for the thirty-three items in the MOS PAQ baseline sample ranged from 0.64 ("thinking about taking own life") to 1.71 ("love relationships full, complete"). The percentage missing ranged from 1.9 to 3.8.

The cognitive functioning items, which are all worded negatively, were skewed indicating fewer problems. The percentage that reported any problems ranged from 38% ("become confused") to 64% ("forgetful"). Standard deviations ranged from 0.91 to 1.13. The percentage missing ranged from 2.7 to 3.6.

Scale Construction In the 6-scale model, all items met the stringent convergent validity criterion of 0.40, that is, correlated at least 0.40 with their own scale, corrected for overlap (Table 7–5). Thirty of the thirty-nine items met our criterion for discriminant validity. One anxiety item (MHAO 5—anxious and worried) correlated as highly with the depression scale as with the anxiety scale. Only three of the eight behavioral-emotional control items met our criterion of discriminant validity. Of the remaining five items, one (MHCO 4—felt like crying) correlated significantly higher with the depression scale, four correlated within two standard errors (MHCO 1—down in the dumps; MHCO 2—nothing to look forward to; MHCO 7—emotionally stable; MHCO 8—think about taking own life). However, all of the depression items discriminated well from all of the other constructs. Two of the belonging/loneliness items (LNLY 5—feeling isolated, and LNLY 1—feeling left out) correlated within two standard errors with the depression scale. One behavioral-emotional control item (MHCO 6—losing mind, losing control over way you act, talk, think, feel, or of your memory) correlated within two standard errors with the cognitive functioning scale.

Most of the behavioral-emotional control items did not discriminate well from depression. We then looked at the results regarding these two scales from the HIE (Ware, Veit, and Sherbourne, 1985). In results for the 5,089 respondents in that general population, MHCO 4 ("felt like crying") and MHCO 2 ("down in the dumps") also correlated higher with the depression scale, although the differences were within two standard errors. The other three problem items discriminated in that sample.

Based on MOS and HIE results and on the evaluation of the content of items in these two subscales, the 5-scale model in which these are combined (see above) was tested next. We tested the 5-scale model with all other hypothesized groupings intact to determine whether some of the other scaling problems would be corrected. Again, all items met the convergent validity criterion of 0.40. Thirty-four of the thirty-nine items met the criterion of discriminant validity. The same anxiety item (MHAO 5—anxious or worried) still correlated equally with the depression/behavioral-emotional control scale. The same depression/behavioral-emotional control item (MHCO 6—losing mind, losing control over way you act, talk, think, feel, or of your memory) still correlated within two standard errors of the cognitive functioning scale. Two loneliness items (LNLY 5—feeling isolated, and LNLY 1—feeling

Table 7–4 Percentage Distribution of Psychological Distress/Well-Being and Cognitive Functioning Items: PAQ Baseline Sample (*N* = 3,053)

Abbreviated Item Content	Item Variable Name
Anxiety	
Very nervous person	MHA01[c]
Bothered by nervousness, nerves	MHA02
Tense, high strung	MHA03[d]
Difficulty trying to calm down	MHA04
Anxious or worried	MHA05[d]
Rattled, upset, flustered	MHA06
Restless, fidgety, impatient	MHA07[d]
Depression	
Low or very low spirits	MHD01[d]
Downhearted and blue	MHD02[c]
How depressed at worst	MHD03
Feel depressed	MHD04[d]
Moody, brooded	MHD05[d]
Feeling depressed interfered	MHD06
Behavioral/emotional control	
So down in dumps, nothing could cheer you up	MHC01[c]
Nothing to look forward to	MHC02[d]
Firm control of behavior, thoughts, emotions, feelings	MHC03[d]
Felt like crying	MHC04
Others better off if you were dead	MHC05
Losing mind, losing control of way act, talk, think, feel, or of memory	MHC06
Emotionally stable	MHC07[c]
Think about taking own life	MHC08
Positive affect	
Been a happy person	MHP01[c]
Generally enjoyed things	MHP02
Felt calm, peaceful	MHP03[c]
Happy, satisfied, pleased	MHP04
Living a wonderful adventure	MHP05
Felt cheerful, lighthearted	MHP06[d]
Daily life full of interesting things	MHP07[d]
Loneliness/belonging	
Feel left out	LNLY1
Love relationships full, complete	LNLY2
Felt loved, wanted	LNLY3
People you were close to	LNLY4
Feel isolated	LNLY5
Cognitive functioning	
Become confused, start several actions at a time	COG1
React slowly to things said, done	COG2
Difficulty reasoning, solving problems	COG3

Response Choice[a]	ITEM RESPONSE[b]					
	1	2	3	4	5	6
AT	2.0	6.2	9.8	17.7	30.7	33.6
U	0.5	4.1	7.4	15.4	33.9	38.6
AT	1.4	4.9	10.5	19.3	36.2	27.2
AL	0.4	2.7	4.8	21.6	34.2	36.3
AT	1.4	6.9	11.6	18.6	41.2	20.2
AL	0.4	3.9	6.6	31.4	37.0	20.7
AT	0.9	3.8	8.5	19.0	41.4	26.4
AT	0.9	4.4	8.1	15.9	36.9	33.7
AT	1.1	4.9	7.9	17.1	36.4	32.6
U	4.9	5.7	8.9	13.8	32.0	34.6
AT	1.5	4.6	7.9	17.8	34.0	34.2
AT	0.9	3.8	7.7	17.5	33.7	36.3
AL	1.4	4.4	6.4	23.4	26.4	37.9
AT	0.5	2.5	3.7	8.9	21.4	63.0
AT	1.3	4.4	5.8	11.0	19.0	58.5
AT	32.1	42.7	10.8	9.1	4.2	1.1
AL	0.7	4.2	5.9	21.6	26.2	41.4
AL	0.5	1.6	1.2	5.4	9.1	82.0
U	62.4	17.3	9.7	7.3	2.2	1.2
AT	36.3	35.3	10.8	8.7	6.5	2.4
U	0.2	0.7	0.9	3.3	4.3	90.6
AT	9.9	44.2	15.7	15.5	22.3	2.4
AT	14.0	44.3	15.5	17.8	7.5	1.1
AT	9.1	39.0	15.8	17.1	14.7	4.3
U	8.9	25.4	30.5	24.5	7.0	3.6
AT	19.8	29.5	11.9	14.7	14.1	10.1
AT	6.1	39.9	17.1	18.7	14.7	3.5
AT	8.2	38.2	20.8	20.3	10.3	2.2
AT	0.9	3.7	5.5	12.6	25.3	51.9
AT	27.5	30.4	7.8	12.0	11.1	11.2
AT	34.4	30.3	11.1	12.8	8.4	3.0
AL	41.3	24.0	15.4	14.4	3.8	1.1
AL	1.1	4.9	5.8	18.2	26.1	43.8
AT	0.3	1.2	3.8	8.7	23.4	62.5
AT	0.4	2.6	4.5	15.2	32.8	44.5
AT	1.2	3.2	5.7	14.3	26.6	49.0

Table 7–4   (*Cont.*)

Abbreviated Item Content	Item Variable Name
Forgetful	COG4
Trouble keeping attention on any activity for long	COG5
Difficulty doing activities involving concentration, thinking	COG6

[a] AT: 1–All of the time; 2–Most of the time; 3–A good bit of the time; 4–Some of the time; 5–A little of the time; 6–None of the time. AL: 1–Always; 2–Very often; 3–Fairly often; 4–Sometimes; 5–Almost never; 6–Never. U: Unique response choices (see appendix).

Table 7–5   Item-Scale Correlation Matrix, Psychological Distress/ Well-Being and Cognitive Functioning Six-Scale Model: PAQ Baseline Sample (*N* = 2,469)

Item	Mean	SD	ANX	DEP	BEHEMO	POS	LNLY
MHA01	2.29	1.28	.80[a]	.65	.62	−.59	.47
MHA02	2.05	1.13	.83[a]	.69	.68	−.62	.51
MHA03	2.33	1.19	.83[a]	.70	.66	−.64	.52
MHA04	2.04	1.03	.78[a]	.67	.66	−.60	.53
MHA05	2.47	1.21	.78[a]	.78	.73	−.71	.61
MHA06	2.38	1.02	.75[a]	.69	.67	−.61	.52
MHA07	2.25	1.10	.76[a]	.68	.64	−.62	.54
MHD01	2.14	1.15	.75	.89[a]	.81	−.78	.69
MHD02	2.18	1.17	.74	.88[a]	.81	−.77	.69
MHD03	2.35	1.43	.72	.86[a]	.78	−.75	.65
MHD04	2.19	1.20	.76	.90[a]	.82	−.77	.68
MHD05	2.12	1.15	.77	.82[a]	.77	−.72	.65
MHD06	2.17	1.21	.70	.81[a]	.76	−.71	.62
MHC01	1.63	1.01	.67	.79	.77[a]	−.68	.63
MHC02	1.81	1.21	.62	.73	.72[a]	−.71	.67
MHC03	2.13	0.14	.61	.62	.65[a]	−.60	.53
MHC04	2.06	1.16	.66	.75	.69[a]	−.64	.58
MHC05	1.33	0.82	.50	.58	.65[a]	−.50	.52
MHC06	1.73	1.14	.58	.61	.65[a]	−.55	.50
MHC07	2.21	1.32	.66	.69	.72[a]	−.67	.61
MHC08	1.18	0.64	.40	.52	.56[a]	−.42	.41
MHP01	4.14	1.29	−.70	−.80	−.76	.89[a]	−.74
MHP02	4.33	1.19	−.63	−.72	−.69	.81[a]	−.65
MHP03	3.95	1.38	−.75	−.75	−.74	.81[a]	−.67

Response	ITEM RESPONSE[b]					
Choice[a]	1	2	3	4	5	6
A T	0.7	1.9	6.0	16.8	38.5	36.2
A T	0.8	2.9	6.0	13.0	31.4	45.9
A T	0.8	3.1	6.2	16.5	29.8	43.6

[b] Percentage of those who responded to each item.
[c] Part of 17-item and 5-item battery.
[d] Part of 17-item battery.

COG	PHYS	SYMP	ROLEMO	ENERGY	CURR	DIST	SOC
−.58	−.18	.39	−.52	−.43	−.37	.47	−.46
−.62	−.18	.43	−.54	−.44	−.39	.50	−.50
−.60	−.12	.40	−.55	−.43	−.34	.46	−.48
−.61	−.14	.37	−.52	−.41	−.35	.47	−.49
−.63	−.14	.40	−.57	−.48	−.40	.54	−.55
−.64	−.13	.40	−.53	−.41	−.35	.45	−.47
−.61	−.15	.41	−.54	−.41	−.35	.44	−.48
−.65	−.13	.39	−.62	−.50	−.43	.54	−.61
−.63	−.12	.37	−.61	−.49	−.41	.53	−.57
−.60	−.07	.37	−.62	−.46	−.38	.49	−.57
−.66	−.13	.41	−.64	−.50	−.43	.55	−.60
−.66	−.09	.38	−.62	−.45	−.37	.51	−.57
−.66	−.19	.40	−.67	−.50	−.43	.58	−.62
−.62	−.13	.34	−.54	−.43	−.36	.50	−.56
−.58	−.16	.34	−.52	−.44	−.38	.48	−.54
−.58	−.11	.29	−.50	−.36	−.30	.40	−.44
−.55	−.10	.38	−.54	−.42	−.31	.45	−.49
−.51	−.13	.26	−.40	−.33	−.28	.40	−.43
−.67	−.16	.35	−.49	−.40	−.36	.45	−.45
−.61	−.11	.35	−.57	−.41	−.33	.44	−.48
−.40	−.02	.17	−.33	−.25	−.19	.32	−.38
−.58	.15	−.37	.59	.53	.46	−.49	.58
−.57	.20	−.39	.55	.56	.46	−.50	.58
−.58	.11	−.38	.58	.50	.39	−.46	.52

Table 7–5 (*Cont.*)

Item	Mean	SD	ANX	DEP	BEHEMO	POS	LNLY
MHP04	3.93	1.20	−.61	−.73	−.67	.77[a]	−.69
MHP05	3.93	1.63	−.57	−.66	−.63	.79[a]	−.66
MHP06	3.91	1.31	−.67	−.76	−.72	.86[a]	−.70
MHP07	4.05	1.23	−.57	−.64	−.63	.77[a]	−.63
LNLY1	1.87	1.15	.60	.70	.71	−.66	.73[a]
LNLY2	2.81	1.71	.49	.59	.58	−.67	.76[a]
LNLY3	2.41	1.43	.49	.60	.61	−.69	.83[a]
LNLY4	2.20	1.28	.44	.52	.53	−.59	.71[a]
LNLY5	2.05	1.21	.64	.73	.72	−.69	.72[a]
COG1	5.41	0.91	−.56	−.52	−.59	.46	−.45
COG2	5.11	1.03	−.46	−.47	−.49	.40	−.40
COG3	5.09	1.13	−.61	−.66	−.67	.57	−.51
COG4	5.00	1.00	−.44	−.39	−.46	.36	−.33
COG5	5.09	1.08	−.63	−.62	−.62	.53	−.51
COG6	5.02	1.11	−.67	−.66	−.68	.58	−.50

Note: Standard error of correlation = 0.02. ANX = Anxiety; DEP = Depression; BEHEMO = Behavioral-emotional control; POS = Positive affect; LNLY = Feelings of belonging/loneliness; COG = Cognitive functioning; PHYS = Physical functioning; SYMP = Physical/psychophysiological symptoms; ROLEMO = Role limitations due to emotional problems; ENERGY = Energy/fatigue; CURR = Current health perceptions; DIST = Health distress; SOC = Social activity limitations due to health.

left out) correlated within two standard errors of the depression/behavioral-emotional control scale. All but one of the cognitive functioning items correlated higher with their own scale than with any of the other scales in the matrix. One item (COG3—difficulty reasoning, solving problems) correlated within two standard errors of the depression/behavioral-emotional control scale.

The belonging/loneliness scale is thus splitting between the positively worded belonging items and the negatively worded loneliness items. In the development of subscales in the HIE, the same problem was found. That is, an item assessing "feeling lonely" tended to correlate higher with behavioral-emotional control than with the two positively worded belonging (emotional ties) items. To see if the loneliness items would discriminate from the depression/behavioral-emotional control scale when scored separately, we tried to score the two loneliness items as a separate scale and the three belonging items as a separate scale. The two loneliness items still correlated equally with loneliness and with depression.

COG	PHYS	SYMP	ROLEMO	ENERGY	CURR	DIST	SOC
−.51	.18	−.38	.54	.49	.45	−.47	.55
−.47	.12	−.31	.49	.48	.37	−.39	.50
−.57	.15	−.37	.56	.53	.43	−.47	.50
.49	.17	−.35	.47	.50	.40	−.44	.52
−.57	−.10	.33	−.51	−.38	−.31	.42	−.51
−.44	−.05	.28	−.44	−.36	−.28	.31	−.39
−.45	−.07	.25	−.43	−.35	−.29	.32	−.40
−.40	−.06	.25	−.40	−.31	−.26	.31	−.37
−.61	−.11	.34	−.54	−.42	−.34	.44	−.55
.69[a]	.15	−.34	.46	.34	.27	−.36	.40
.60[a]	.20	−.32	.39	.34	.32	−.37	.40
.72[a]	.22	−.39	.56	.45	.38	−.49	.54
.59[a]	.25	−.36	.35	.35	.30	−.34	.32
.71[a]	.18	−.34	.51	.41	.33	−.43	.47
.75[a]	.21	−.40	.55	.47	.38	−.49	.51

[a] Denotes hypothesized item groupings and item-scale correlation corrected for overlap.

Some, but not all, of these problem items were eliminated. The items that were correlating equally or higher with other scales (MHAO5, MHCO6, LNLY5, and LNLY1) were eliminated and the analysis was rerun. Results are shown in Table 7–6. All items correlated 0.55 or greater with their hypothesized scales, and all items now met the MOS criterion of discriminant validity. Item-scale correlations ranged from 0.74 to 0.83 for anxiety, 0.55 to 0.89 for depression/behavioral-emotional control, 0.77 to 0.86 for positive affect, 0.70 to 0.83 for feelings of belonging, and 0.59 to 0.75 for cognitive functioning. The belonging/loneliness scale, which hereafter will be called the feelings of belonging scale, now consists of only positively worded belonging items.

Although the scales constructed in the 5-scale model are good and therefore final subscales, there are situations in which more aggregate measures might be useful. We thus tested the following 3-scale model: (1) psychological distress—anxiety, depression, behavioral-emotional control, loneliness—twenty-three items; (2) psychological well-being—positive affect, feelings of belonging—ten items; and (3) cognitive functioning—six items. First tested was the 3-scale model using all of the items (i.e., including the items that were excluded in the final 5-scale

Table 7–6 Item-Scale Correlation Matrix, Psychological Distress/
Well-Being and Cognitive Functioning Five-Scale Model: PAQ Baseline
Sample (N = 2,459)

Item	Mean	SD	ANX	DEPBC	POS	LNLY
MHA01	4.71	1.28	.80[a]	.66	.59	−.40
MHA02	4.94	1.13	.83[a]	.70	.62	−.44
MHA03	4.66	1.20	.82[a]	.70	.64	−.44
MHA04	4.96	1.03	.77[a]	.68	.60	−.44
MHA06	4.61	1.02	.74[a]	.70	.61	−.44
MHA07	4.74	1.10	.75[a]	.68	.62	−.46
MHD01	4.86	1.15	.72	.88[a]	.78	−.60
MHD02	4.82	1.17	.71	.88[a]	.77	−.60
MHD03	4.65	1.43	.70	.84[a]	.75	−.56
MHD04	4.80	1.21	.74	.89[a]	.77	−.59
MHD05	4.87	1.15	.75	.82[a]	.72	−.55
MHD06	4.82	1.21	.68	.81[a]	.70	−.54
MHC01	5.36	1.01	.65	.81[a]	.69	−.54
MHC02	5.17	1.21	.61	.75[a]	.71	−.59
MHC03	4.86	1.13	.61	.65[a]	.60	−.48
MHC04	4.93	1.16	.64	.75[a]	.64	−.50
MHC05	5.66	0.83	.49	.63[a]	.50	−.43
MHC07	4.78	1.32	.65	.73[a]	.68	−.55
MHC08	5.80	0.64	.39	.55[a]	.42	−.34
MHP01	4.14	1.29	.67	.81	.89[a]	−.69
MHP02	4.33	1.19	.62	.73	.81[a]	−.60
MHP03	3.94	1.38	.73	.77	.81[a]	−.62
MHP04	3.93	1.20	.59	.73	.77[a]	−.66
MHP05	3.93	1.63	.55	.67	.79[a]	−.61
MHP06	3.91	1.31	.65	.77	.87[a]	−.64
MHP07	4.05	1.23	.56	.66	.77[a]	−.60
LNLY2	2.82	1.71	−.47	−.60	−.67	.76[a]
LNLY3	2.42	1.44	−.47	−.62	−.69	.83[a]
LNLY4	2.21	1.28	−.42	−.54	−.59	.70[a]
COG1	5.41	0.91	.57	.56	.46	−.37
COG2	5.11	1.03	.46	.49	.40	−.34
COG3	5.09	1.13	.60	.68	.57	−.43
COG4	5.00	1.00	.44	.42	.36	−.27
COG5	5.09	1.08	.62	.63	.53	−.43
COG6	5.02	1.11	.66	.68	.58	−.42

Note: Standard error of correlation = 0.02. ANX = Anxiety; DEPBC = Depression/behavioral-
emotional control; POS = Positive affect; LNLY = Feelings of belonging/loneliness; COG =
Cognitive functioning; SYMP = Physical/psychophysiological symptoms; ROLEMO = Role limitations due to emotional problems; ENERGY = Energy/fatigue; CURR = Current health perceptions;
DIST = Health distress; SOC = Social activity limitations due to health.

COG	PHYS	SYMP	ROLEMO	ENERGY	CURR	DIST	SOC
.58	.18	−.39	.46	.42	.37	−.47	.46
.62	.18	−.43	.49	.45	.39	−.51	.51
.60	.12	−.40	.49	.43	.34	−.46	.48
.62	.14	−.37	.47	.41	.35	−.47	.49
.64	.13	−.39	.47	.41	.34	−.46	.47
.61	.15	−.40	.48	.42	.35	−.45	.48
.65	.13	−.39	.57	.50	.43	−.54	.61
.63	.12	−.37	.57	.49	.41	−.53	.57
.60	.06	−.37	.57	.46	.37	−.49	.57
.66	.13	−.41	.61	.51	.43	−.56	.60
.66	.09	−.38	.57	.45	.37	−.51	.57
.66	.19	−.40	.64	.51	.43	−.58	.62
.62	.13	−.35	.52	.44	.36	−.51	.56
.58	.16	−.35	.49	.44	.39	−.48	.54
.59	.10	−.30	.47	.37	.31	−.40	.45
.55	.10	−.38	.50	.42	.32	−.45	.49
.51	.13	−.26	.39	.33	.28	−.40	.43
.61	.11	−.35	.54	.42	.33	−.45	.48
.40	.02	−.17	.33	.25	.19	−.32	.38
.58	.15	−.37	.54	.53	.46	−.49	.58
.57	.20	−.39	.52	.56	.46	−.50	.58
.58	.11	−.38	.53	.50	.39	−.47	.52
.51	.18	−.38	.51	.49	.45	−.47	.55
.47	.12	−.31	.46	.48	.37	−.39	.50
.57	.15	−.37	.52	.53	.43	−.48	.56
.49	.17	−.35	.44	.50	.40	−.44	.52
−.44	−.05	.28	−.41	−.36	−.28	.31	−.39
−.45	−.07	.25	−.41	−.35	−.29	.32	−.40
−.41	−.06	.25	−.38	−.32	−.26	.31	−.37
.69[a]	.15	−.34	.43	.34	.27	−.36	.40
.60[a]	.20	−.32	.39	.34	.32	−.37	.40
.72[a]	.22	−.39	.55	.45	.38	−.49	.54
.59[a]	.25	−.36	.34	.36	.30	−.34	.32
.72[a]	.18	−.33	.49	.41	.33	−.43	.47
.75[a]	.21	−.40	.53	.47	.38	−.49	.51

[a] Denotes hypothesized item groupings and item-scale correlation corrected for overlap.

model). Based on these results, the same depression/behavioral-emotional control item (MHCO6), which correlated higher with the cognitive functioning scale, was eliminated. Thus, two additional aggregate indexes were added to the set of final MOS measures: psychological distress (twenty-two items) and psychological well-being (ten items).

After determining the best subscale structure based on the full battery, the same structure was tested using the 17-item battery (Table 7–2). The following indexes and scales, which paralleled results from the long-form battery, were constructed:

Psychological distress (anxiety, depression/ behavioral-emotional control)	12 items
Anxiety	3 items
Depression/behavioral-emotional control	8 items
Psychological well-being (positive affect, feelings of belonging)	5 items
Positive affect	4 items

The final goal was to test an overall psychological distress and well-being index comprising all of the components, for each battery (33-item, 17-item, and 5-item). In the multitrait scaling analysis, item-total correlations ranged from 0.50 to 0.87 for the 33-item battery. One depression/behavioral-emotional control item (MHC6-losing mind, losing control over way you act, talk, think, feel, or of your memory) again correlated higher (although not significantly) with the cognitive functioning scale as earlier. Because the item was not necessary for purposes of reliability and because it appears to tap cognitive functioning, it was eliminated from the overall index, thus making sure that the overall index was clearly distinct from the cognitive functioning scale. In the resulting 32-item index, item-scale correlations still ranged from 0.50 to 0.87.

Item-total correlations for the 17-item battery ranged from 0.65 to 0.86 in the MOS sample and from 0.55 to 0.84 in the ECA sample. All items discriminated from all other measures in the MOS sample (no discriminant validity analysis was possible in the ECA). We concluded that an overall index was warranted from all seventeen items.

A summary of item-scale correlations for the MHI-5 is presented in Table 7–7. For comparative purposes, Table 7–7 also includes correlations from three additional samples. Item-scale correlations ranged from 0.54 to 0.81 across all four samples.

Table 7–7 Item-Scale Correlations Correlated for Overlap for the MHI-5: Four Samples

Abbreviated Item Content	Item Variable Name	MOS Baseline Sample (N = 2,862)	MOS Screening Sample[a] (N = 10,771)	ECA (N = 229)	U.S. Adults[b] (N = 2,008)
Nervous person[c]	MHA01	.65	.67	.65	.60
Felt calm and peaceful	MHP03	.78	.73	.71	.65
Felt down-hearted and blue[c]	MHD02	.81	.76	.79	.65
Happy person	MHP01	.80	.75	.72	.64
Down in the dumps[c]	MHC01	.73	.69	.56	.54

[a] See Stewart, Hays, and Ware, 1988.
[b] See chapter 16.
[c] Reversed so that a high score indicates less negative affect.

The three indexes reflect different proportions of the various components. A summary of the number (k) and percentage of items comprising each of the indexes is given in Table 7–8. Another way to look at these is to examine the proportion of items assessing psychological distress and psychological well-being in each of the indexes (see Table 7–8). All indexes are weighted more heavily in the direction of distress. The MHI-5 is the most balanced and the MHI-17 the least balanced, a fact that can be confirmed by examining the correlations of the three indexes with various long-form subscales in Table 7–9. The correlations parallel the proportion of items in each of the indexes. All correlations are significant ($p < .001$) and, except for the correlation with feelings of belonging, are moderate to high.

Scoring Rules Scales and indexes were constructed as shown in Table 7–10. All subscale items were recoded so that a high score indicated more of the subscale name (e.g., a high score on anxiety indicated more anxiety). Total index scores were scored so that a high score indicated more positive feelings. All scales were scored by computing the average for items that were answered. If a respondent was missing half or more of the items in a scale, he or she was assigned a missing value on the

Table 7–8 Proportion of Components of Psychological Distress/Well-Being Represented in Three Summary Indexes

	MHI-32		MHI-17		MHI-5	
	k	%	k	%	k	%
Anxiety	7	22	4	24	1	20
Depression/behavioral-emotional control	13	41	8	47	2	40
Positive affect	7	22	4	24	2	40
Belonging/loneliness	5	16	1	6	0	0
Psychological distress	22	69	12	71	3	60
Psychological well-being	10	31	5	30	2	40

Table 7–9 Correlations of MHI-5 and MHI-17 with Measures of Cognitive Functioning and Psychological Distress/Well-Being Subscales and Indexes

Scale[a]	# of Items	MHI-5	MHI-17
Cognitive functioning (+)	6	.69	.73
Mental health index I (+)	32	.96	.99
Psychological Distress I (−)	22	−.94	−.96
Depression/behavioral-emotional control I (−)	13	−.92	−.96
Anxiety I (−)	6	−.86	−.86
Psychological well-being I (+)	10	.88	.91
Positive affect I (+)	7	.90	.92
Feelings of belonging (+)	3	.66	.72

Note: All correlations are significant ($p < .001$).
[a] A (+) high score indicates better health. A (−) high score indicates poor health.

scale. As described in chapter 5 on methods of scale construction, most of the people excluded due to this missing value rule were missing all of the items in the scale. All scores were then transformed to a 0–100 scale. Because item variances and item-scale correlations were generally comparable within each scale, we did not standardize or weight items before scoring. Scoring rules for the subscales and indexes are summarized in Table 7–11.

Table 7-10 Summary of Number of Items in Final Psychological Distress/
Well-Being and Cognitive Functioning Scales and Indexes

	# OF ITEMS		
Scale	Full Battery	17-Item Battery	5-Item Battery
Cognitive functioning	6		
Mental health index	32	17	5
Psychological distress	22	12	—
Anxiety	6	3	—
Depression/behavioral-emotional control	13	8	—
Psychological well-being	10	5	—
Feelings of belonging	3	—	—
Positive affect	7	—	—

Characteristics of Measures

Descriptive Statistics Descriptive statistics for the psychological
distress/well-being and cognitive functioning scales and indexes are
shown in Table 7-12 for the PAQ baseline sample. Indicated in the table
are the number of items in each scale, the percentage who obtained a
perfect score (e.g., completely positive feelings, completely negative
feelings, no problems in cognitive functioning), the observed range (the
possible range was 0-100), the means and standard deviations, and the
percentage missing (less than 1 in nearly all cases).

Variability The full range of scores was observed for cognitive
functioning, both of the anxiety scales, positive affect, feelings of
belonging, psychological well-being, and the MHI-5. Nearly the full
range of scores was observed for the remaining scales. Cognitive
functioning and depression/behavioral-emotional control were the
most skewed toward better health, both with skewness coefficients of
1.3, absolute value. The other measures were skewed, but less so, with
the majority of patients experiencing less distress.

Reliability A summary of the internal-consistency reliability of the
various subscales and indexes for the MOS PAQ baseline sample and the
ECA sample are shown in Table 7-13. In both samples, reliabilities
range from 0.85 to 0.98. The reliability of selected subscales in subgroups of those over age seventy, those with less than a high school
education, and those with depressive symptoms was tested and compa-

Table 7–11 Content and Scoring of Final Psychological Distress/Well-Being and Cognitive Functioning Scales and Indexes

Abbreviated Item Content	Item Variable Name	FULL BATTERY MEASURES					
		ANX6	DBC13	POS7	BEL	COG	DIS22
Number of Items		6	13	7	3	6	22
Anxiety							
Very nervous person	MHA01	R					R
Bothered by nervousness	MHA02	R					R
Tense, high strung	MHA03	R					R
Difficulty calming down	MHA04	R					R
Anxious or worried	MHA05	—					R
Rattled, upset	MHA06	R					R
Restless, fidgety	MHA07	R					R
Depression/behavioral-emotional control							
Low or very low spirits	MHD01		R				R
Downhearted and blue	MHD02		R				R
How depressed at worst	MHD03		R				R
Feel depressed	MHD04		R				R
Moody, brooded	MHD05		R				R
Depression interfered	MHD06		R				R
Down in dumps	MHC01		R				R
Nothing to look forward to	MHC02		R				R
Firm control of behavior	MHC03		NR				NR
Felt like crying	MHC04		R				R
Better off if dead	MHC05		R				R
Losing mind, control	MHC06		—				—
Emotionally stable	MHC07		NR				NR
Think about taking life	MHC08		R				R
Positive affect							
Been a happy person	MHP01			R			
Generally enjoyed things	MHP02			R			

| | | 17-ITEM | | | | | | 5-ITEM |
| | | BATTERY MEASURES | | | | | | MEASURE |
PWB10	MHI32	ANX3	DBC8	POS4	DIS12	PWB5	MHI17	MHI5
10	32	3	8	4	12	5	17	5
	NR	R			R		NR	NR
	NR							
	NR	R			R		NR	
	NR							
	NR	—			R		NR	
	NR							
	NR	R			R		NR	
	NR		R		R		NR	
	NR		R		R		NR	NR
	NR							
	NR		R		R		NR	
	NR		R		R		NR	
	NR							
	NR		R		R		NR	NR
	NR		R		R		NR	
	R		NR		NR		R	
	NR							
	NR							
	—							
	R		NR		NR		R	
	NR							
R	R			R		R	R	NR
R	R							

Table 7–11 (*Cont.*)

Abbreviated Item Content	Item Variable Name	FULL BATTERY MEASURES					
		ANX6	DBC13	POS7	BEL	COG	DIS22
Felt calm, peaceful	MHP03			R			
Happy, satisfied, pleased	MHP04			R			
Living an adventure	MHP05			R			
Cheerful, light-hearted	MHP06			R			
Daily life interesting	MHP07			R			
Belonging/loneliness							
Feel left out	LNLY1				—		R
Love relationships full	LNLY2			R			
Felt loved, wanted	LNLY3			R			
People close to	LNLY4			R			
Feel isolated	LNLY5				—		R
Cognitive functioning							
Became confused	COG1					NR	
React slowly to things	COG2					NR	
Difficulty reasoning	COG3					NR	
Forgetful	COG4					NR	
Trouble keeping attention	COG5					NR	
Difficulty concentrating	COG6					NR	

Note: NR = not reversed before averaging; R = reversed before averaging; — = item not included in scale.

rable reliabilities for all subgroups were found. Reliabilities for the shortest index, the MHI-5, were 0.90 and 0.86 in these two samples. Reliabilities for all measures in all groups are excellent, far exceeding the 0.50 criterion for group comparisons.

Validity A matrix of correlations among the different subscales is shown in Table 7–14. Cognitive functioning is moderately related to all other measures, although as expected it is more highly related to psychological distress ($-.76$) than to psychological well-being ($.60$). The absolute magnitude of the correlations among the psychological distress and well-being subscales range from 0.50 (between feelings of

	17-ITEM BATTERY MEASURES							5-ITEM MEASURE
PWB10	MHI32	ANX3	DBC8	POS4	DIS12	PWB5	MHI17	MHI5
R	R			R		R	R	NR
R	R							
R	R							
R	R			R		R	R	
R	R			R		R	R	
—	NR							
R	R							
R	R					R	R	
R	R							
—	NR							

belonging and anxiety) to 0.83 (between depression/behavioral-emotional control and positive affect). For scales that parallel those from the original MHI administered in the HIE general population, correlations tend to be higher in this patient sample, but the pattern of correlations is remarkably similar (Ware, Veit, and Sherbourne, 1985). For example, the lowest correlation in the HIE was also between anxiety and emotional ties (absolute magnitude .39). Depression was correlated 0.76 with anxiety in the HIE, compared with 0.80 in this sample, and −0.68 with positive affect, compared with −0.83 in this sample.

Table 7–12 Descriptive Statistics for Psychological Distress/Well-Being and Cognitive Functioning Scales and Indexes: PAQ Baseline Sample (*N* = 3,053)

Scale[a]	*k*	Mean	SD	% Perfect Score	Observed Range	% Missing
Cognitive Functioning (+)	6	82.4	16.5	15.8	0–100	0.3
Mental Health Index I (+)	32	70.3	16.2	0.0	9–96	0.2
Psychological distress I (−)	22	26.8	14.8		4–91	0.3
Depression/behavioral-emotional control I (−)	13	19.3	18.3	9.5	0–98	0.2
Anxiety I (−)	6	24.5	19.3	8.8	0–100	0.6
Psychological well-being I (+)	10	64.0	22.3	0.0	0–100	0.3
Positive affect I (+)	7	61.2	22.8	1.6	0–100	0.5
Feelings of belonging (+)	3	70.6	26.3	0.4	0–100	1.0
Mental Health Index II (+)	17	72.8	19.5	0.1	7–100	0.3
Psychological distress II (−)	12	23.0	19.2	6.1	0–98	0.6
Anxiety II (−)	3	25.8	21.3	15.2	0–100	0.6
Depression/behavioral emotional control II (−)	8	21.1	19.6	12.4	0–98	0.3
Psychological well-being II (+)	5	63.0	22.9	0.2	4–100	0.8
Positive affect II (+)	4	60.7	23.3		0–100	0.5
Mental Health Index III (+)	5	72.0	20.8	4.7	0–100	0.5

[a] A (+) high score indicates better health; a (−) high score indicates poorer health.

The MHI-5 and the MHI-17 were evaluated in relation to the various subscales and the overall 32-item index (MHI-32) to determine the extent of information on each contained in the respective short versions (Table 7–9). The correlations were all significant ($p < .001$). The MHI-17 correlated 0.99 with the MHI-32, which is remarkable. The MHI-5 correlates 0.96 with the MHI-32, which is very high considering the amount of reduction in the number of items. It is notable that the correlations are nearly identical with each of the subscales.

Resolution of Issues and Future Directions

Measures of psychological distress and well-being and cognitive functioning were successfully developed that discriminate from one another

Table 7–13 Internal Consistency Reliability for Psychological Distress/Well-Being and Cognitive Functioning Scales and Indexes

Index/Scale[a]	Variable Name	# of Items	RELIABILITY	
			PAQ Baseline Sample ($N = 2,862$)	ECA Sample ($N = 229$)
Cognitive functioning (+)	COG	6	.87	—
Mental health index I (+)	MHI 32	32	.98	—
Psychological distress I (−)	DIS 22	22	.97	—
Depression/behavioral-emotional control I (−)	DBC 13	13	.95	—
Anxiety I (−)	ANX 6	6	.92	—
Psychological well-being I (+)	PWB 10	10	.94	—
Positive affect I (+)	POS 7	7	.94	—
Feelings of belonging (+)	BEL	3	.87	
Mental health index II (+)	MHI 17	17	.96	.94
Psychological distress II (−)	DIS 12	12	.95	.93
Anxiety II (−)	ANX 3	3	.86	.85
Depression/behavioral emotional control II (−)	DBC 8	8	.94	.90
Psychological well-being II (+)	PWB 5	5	.91	.86
Positive affect II (+)	POS 4	4	.92	.85
Mental health index III (+)	MHI 5	5	.90	.86

[a] A (+) high score means better health; a (−) high score means poorer health.

and from other related concepts and that are reliable in this patient population. In doing so, several issues were addressed: the dimensionality of psychological distress and well-being was generally confirmed; shorter measures of psychological distress and well-being than have previously been available were provided, although with some caveats; the assessment of feelings of belonging/loneliness was slightly improved, although some problems were encountered raising new issues; and a self-administered measure of cognitive functioning was developed that shows promise as a supplement to more traditional measures.

Two issues for future study are whether additional concepts of psychological distress should be added to the battery and the extent of responses bias in all of these measures.

Table 7–14 Correlations Among Psychological Distress/Well-Being and Cognitive Functioning Scales

Measure[a]	COG	DBC	ANX	POS	BEL
Cognitive functioning (COG) (+)	(.87)				
Depression/behavioral-emotional control I (DBC) (−)	−.73	(.95)			
Anxiety I (ANX) (−)	−.70	.80	(.92)		
Positive affect I (POS) (+)	.60	−.83	−.71	(.94)	
Feelings of belonging (BEL) (+)	−.47	.65	.50	−.72	(.87)

Note: All coefficients significant (*p* < .001). N ranges from 3,004 to 3,034. Internal consistency reliabilities are on the diagonal.
[a] A (+) high score indicates better health; a (−) high score indicates poorer health.

Dimensionality of Psychological Distress and Well-Being The results generally confirmed the structure of psychological distress and well-being observed in the development of the MHI (Veit and Ware, 1983). Consistent with previous studies, depression and behavioral-emotional control are highly related concepts. After applying fairly stringent criteria for item discrimination and considering carefully the item content of the originally distinguished measures, they were combined into a single measure. A high priority for future work is to explore this dimensionality separately for depressed patients and for patients with only medical conditions.

Emotional stability, emotional control, and behavioral control might still be important to measure separately from depression. These were originally hypothesized as separate (Dupuy, 1973), but the HIE scaling studies resulted in a behavioral-emotional control scale that included several severe depression items in addition to the control and stability items. Possibly the lack of control and emotional instability are simply indicators of severe depression, which would explain why these couldn't be scored separately. However, the current items are complex: losing control of one's mind, thoughts, feelings, and behavior are all mentioned in one item. The addition of several additional simplified control and stability items could possibly allow this concept to discriminate from depression.

The resulting depression/behavioral-emotional control scale is a conceptually rich measure of depression and will be useful as an additional measure of severity of depression for purposes of evaluating those with major depressive disorder in the MOS. Although the two loneliness items were not included in this scale, they could be included later if future studies confirm that depression and behavioral-emotional control cannot be distinguished in groups of depressed and non-depressed patients.

The scaling results indicated a psychometric basis for scoring a number of subscales separately and for scoring psychological distress and well-being separately. Other studies are finding that the different dimensions of distress and well-being might have different meanings, at least in relation to subsequent utilization of mental health services. For example, a one-point difference in distress is associated with a larger change in the use of mental health services than a one-point change in psychological well-being (Ware, Manning, Duan, et al., 1984). A different approach to the same data indicated comparable findings— that each dimension of psychological distress had separate and signifi-cant effects on the probability of outpatient mental health care, but psychological well-being had little effect (Keeler, Wells, Manning, et al., 1986). All of these findings strongly emphasize the importance of using disaggregated scores wherever possible. At the least, investigators should include the separate psychological distress and psychological well-being scales.

Options for Shorter Measures The development of more practical measures advanced in several ways. First, respondent burden was reduced for the entire psychological distress and well-being battery from thirty-eight to thirty-two items without sacrificing reliability. Second, a promising battery of seventeen items is offered. All but one of the subscales in this battery have reliabilities above 0.90 as well. The overall 17-item index correlated nearly perfectly with the 32-item index, lending evidence that this shorter version contains much of the original information. Third, the MHI-5 is reliable in this chronically ill sample and contains a great deal of the information available in the long-form index.

Shorter measures should be used with caution. Although the 17-item index might be as sensitive and valid as the 32-item index, this may not be true for the subscales scored from the 17-item version. For example, the long-form anxiety scale may be sensitive to clinically relevant changes, but the short form might not be. Such findings are important to determine before investigators choose short-form measures over the long for reasons of practicality. We know that the shorter measures are less sensitive to relevant changes. The question that must be addressed empirically is whether the shorter measures are sufficiently sensitive.

Assessing Belonging/Loneliness We initially thought that a measure of belonging/loneliness could be developed that contained both negative (loneliness) and positive (belonging) affective items. Even though loneliness is a symptom of depression, feelings of belonging/loneliness are somewhat distinct from depression and have different implications for care. We hoped that by including a substantial number of items we could construct an independent measure. However, the loneliness items would not discriminate from depression/behavioral-emotional control, although feelings of belonging did discriminate from positive affect. These same findings occurred in the studies of the MHI in a general population (Ware, Veit, and Sherbourne, 1985). Apparently, a variety of negative emotions go together to define depression, including loneliness. However, people can feel positive feelings such as cheerfulness or interest in life without necessarily having feelings of belonging. The two loneliness items were not included in the depression/behavioral-emotional control scale at this time; further analyses must be undertaken that explore the usefulness of retaining belonging/loneliness as a separate concept.

New Measure of Cognitive Functioning A highly reliable self-administered measure of cognitive functioning was developed based on the Sickness Impact Profile. Although cognitive impairment is a symptom of depression and is highly correlated with psychological distress, this measure was easily constructed to be distinct from distress. In order to achieve adequate discrimination, however, it was necessary to delete one item that included the phrases "losing your mind" and "losing control over your memory" from the original MHI that appears to have been tapping cognitive functioning. Although the cognitive functioning measure is skewed with more patients reporting better functioning, the full range of scores was observed. Evaluating the validity of this measure in relation to observer ratings of cognitive functioning will be especially useful. Our main purpose in constructing this measure was to identify a range of less severe, day-to-day problems in cognitive functioning that might be associated with various chronic conditions and their treatments. Even if this measure is not correlated with other measures of severe impairments, it could be valid in detecting less severe problems.

Adding Concepts of Psychological Distress Some aspects of depression defined by others are not represented in the MOS depression measure. We already noted that we could incorporate the two loneliness items, because loneliness has been considered a symptom of depression. Depression has been defined in terms of feelings of worthlessness, helplessness, hopelessness, meaninglessness, and loss of interest in people and things (Beck, 1967a, 1967b; see also Wells, 1985). The MOS measure includes only one item that could be considered indicative of loss of interest (nothing to look forward to) but does not directly tap these other feelings. Determining whether these additional concepts are part of depression or can be developed as separate measures might be helpful in finding out how to help people with depression. Although some measures of some of these concepts exist (e.g., Beck, Weissman, Lester, and Trexler, 1974; Rosenberg, 1965), they were not developed to be independent from depressed mood.

Anger has been increasingly considered an important component of psychological distress and a concept with important health consequences (Chesney and Rosenman, 1985; Diamond, 1982; Johnson and Broman, 1987). The next generation of these measures should include a test of whether an additional subscale of anger could be incorporated that would discriminate from the other components. Anger can range from mild irritation to rage and has been distinguished from hostility, which is more an attitude motivating aggressive behavior (Spielberger, Johnson, Russell, et al., 1965).

Response Bias The extent of response bias present in these measures is of some concern. All measures had low but significant correlations with socially desirable responding. Some people underreport distress, either because they are unaware of distressing feelings or unwilling to report them (e.g., it is commonly known that women report more psychological distress than men, but the reason for this is unclear). Others may overreport distress, exhibiting a tendency to complain.

The possibility of an acquiescence response set is exacerbated by the fact that none of the subscales contains a balance of positively and negatively worded items. Apparently, developing such balanced measures of emotional status is difficult; nearly all attempts have failed. In the MHI studies, although the "relaxed and calm" item was originally hypothesized as a positively worded aspect of anxiety, this item in fact correlated with the other positively worded items on the general positive affect scale (Veit and Ware, 1983). The same problem occurred in a study of the General Health Questionnaire (Berwick, Budman, Damico-White, et al., 1987). Also, people's level of distress or well-being at the time they complete the questions can affect how they report their states over the prior four weeks. More attention on response bias issues is warranted.

8. Health Perceptions, Energy/Fatigue, and Health Distress Measures

Anita L. Stewart, Ron D. Hays,
and John E. Ware, Jr.

The MOS measures of general health perceptions, energy/fatigue, and health distress are combined because all substantially reflect both physical and mental health, and because the approach to scale construction and validation was very similar.

Definitions and Issues: Health Perceptions and Health Distress

Health perceptions are personal beliefs and evaluations of general health status. These perceptions focus on health in general rather than on either physical or mental components specifically. People's perceptions of their health are important for at least two reasons. Health perceptions integrate the available information about people's health, taking into account differences in health preferences, values, needs, and attitudes. For example, two persons with the same objective levels of physical and mental health might rate their overall health differently because they experience or evaluate those states differently. Measures of health perceptions are also among the best predictors of utilization of general medical services and mental health services (Manning, Newhouse, and Ware, 1982; Wells, Manning, Duan, et al., 1984; Berki and Ashcraft, 1979).

The most widely used battery of measures of health perceptions is the Health Perceptions Questionnaire (HPQ) developed by Ware and Karmos (1976a; Ware, 1976). The HPQ was studied extensively in the Health Insurance Experiment (HIE), which contained twenty-six HPQ items (Ware, Davies-Avery, and Donald, 1978; Davies and Ware,

1981). The HPQ items were originally developed for the general population and can be self-administered, administered in person, or administered by telephone. The original HPQ assesses six components of health perceptions: (1) current health, (2) prior health, (3) health outlook, (4) resistance to illness, (5) sickness orientation, and (6) health worry/concern. A 22-item General Health Rating Index (GHRI) aggregated information across components, except sickness orientation, into a summary measure.

Of the six health perceptions components, the face validity of items in current health and prior health suggests they are fairly direct indicators of health status. Sickness orientation appears to pertain to a general attitude or personality construct, and the other three components—resistance to illness, health outlook, health worry/concern—appear to tap a mixture of health-related concepts.

Current health perceptions refer to ratings of health "now" and most directly indicate health. In the HIE, the current health subscale was more highly correlated with measures of physical and mental health than the other HPQ subscales; current health correlated about equally (0.40) with physical and mental health validity variables (Davies and Ware, 1981), indicating that it is indicative of both physical and mental health. Davies and Ware concluded that the current health subscale provides a better summary of the information about health status contained in the HPQ than any other HPQ subscale. The reliability of the current health scale is high (0.88), so this 9-item scale could probably be shortened.

Prior health refers to health in the past, without a particular time frame. Because prior health shows little or no change over time, it is not as useful as an outcome of care, but it can be useful as a control variable in predictive studies.

Health outlook refers to personal expectations regarding future health status. Such expectations appear in part to be a projection of a person's current and prior health experience. Health outlook may also reflect inherent optimism or pessimism or perhaps a sense of hopefulness or hopelessness.

A person's sense of susceptibility or resistance to illness is primarily a health belief (Jette, Cummings, Brock, et al., 1981; Weissfeld, Brock, Kirscht, et al., 1987). To the extent that a sense of susceptibility is based on a person's current and prior experiences with health problems, it also reflects health status. Susceptibility is a major component of the Health Belief Model, one of the earliest comprehensive attempts to explain differences in health-related behavior from a value-expectancy theoretical framework (Becker, 1974; Becker and Maiman, 1975; Janz and Becker, 1984; Jette, Cummings, Brock, et al., 1981; Kirscht, Becker, and Eveland, 1976; Rosenstock, 1974).

Sickness orientation refers to a tendency to accept sickness as a part of life (Davies and Ware, 1981) and is more a reaction to health status, appearing to be the least direct of the HPQ indicators of health. Accordingly, the sickness orientation measure was only weakly related to other health measures and was excluded from the MOS battery of health perceptions.

Health worry/concern refers to the extent to which health problems cause people to worry or be greatly concerned about health. The content of health worry/concern measures is similar to measures of health motivation, a concept added to the health belief model by Becker and Maiman (1975). Health motivation has been defined as a desire for good health (Becker, Maiman, Kirscht, et al., 1977). Concern about health may also reflect the value placed on health (Lau, Hartman, and Ware, 1986). Some contend that people are not concerned about their health until good health is threatened in some way (Herzlich, 1973). Thus, health concern could be indicative of health problems rather than simply a day-to-day concern for behaviors to promote optimal health.

Davies and Ware (1981) distinguished between worry about health and concern about health and called into question the appropriateness of combining these into one scale. In the HIE, items in this scale barely met standards of convergent validity (corrected item-scale correlations were all less than 0.40) and one item (worry or concern about health) correlated significantly higher with the current health scale than the worry/concern scale (Davies and Ware, 1981). This scaling failure is particularly noteworthy given the face validity of this item. Items in this scale exhibited more scaling problems than any other general health perceptions scale in the HIE. Additional scaling studies confirmed that the three worry items could be combined into a single scale, but that the concern items could not be combined into their own scale (i.e., they needed to be combined with the worry items to form an adequate scale). It would thus be useful to try to enhance their distinction and develop separate measures for each concept.

Measures of health worry focus on only the worry component of a broad range of negative emotions resulting from health problems such as frustration, despair, and discouragement. Thus, there is a need to develop a measure that assesses these other aspects of distress that are attributable to health problems. Because distress about health is likely to cause a person to visit the doctor, such a measure can prove useful in predicting subsequent ulilization of health care services. If the distress reflects fear about harmful consequences of various symptoms (Mc-Whinney, 1972), then adequate reassurance can alleviate it, making health distress a useful measure of the outcome of the quality of interpersonal care.

The General Health Rating Index (GHRI) was developed from the HPQ to achieve a single summary measure with a high degree of reliability and validity (Ware, Davies-Avery, and Donald, 1978; Davies and Ware, 1981). The GHRI has been shown to be a sensitive indicator of individual differences in disease status, self-reported limitations in physical and role functioning due to poor health, self-reported acute physical and psychosomatic symptoms, and self-reported psychological distress and well-being (Davies and Ware, 1981). The validity of the GHRI has been investigated extensively (Ware, 1984). The GHRI has also been shown to be substantially related to subsequent use of general medical and mental health services in the ambulatory system (Manning, Leibowitz, Goldberg, et al., 1984; Manning, Wells, Duan, et al., 1984). Previous studies also suggested that an aggregate health perceptions score (the GHRI) was better than the current health scale in predicting utilization, but not better than a multivariate model in which all of the subscales were used separately (Manning, Leibowitz, Goldberg, et al., 1984). Finally, unpublished data from the HIE indicate that the GHRI predicts length of survival.

Although the usefulness of the GHRI is apparent, it is important to continue to determine the best method for aggregating information into an overall health perceptions index. This future work is especially important because of the differences in interpretation of the six components of health perceptions and given the potential modifications in these components in the MOS.

Definition and Issues: Energy/Fatigue

Fatigue, a common complaint even among those who are relatively healthy (Atkinson, 1985; Hennen, 1987, cited in Saultz, 1988; Morrison, 1980; Solberg, 1984), is associated with nearly all chronic illnesses, providing "an added drain on the ill person" (Kerson and Kerson, 1985). Chronic illness can cause fatigue directly (i.e., from the physical and emotional demands of the illness) and indirectly (i.e., as a side effect of its treatment). Fatigue often has no underlying physical basis and is often attributed to psychological or emotional problems or to coping with extensive life changes (Hargreaves, 1977; Saultz, 1988; Sugarman and Berg, 1984). For example, Sugarman and Berg (1984) found that 50% of patients with fatigue were identified as having a diagnosis that was "psychosocial" in nature, 22% had a biomedical diagnosis, and for 33% no diagnosis was reached. Similarly, Valdini (1985) found psychological causes in 57% of patients with fatigue and physical causes in 37%. Fatigue is a common symptom of depression and can also represent a somatic expression of psychological distress. For example, fatigued patients were more likely than controls to have elevated scores on the Beck Depression Inventory (Kroenke, Wood, Mangelsdorff, et al., 1988). Thus, fatigue can be considered an aspect of both physical and mental health. Empirical support for this conclusion is provided by Ware, Davies-Avery, and Brook (1980), who found that a measure of vitality or energy/fatigue correlated 0.60 with a mental health factor and 0.47 with a factor defined by perceptions of physical health.

There is some disagreement on how fatigue should be defined. As Phillips (1980) noted, terms such as tiredness and weakness are often used interchangeably. Fatigue has been conceptualized in terms of general feelings (e.g., overall unpleasantness, feeling tired) and specific symptoms (e.g., yawning) (Haylock and Hart, 1979). Physical symptoms that correlated significantly with feelings of fatigue in the Haylock and Hart study included the following: tired in whole body, tired legs, heavy head, eyestrain, yawning, wanting to lie down, and feeling ill. Symptoms of fatigue were grouped into three categories in Japanese studies: drowsiness or sleepiness, difficulty concentrating (e.g., difficulty thinking, inability to concentrate, forgetfulness), and bodily complaints (e.g., headache, feeling ill) (Yoshitake, 1971).

The main issue in developing a measure of energy/fatigue as part of a battery of health status measures is defining both positive (energy) and negative (fatigue) states that are conceptually and empirically distinct from similar concepts such as depression, positive affect, cognitive functioning, and sleep problems.

Although some good measures were available to review, none was without problems. A vitality scale was included in preliminary evaluations of the HIE Mental Health Index (Ware, Johnston, Davies-Avery, et al., 1979), which was adopted from the National Center for Health

Statistics General Well-Being Schedule (Dupuy, 1969, 1973, 1984). The four HIE items represented both the positive and the negative ends of the energy/fatigue continuum. The HIE vitality scale was originally hypothesized as a measure of mental health. Results from the HIE led to exclusion of the scale from the Mental Health Index because it "did not clearly appear to assess primarily mental health or illness" (Ware, Johnston, Davies-Avery, et al., 1979, p. 79). After its exclusion from the Mental Health Index, the measure was not used again in the HIE despite its adequate internal-consistency reliability in that study (alpha = 0.81).

The HIE vitality scale exhibited adequate reliability in a study reported by Nelson, Conger, Douglass, et al. (1983). In a clinical trial of antihypertensive drugs, one drug was associated with significantly higher scores on this vitality measure, indicating that the measure can be useful in monitoring side effects of such drugs (Levine, Croog, Sudilovsky, et al., 1987). The same measure predicted subsequent utilization and new diagnoses in a one-year longitudinal study (Valdini, Steinhardt, Valicenti, et al., 1988).

Despite these promising characteristics of the HIE vitality scale, three problems exist: more than one construct is represented in each item (e.g., "active," "vigorous," "dull," and "sluggish" are all included in one item); response choices for two of the items confound intensity with frequency; and it is unclear whether the measure is distinct from similar measures. In the HIE, some of the energy items tended to correlate with measures of general health and mental health (Ware, Johnston, Davies-Avery, et al., 1979).

Comrey (1970) developed a 4-item scale of energy and activity which was balanced in terms of positive and negative items. Items pertain to "having drive to get things done," "having vim and vigor," and "being energetic." This was one of five scales that formed an activity/lack of energy factor in a test of the structure of Comrey's scales (Montag and Comrey, 1982). The factor also included measures of exercise (e.g., "I enjoy doing things that involve quite a bit of physical exercise"), need to excel (e.g., "I am willing to work very hard to get ahead of the next fellow"), liking for work (e.g., "I like to work hard"), and stamina (e.g., "I can work a long time without feeling tired"). The main problem with this scale is that it defines a personality characteristic rather than health, is slightly confounded with drive, and is defined too much in relation to other people.

The Profile of Mood States (McNair, Lorr, and Doppleman, 1981) includes a fatigue/inertia scale and a vigor/activity scale as two of its six component scales (e.g., Norcross, Guadagnoli, and Prochaska, 1984). Coefficient alpha (internal-consistency reliability) ranged from 0.87 to 0.92 for the vigor/activity scale and from 0.90 to 0.91 for the fatigue/ inertia scale in three samples (Reddon, Marceau, and Holden, 1985). However, Reddon et al. suggest that the scales may not demonstrate discriminant validity.

Belloc, Breslow, and Hochstim (1971) assessed energy/fatigue in terms of energy, trouble sleeping, how tired people feel if they only get four or five hours of sleep, and frequency of feeling worn out at the end of the day. This measure is difficult to interpret because it confounds sleep problems with energy.

Content and Measurement Strategy

Pilot Studies Three pilot studies were conducted that attempted to resolve some of the problems of the HPQ and energy/fatigue measures. Items from all HPQ concepts were included, but over thirty new items pertaining to health concern, worry, and other types of distress due to health were added. The pilot studies included primarily adults visiting ambulatory clinics.

As a result of the pilot studies, the 9-item current health scale was shortened to six items while achieving an improved internal-consistency reliability (0.93). A modified single-item overall health rating, as recommended by Davies and Ware (1981), was tested, adding a "very good" response option to increase the number of choices to five (excellent, very good, good, fair, poor). Because the response distribution was good, the modified item was used for the final battery.

Additionally, two new prior health items were tested and one was added to the existing HPQ prior health scale, increasing the number of items from three to four. Nine health outlook items (six HPQ items and three new ones) were tested and seven were selected which had an internal-consistency reliability of 0.86. One more item was eliminated in the third pilot study, leaving six items (three original HPQ items and three new ones). Six resistance to illness items (four HPQ items and two new ones) were piloted and four of the six items retained (three original HPQ items and one new item).

In the first pilot, the MOS tested nine new health worry items (some adapted from the HPQ worry/concern items), the two original HPQ health concern items, six new health concern items, and eighteen new health distress items that assessed feelings of frustration, despair, and fear resulting directly from health problems. From this set, a 4-item health concern scale was constructed that was distinct from the other concepts as well as from health value (internal-consistency reliability of 0.75 in the second pilot). The health worry and health distress items defined a single health factor. Thus, the hypothesis of a single health distress concept was tested in the next pilot study. Thirteen of the twenty-seven health distress and health worry items from the first pilot were included in the second pilot (three worry and ten distress items). The new hypothesis was confirmed. Seven items were selected to represent a spectrum of severity, ranging from relatively minor distress (e.g., frustration) to severe distress (e.g., weighed down by health problems). The reliability of this 7-item scale was 0.92. One more item was eliminated based on a third pilot study, and a 6-item health distress scale was then adopted.

The HIE vitality scale was considered sufficiently good to use as a basis for developing the energy/fatigue measure. Seven items were written to capture the different concepts in the four HIE items (i.e., disentangling the HIE items) and four new items were written to assess additional concepts. Items were written in such a way as to be confounded as little as possible with closely related concepts (e.g., sleepiness during the day, cognitive functioning, depression). The response choices were limited to a frequency dimension and represented intensity in the item stems (e.g., ranging from "feeling tired" to "feeling exhausted"). Six negatively worded items ("tired") and five positively worded items ("full of pep") were included in the initial pilot study. In the first pilot, the eight best items were selected, which had a reliability of 0.91.

The eight items were administered to the second pilot sample for cross-validation and further evaluation. Six items were selected that discriminated best from measures of sleep (internal-consistency reliability of 0.85). One additional item was eliminated based on the third pilot study.

Final Items Thirty-one items assessing health perceptions, six items assessing health distress, and five items assessing energy/fatigue were selected for the final set. The actual health perceptions questions appear on pages 373 and 397–399 in the Appendix. The health distress and energy/fatigue questions appear on pages 377–378. A summary of the MOS health perceptions items is shown in Table 8–1, along with information about which ones were carried over from the HIE version of the HPQ. Energy/fatigue and health distress items are summarized in Table 8–3.

For the health perceptions items, respondents were asked to rate the extent to which the item was true, with five response choices (ranging from definitely true to definitely false). This method was used successfully in the HPQ and in the MOS pilot tests of these scales. For the energy/fatigue and health distress items, respondents were asked how often during the past four weeks the statements applied. One of the current health items asked respondents to rate their health in general, with five response choices (excellent, very good, good, fair, and poor).

Construction and Evaluation of Measures

Analysis Plan The general MOS goals were to develop scores for each separate hypothesized scale and a summary health perceptions index. To test the discriminant validity of items in the subscales, items from seven measures were included in the multitrait scaling matrix: sleep somnolence, anxiety, positive affect, value placed on health, physical functioning, role limitations due to physical health, and role limitations due to emotional problems. We were especially interested that the energy/fatigue items discriminate from sleep somnolence, that the health distress items discriminate from the two psychological distress subscales, and that the health concern items discriminate from health value.

The goal in constructing an overall health perceptions index was to select items from the full battery that best represented an underlying construct of health perceptions. Although most of the subscale concepts are highly correlated and are fairly indicative of health in general, we wanted the index to represent general health as purely as possible and to detect changes in health over time. Because some of the subscale constructs were more direct indicators of general health than others, we tested four possible combinations of constructs. The four potential indexes are given in Table 8–2.

Current health was included in all potential indexes because it is the best of the health perception concepts. Health concern was excluded, as was done in the HIE (Davies and Ware, 1981). Because prior health shows little or no change over time and because the prior health items contributed little to the first unrotated component in prior studies (Davies and Ware, 1981), it was excluded from all MOS indexes.

Table 8–1 General Health Perception Items Studied in the Health Insurance Experiment (HIE) and the MOS

Subscale/Abbreviated Item Content	HIE		MOS	
	Full Battery	Index GHRI	Full Battery	20-Item Short Form
Number of items	34	22	31	5
Current health				
Overall health in general	x		x	x
Health is excellent	x	x	x	x
Feel as good now as ever	x	x	x	
Doctors say health is now excellent	x	x		
Not as healthy now as used to be	x	x		
Healthy as anybody I know	x	x	x	x
I am somewhat ill	x	x	x	x
Been feeling bad lately	x	x	x	x
Feel better now than ever	x	x		
Doctors say now in poor health	x	x		
I am in poor health			x	
Prior health				
Never been seriously ill	x	x	x	
Never had a long illness	x	x	x	
So sick once thought I might die	x	x	x	
Sickly for a long time			x	
Health outlook				
Health worse in future than now	x	x	x	
Expect a healthy life	x	x	x	
Probably sick a lot in future	x	x		
Expect to have better health than others	x	x	x	
Future will be unhealthy			x	
Good health in my future			x	
Expect my health to get worse			x	
Resistance				
Body resists illness	x	x	x	
Something going around, catch it	x	x	x	
Get sick easier than others	x	x	x	
People get sick easier than I do	x	x		
Usually last one to catch a cold			x	
Health worry/concern				
Worry about health more than others	x	x		
Never worry about my health	x	x		
Health is a concern	x		x	
Others more concerned about health	x			
Worry or concern about health	x			

Table 8–1 (*Cont.*)

Subscale/Abbreviated Item Content	HIE		MOS	
	Full Battery	Index GHRI	Full Battery	20-Item Short Form
Health concern				
Concerned about my health			x	
Only think about health when see doctor			x	
Often think about my health			x	
Sickness orientation				
Getting sick part of life	x			
Accept that sometimes I'm sick	x			
Not included in subscales				
Avoid letting illness interfere	x			
Don't like to go to doctor	x			
Try to keep going as usual	x			
When sick, try to keep it to self	x			
Doesn't bother me to go to doctor	x			
When I think I'm sick, I fight it	x			

Table 8–2 Number of Items from Scales in Each Hypothesized Index

Scale	INDEX			
	MOSGHP23	MOSGHP19	MOSGHP13	GHRI19
Current health	7	7	7	6
Prior health				3
Health outlook	6	6		6
Resistance to illness	4			3
Health concern				
Health distress	6	6	6	1

Only one of the three potential MOS indexes included the resistance to illness items, because resistance has been shown to contribute negligibly to overall general health in previous studies (Davies and Ware, 1981) and is also very stable (thus possibly decreasing the sensitivity of the overall index to changes in health). One index without the health outlook items was tested, because these items might be more indicative of optimism than health.

The MOS tested one index that approximated as closely as possible the GHRI constructed for the HIE because it has been extensively used and validated. To match the GHRI, all six current health items (not the overall item), four health outlook items, three prior health items (only the three old HIE items), three resistance to illness items (only the three old HIE items), and one health worry item from the health distress scale intended to match the HIE health worry item were included.

The MOS analyses of the items in the subscales earmarked for the four potential indexes included the following to determine which best reflected the underlying general health construct:

1) factor analysis of items in each potential index and subscales included in each potential index to determine the percentage of variance explained by each possible index and to assure that each item and subscale correlated at least 0.30 with the first unrotated factor;

2) correlations with a set of validity variables to determine which, if any, subscales correlated in the opposite direction with any validity variable and hence should not be combined into an overall index. Validity measures included number of chronic conditions; number of doctor visits in previous two weeks; number of nights in a hospital during past year; pain index; physical/psychophysiologic symptoms; energy/fatigue; physical functioning; mental health index; social activity limitations due to health; role limitations due to physical health; and role limitations due to emotional problems;

3) multitrait scaling analyses for each potential index to determine the convergent and discriminant validity. Because the health distress items had six and the others five response choices, we standardized all items for these analyses; and

4) correlations of each of the indexes with the validity variables outlined above to determine which had the highest correlations.

Item Variability The means and standard deviations for the energy/fatigue, health perceptions, and health distress items are shown in the first multitrait analysis. Item frequencies are shown in Table 8–3.

The energy/fatigue items exhibited the most normal distributions, followed by the current health items. The percentage of responses in the "don't know" (neutral) category was greater for health outlook than for prior health, confirming that people feel more uncertain about the future than the past. Responses, excluding "don't know" for health outlook, were skewed, with the majority of patients expecting good

Table 8–3 Percentage Distribution of Health Perceptions, Energy/Fatigue, and Health Distress Items: PAQ Baseline Sample (N = 3,053)

Abbreviated Item Content	Item Variable Name	Response Choice[a]	ITEM RESPONSE[b]					
			1	2	3	4	5	6
Energy/fatigue								
Feel full of pep	EFT01	AT	2.6	20.3	15.3	25.9	19.4	16.5
Have a lot of energy	EFT02	AT	4.1	23.8	19.1	29.6	18.0	8.5
Feel worn out	EFT03	AT	2.9	8.5	15.2	28.4	32.6	12.5
Feel tired	EFT04	AT	4.0	9.9	14.1	34.5	30.1	7.5
Have enough energy to do things	EFT05	AT	15.9	35.8	12.8	20.9	9.7	4.9
Current health								
Somewhat ill	GHP01	DT	12.7	25.4	8.8	25.1	28.1	—
My health is excellent	GHP02	DT	7.5	41.9	11.9	22.6	16.1	—
I am in poor health	GHP03	DT	4.4	12.9	8.8	32.1	41.7	—
As healthy as anybody I know	GHP04	DT	11.6	34.8	20.0	20.7	12.9	—
Feeling bad lately	GHP05	DT	9.5	23.8	3.0	33.6	30.1	—
Feel as good as ever have	GHP06	DT	11.5	35.6	3.7	29.2	20.0	—
Health excellent, very good, etc.	GHP31	U	6.1	27.9	42.7	20.3	3.0	—
Prior health								
Never been seriously ill	GHP17	DT	24.9	23.4	2.7	15.5	33.4	—
So sick once thought I might die	GHP18	DT	22.2	13.1	4.1	16.0	44.5	—
Never had illness that lasted	GHP19	DT	37.3	22.9	2.1	13.9	23.8	—
Been sickly for long time	GHP20	DT	6.0	15.0	3.1	29.9	45.9	—
Health outlook								
Future will be unhealthy	GHP11	DT	2.3	7.5	47.7	19.5	23.0	—
Good health in my future	GHP12	DT	19.6	24.7	45.5	6.1	4.0	—
Health worse in future	GHP13	DT	14.2	19.8	42.3	10.6	13.0	—
Expect to have healthy life	GHP14	DT	19.9	36.2	30.5	9.0	4.4	—

Table 8–3 (*Cont.*)

Abbreviated Item Content	Item Variable Name	Response Choice[a]	ITEM RESPONSE[b]					
			1	2	3	4	5	6
Expect better health than others	GHP15	DT	14.9	28.9	41.5	9.9	4.8	—
Expect health to get worse	GHP16	DT	5.0	14.6	36.9	21.1	22.5	—
Resistance to illness								
Get sick easier than others	GHP07	DT	3.8	9.7	11.2	30.6	44.7	—
Body resists illness	GHP08	DT	16.6	46.7	14.4	14.9	7.4	—
When illness, usually catch it	GHP09	DT	2.8	10.1	7.4	48.7	31.0	—
Usually last one to catch cold	GHP10	DT	19.4	39.2	11.9	22.1	7.4	—
Health concern								
Concerned about my health	GHP21	DT	43.8	33.0	2.1	14.0	7.1	—
Only think about health when see doctor	GHP22	DT	5.9	18.7	3.2	40.1	32.0	—
Health is a big concern	GHP23	DT	25.7	40.6	5.8	20.9	6.9	—
Often think about health	GHP24	DT	18.1	42.0	5.2	27.2	7.5	—
Health distress								
Frustrated about health	HD1	AT	3.0	5.9	7.3	14.3	21.5	48.0
Weighed down by health	HD2	AT	2.3	4.9	6.6	15.1	23.3	47.6
Discouraged by health	HD3	AT	2.8	5.8	7.3	17.9	25.2	41.1
Feel despair over health	HD4	AT	2.2	3.8	4.4	9.7	16.5	63.5
Afraid because of health	HD5	AT	1.8	3.5	4.2	12.2	20.1	58.2
Health a worry	HD6	AT	3.1	4.4	6.0	14.8	26.6	45.1

[a] AT: 1–All of the time; 2–Most of the time; 3–A good bit of the time; 4–Some of the time; 5–A little of the time; 6–None of the time. DT: 1–Definitely true; 2–True; 3–Don't know; 4–False; 5–Definitely false. U: 1–Excellent; 2–Very good; 3–Good; 4–Fair; 5–Poor.
[b] Percentage of those who responded to each item.

health. All six health distress items were very skewed: from 41% to 64% reporting never feeling distressed during the past four weeks. The four health concern items were skewed, with the majority reporting "some" concern. The lowest standard deviation (0.90) was for the single overall health item, which had different response choices from the other items (excellent, very good, good, fair, poor). The remaining standard deviations ranged from 1.00 to 1.65. The percentage missing on any one item ranged from 1% to 4%.

Construction of Scales The seven hypothesized scales as outlined in Table 8–3, were evaluated. When the multitrait correlation matrix was evaluated, the new prior health item (GHP 20—I have been sickly for a long time) correlated 0.72 with the current health scale and only 0.41 with the prior health scale. Closer attention to the item content suggested that this item implies that the person has been sick for a long time and is still sick, hence its correlation with the current health scale. We thus eliminated the item.

The multitrait correlation matrix for the remaining thirty-five items is presented in Table 8–4. In this matrix, row entries represent correlations between each item and the sum of the items in each scale grouping. Footnote "a" indicates the hypothesized scale placement of each item as well as item-scale correlations that were corrected for overlap (i.e., each item is correlated with the sum of the other items in the scale).

All but one of the thirty-five items correlated 0.50 or greater with its hypothesized scale, thus exceeding our stringent convergent validity criterion. Correlations between the items and their hypothesized scales ranged from 0.64 to 0.76 for current health, 0.56 to 0.74 for health outlook, 0.50 to 0.61 for prior health, 0.76 to 0.87 for health distress, 0.36 to 0.62 for health concern, 0.55 to 0.64 for resistance to illness, and 0.68 to 0.78 for energy/fatigue.

All but one item met the criterion of item discrimination—that is, it correlated significantly higher with its own scale than with any other scale. One current health item (GHP 5—I have been feeling bad lately) had three instances where its correlations with other scales were within two standard errors of its correlation with current health—health distress, energy/fatigue, and social functioning. Because we expect the health perceptions items to correlate with other measures of health, these three probable scaling errors were not considered to be serious and the item was retained in the scale.

Construction of Overall Health Perceptions Index In the principal components analysis of the items for each of the four potential indexes,

Table 8–4 Item-Scale Correlation Matrix, Health Perceptions, Energy/ Fatigue, and Health Distress: PAQ Baseline Sample (N = 2,389)

Item	Mean	SD	CURR	OUT	PRIOR	DIST	CONCRN	RESIST
GHP31	3.16	.89	.69a	.42	.36	−.51	−.26	.34
GHP01	3.32	1.41	.73a	.39	.42	−.56	−.37	.35
GHP02	3.02	1.25	.76a	.51	.43	−.52	−.29	.44
GHP03	3.94	1.18	.75a	.47	.41	−.59	−.31	.39
GHP04	3.10	1.22	.67a	.49	.41	−.43	−.28	.42
GHP05	3.51	1.37	.64a	.32	.29	−.64	−.26	.37
GHP06	2.87	1.36	.64a	.37	.29	−.46	−.25	.28
GHP11	3.53	.99	.48	.71a	.27	−.32	−.14	.31
GHP12	3.48	.99	.45	.73a	.23	−.26	−.05	.26
GHP13	2.88	1.17	.29	.58a	.10	−.19	−.07	.15
GHP14	3.57	1.03	.57	.70a	.32	−.36	−.14	.31
GHP15	3.37	1.00	.37	.56a	.21	−.22	−.08	.24
GHP16	3.41	1.12	.38	.74a	.19	−.25	−.08	.20
GHP17	2.92	1.64	.34	.18	.61a	−.20	−.18	.22
GHP18	3.50	1.65	.35	.21	.50a	−.30	−.20	.25
GHP19	3.34	1.63	.47	.29	.58a	−.33	−.20	.30
HD1	2.09	1.36	−.62	−.32	−.30	.87a	.33	−.33
HD2	2.04	1.30	−.63	−.31	−.29	.81a	.32	−.34
HD3	2.18	1.33	−.65	−.32	−.31	.81a	.32	−.34
HD4	1.72	1.20	−.56	−.27	−.28	.84a	.32	−.32
HD5	1.78	1.18	−.52	−.26	−.26	.76a	.35	−.29
HD6	2.05	1.29	−.56	−.30	−.32	.77a	.39	−.31
GHP21	3.91	1.28	−.40	−.15	−.22	.36	.52a	−.17
GHP22	3.76	1.23	−.16	−.05	−.14	.13	.36a	−.08
GHP23	3.55	1.25	−.25	−.05	−.15	.31	.62a	−.14
GHP24	3.34	1.25	−.29	−.11	−.19	.36	.62a	−.18
GHP07	4.02	1.12	.49	.31	.31	−.43	−.18	.60a
GHP08	3.49	1.14	.50	.30	.32	−.37	−.20	.64a
GHP09	3.92	1.02	.28	.22	.21	−.25	−.14	.63a
GHP10	3.38	1.22	.22	.15	.16	−.13	−.08	.55a
EFT01	3.10	1.41	.58	.33	.25	−.45	−.15	.32
EFT02	3.44	1.34	.53	.30	.23	−.42	−.14	.31
EFT03	4.16	1.23	.58	.30	.24	−.58	−.17	.34
EFT04	3.98	1.20	.55	.30	.22	−.56	−.19	.32
EFT05	4.13	1.41	.55	.28	.24	−.51	−.17	.27

Note: Standard error of correlation = 0.02. CURR = Current health; OUT = Health outlook; PRIOR = Prior health; DIST = Health distress; CONCRN = Health concern; RESIST = Resistance to illness; ENERGY = Energy/fatigue; SLPSOM = Sleep somnolence; ANX = Anxiety; POS = Positive affect; HVALUE = Health value; PHYS = Physical functioning; ROLPHY = Role limitations due to physical health; ROLEMO = Role limitations due to emotional problems.
aDenotes hypothesized item groupings and item-scale correlations corrected for overlap.

ENERGY	SLPSOM	ANX	POS	HVALUE	PHYS	ROLPHY	ROLEMO
.53	−.33	.26	.30	.02	.58	.51	.27
.50	−.33	.32	.32	.06	.47	.48	.31
.53	−.35	.30	.35	.08	.49	.46	.29
.55	−.35	.32	.37	.04	.53	.51	.33
.45	−.25	.24	.32	.09	.41	.38	.24
.63	−.38	.51	.55	.08	.40	.53	.47
.53	−.31	.31	.43	.07	.40	.44	.31
.31	−.22	.24	.27	.12	.28	.27	.19
.30	−.20	.19	.26	.17	.28	.24	.15
.20	−.14	.13	.15	.11	.18	.17	.12
.39	−.23	.24	.34	.19	.35	.32	.22
.26	−.12	.14	.23	.09	.22	.20	.15
.25	−.18	.16	.21	.17	.24	.23	.14
.17	−.13	.05	.05	.02	.25	.19	.05
.24	−.18	.19	.16	.02	.25	.27	.17
.28	−.19	.19	.20	.10	.28	.26	.15
−.57	.39	−.51	−.51	−.03	−.40	−.50	−.47
−.57	.38	−.47	−.47	.01	−.46	−.54	−.45
−.62	.40	−.50	−.51	−.03	−.48	−.56	−.47
−.50	.36	−.51	−.49	.03	−.35	−.44	−.46
−.43	.33	−.41	−.37	.07	−.33	−.41	−.39
−.46	.32	−.44	−.42	.04	−.33	−.40	−.40
−.20	.15	−.13	−.11	.15	−.23	−.23	−.16
−.09	.04	−.06	−.05	.15	−.07	−.06	−.07
−.12	.14	−.12	−.08	.38	−.17	−.16	−.15
−.18	.16	−.17	−.14	.28	−.16	−.18	−.18
.38	−.23	.36	.35	.07	.22	.31	.30
.38	−.25	.30	.30	.02	.26	.29	.22
.26	−.18	.30	.29	.04	.09	.19	.22
.17	−.11	.15	.14	.03	.10	.11	.11
.78[a]	−.37	.37	.51	.08	.45	.52	.40
.76[a]	−.37	.35	.47	.07	.43	.50	.37
.70[a]	−.48	.54	.53	.11	.42	.53	.46
.68[a]	−.46	.47	.50	.08	.41	.49	.44
.68[a]	−.39	.37	.43	.04	.52	.57	.39

all but one item correlated at least 0.30 with the first unrotated component, indicating that they could appropriately be combined into an index score. The percentage of variance explained by the first unrotated factor of each set of items and scales is summarized in Table 8–5. As the concepts included in the index become more homogeneous, the percentage of variance explained increases.

The correlations of each of the scales with the set of validity variables (Table 8–6) were examined to see if any scales correlated in the opposite direction with any validity variable and thus should be excluded from an index. There were fairly distinct patterns of correlations of each scale with the validity variables, indicating that each scale contains somewhat unique information. For example, the mental health index correlates −0.59 with health distress and 0.48 with current health but only 0.28 with health outlook and only 0.19 with prior health. The pain index correlates highest with current health (−0.58), next highest with health distress (0.54), and −0.30 with prior health. Current health and health distress tended to correlate highest with all other health variables (correlations ranged from 0.42 to 0.68 absolute magnitude). These results suggest that some information will be lost by aggregating across scales, depending on the particular aggregation scheme.

In the multitrait scaling analysis (not presented), one item (GHP10— usually the last one to catch a cold) did not correlate 0.30 with the overall MOSGHP23 index. Item-total correlations for the remaining items ranged from 0.38 to 0.73. For MOS GHP19, item-scale correlations ranged from 0.40 to 0.74. For MOS GHP13, item-scale correlations ranged from 0.59 to 0.79. All items met our discriminant validity criterion. For GHR119, item-scale correlations ranged from 0.38 to 0.74. The correlation of GHP5 ("feeling bad lately") with depression/ behavioral-emotional control, positive affect, energy/fatigue, and social functioning were all within two standard errors of its correlation with the index. The correlation of GHP6 ("feel as good as ever") with energy/ fatigue was within two standard errors of its correlation with the index. All of the indexes had an abundance of scaling successes, although the most problems were observed in the GHR119.

Regarding the correlations of indexes with validity variables, all indexes correlated roughly the same with number of doctor visits, number of nights in the hospital, and the number of chronic conditions (Table 8–7). MOSGHP13 tended to correlate the highest and GHR119 the lowest with the remaining ten health measures, suggesting that the

Table 8–5 Common Variance of Items and Subscales and Number of Items from each Subscale in Potential Indexes

	INDEX			
Subscale	MOSGHP23	MOSGHP19	MOSGHP13	GHRI19
Current health	7	7	7	6
Prior health				3
Health outlook	6	6		6
Health distress	6	6	6	1
Resistance to illness	4			3
Common variance				
items	42	46	57	39
subscales	60	68	77	—

Table 8–6 Correlations between Health Perceptions and Health Distress Scales in Potential Indexes and Validity Variables[a]

Validity Variables	Current Health (+)	Health Outlook (+)	Prior Health (+)	Health Distress (−)	Resistance (+)
Physical/psychophysiologic					
symptoms (−)	−.57	−.27	−.30	.52	−.40
Energy/fatigue (+)	.68	.37	.29	−.60	.38
Physical functioning (+)	.59	.32	.31	−.45	.22
Mental health index (+)	.48	.28	.19	−.59	.36
Social activity limitations					
due to health (−)	−.61	−.30	−.26	.63	.35
Role limitations due to					
physical health (−)	−.60	−.30	−.30	.54	−.29
Role limitations due to					
emotional problems (−)	−.42	−.21	−.16	.50	−.27
Pain index (−)	−.58	.27	−.30	.54	−.33

Note: All coefficients are significant ($p < .001$); N ranged from 2,866 to 3,021.

[a] A (+) high score is better health; a (−) high score is poorer health.

most homogeneous index (MOSGHP13) might contain the most information on health status.

The only finding that emerges from these results is that all potential indexes show good validity. The GHRI19 tends to do the worst, but it still does quite well. The shortest index, which is also the most homogeneous (MOSGHP13), is better in relation to these criteria. Until more information on the predictive power of these indexes in terms of subsequent utilization and their ability to discriminate changes in clinical status over time is obtained, we cannot make a final decision regarding which is best. The three MOS indexes were retained for further study.

Scoring Rules All subscale items were recoded so that a high score indicated more of the subscale name (e.g., a high score on health concern indicated more concern). We scored all scales by computing the average for items that were answered. If a respondent was missing half or more of the items in a scale, he or she was assigned a missing value on

Table 8–7 Correlations between Potential Health Perceptions Indexes and Validity Variables

Validity Variable	MOSGHP23	MOSGHP19	MOSGHP13	GHRI19
Number of chronic conditions	−.15	−.17	−.15	−.18
Number of doctor visits (past 2 wks)	−.20	−.20	−.21	−.19
Number of nights in hospital (past yr)	−.22	−.21	−.23	−.22
Pain index	−.57	−.57	−.61	−.52
Physical/psychophysiologic symptoms	−.58	−.56	−.59	−.53
Energy/fatigue	.68	.68	.70	.62
Physical functioning	.54	.56	.57	.52
Mental health index	.56	.55	.58	.48
Social activity limitations due to health	−.63	−.63	−.67	−.55
Role limitations due to physical health	−.58	−.59	−.62	−.53
Role limitations due to emotional problems	−.46	−.46	−.49	−.39

Note: All coefficients are significant ($p < .001$); N ranged from 761 to 3,019.

the scale. All scores were then transformed to a 0–100 scale. Because item variances and item-scale correlations were generally comparable within each scale, we did not standardize or weight items before scoring, thus simplifying the scoring algorithms.

The scoring rules for the general health scales are shown in Table 8–8. An "R" indicates items needing to be reversed before they are combined into either the scale or the index, and an "NR" indicates items it is not necessary to reverse.

Characteristics of the Measures

Descriptive Statistics Descriptive statistics for the scales are shown in Table 8–9. The full range of scores was observed for all measures. The percentage who received a perfect score was very low for all scales except health distress and prior health.

Variability All possible scale levels were observed for all scales. Scores were fairly well distributed for most of the scales, although they were not perfectly normal in all cases. Prior health had a bimodal distribution, with 10% receiving the worst score and 16% receiving the best possible score. Health distress was skewed, with 27% receiving a score of 0 (no distress) and half the sample receiving a score of 12 or less. Health concern was slightly skewed, with more people tending to report greater concern (8% received a score of 100).

Reliability Internal-consistency reliability coefficients are shown in Table 8–9. All three indexes had a reliability of 0.90 or greater. Internal-consistency coefficients of the subscales ranged from 0.74 to 0.94, which are more than adequate for purposes of group comparisons (for which the minimum standard is 0.50). The reliability of the 7-item current health scale is identical to that for the original 9-item scale in the HIE. Although prior health was identical to that fielded in the HIE, the reliability increased from 0.65 in the HIE to 0.74 in this sample. This could be because of the increased variation in prior health items in this patient sample. For all other scales, reliabilities increased substantially over those in the HIE.

Validity To begin to understand the validity of the subscales, we evaluated correlations among the scales as well as a principal components analysis of the seven scales. Table 8–10 presents the correlations among the seven scales. The highest correlations are between current

Table 8–8 Content and Scoring of Health Perceptions, Energy/Fatigue, and Health Distress Scales and Indexes

Item Content	Item Variable Name	EF	CH	RI
Number of Items		5	7	4
Energy/fatigue				
How often during the past 4 weeks did you feel full of pep?	EFT01	R		
How often during the past 4 weeks did you have a lot of energy?	EFT02	R		
How often during the past 4 weeks did you feel worn out?	EFT03	NR		
How often during the past 4 weeks did you feel tired?	EFT04	NR		
How often during the past 4 weeks did you have enough energy to do the things you wanted to do?	EFT05	R		
Current health				
I am somewhat ill.	GHP01[b]		NR	
My health is excellent.	GHP02[b]		R	
I am in poor health.	GHP03		NR	
I am as healthy as anybody I know.	GHP04[b]		R	
I feel about as good now as I ever have.	GHP06		R	
In general, would you say your health is: (excellent, very good, good, fair, poor)	GHP31[b]		R	
I have been feeling bad lately.	GHP05[b]		NR	
Resistance to illness				
I seem to get sick a little easier than other people.	GHP07			NR
My body seems to resist illness very well.	GHP08			R
When there is an illness going around, I usually catch it.	GHP09			NR
I am usually the last one to catch a cold.	GHP10			R

SCALES[a]				INDEXES[a]		
HO	PH	HC	HD	GHP23	GHP19	GHP13
6	3	4	6	23	19	13
				NR	NR	NR
				R	R	R
				NR	NR	NR
				R	R	R
				R	R	R
				R	R	R
				NR	NR	NR
				NR		
				R		
				NR		
				R		

Table 8–8 (*Cont.*)

Item Content	Item Variable Name	EF	CH	RI
Health outlook				
My future will be unhealthy.	GHP 11			
Good health is in my future.	GHP 12			
I think my health will be worse in the future than it is now.	GHP 13			
I expect to have a very healthy life.	GHP 14			
In the future, I expect to have better health than other people I know.	GHP 15			
I expect my health to get worse.	GHP 16			
Prior health				
I have never been seriously ill.	GHP 17			
I was so sick once I thought I might die.	GHP 18			
I have never had an illness that lasted a long period of time.	GHP 19			
I have been sickly for a long time.	GHP 20			
Health concern				
I am concerned about my health.	GHP 21			
I only think about my health when I go to the doctor for an examination.	GHP 22			
My health is a big concern in my life.	GHP 23			
I often think about my health.	GHP 24			
Health distress				
Were you frustrated about your health?	HD 1			
Did you feel weighed down by your health problems?	HD 2			
Were you discouraged by your health problems?	HD 3			
Did you feel despair over your health problems?	HD 4			

SCALES[a]				INDEXES[a]		
HO	PH	HC	HD	GHP23	GHP19	GHP13
NR				NR	NR	
R				R	R	
NR				NR	NR	
R				R	R	
R				R	R	
NR				NR	NR	
	R					
	NR					
	R					
	—					
		R				
		NR				
		R				
		R				
			R	R	R	R
			R	R	R	R
			R	R	R	R
			R	R	R	R

Table 8–8 (*Cont.*)

Item Content	Item Variable Name	EF	CH	RI
Were you afraid because of your health?	HD5			
Was your health a worry in your life?	HD6			

health and energy/fatigue ($r = 0.68$), current health and health distress ($r = -0.68$), and energy/fatigue and health distress ($r = -0.60$). These correlations are well below the reliabilities for these scales, indicating that the scales contain unique reliable variance. Consistent with prior studies (Davies and Ware, 1981), the current health scale best represents all of the general health constructs, as its correlations with the other scales are generally the highest (ranging from 0.37 for health concern to 0.68 for energy/fatigue and health distress, absolute magnitude). The health concern scale is the least related to the other measures, with correlations ranging from 0.13 to 0.39, absolute magnitude. The correlation between health distress and the mental health index was -0.59.

Another approach to understanding the relationships among the scales was to perform a factor analysis of their intercorrelations. Results are shown in Table 8–11. All subscales form only one factor, which explains 48% of the common variance. Correlations between the scales and the factor range from 0.49 to 0.90 (absolute magnitude). The lowest correlation is the health concern scale and the highest is current health. These findings again confirm that current health is the core concept underlying all of the general health measures. Its communality is nearly equal to its reliability, indicating that nearly all of its reliable variance is explained by this common factor. The other concepts depart radically from this finding, suggesting that current health is getting at general health more directly and that other concepts have different validities.

	SCALES[a]			INDEXES[a]		
HO	PH	HC	HD	GHP23	GHP19	GHP13
			R	R	R	R
			R	R	R	R

[a] R = Reversed before averaging; NR = Not reversed before averaging.
[b] Part of Short-Form Current Health Scale (see chapter 16 and introduction to part IV).

Table 8–9 Descriptive Statistics and Reliability Coefficients for Health Perceptions, Energy/Fatigue, and Health Distress Scales and Indexes: PAQ Baseline Sample ($N = 3,053$)

Scale[a]	k	Mean	SD	% Perfect Score	Obs. Range	% Missing	Reliability
Current health (+)	7	56.9	24.6	1.3	0–100	2.3	.88
Health outlook (+)	6	59.6	20.7	3.4	0–100	1.0	.87
Prior health (+)	3	56.2	33.3	15.6	0–100	2.3	.74
Health distress (−)	6	20.0	22.6	27.2	0–100	2.6	.94
Health concern (−)	4	66.2	23.6	0.6	0–100	1.0	.73
Resistance to illness (+)	4	68.0	22.2	6.9	0–100	2.4	.79
Energy/fatigue (+)	5	55.4	22.0	0.8	0–100	2.4	.88
Health perceptions index I (+)	23	64.0	19.2	0.1	0–100	1.0	.93
Health perceptions index II (+)	19	64.7	19.2	0.3	0–100	1.0	.93
Health perceptions index III (+)	13	67.1	22.0	1.0	0–100	1.0	.94

[a] A (+) high score means better health; a (−) high score means poorer health.

Table 8–10 Correlations among Health Perceptions, Health Distress, and Energy/Fatigue Scales

Measure[a]		CH	HO	PH	HD	HC	RI	EF
Current health (+)	CH	(.88)						
Health outlook (+)	HO	.54	(.87)					
Prior health (+)	PH	.47	.28	(.74)				
Health distress (−)	HD	− .68	− .35	− .34	(.94)			
Health concern (−)	HC	− .37	− .13	− .24	.39	(.73)		
Resistance to illness (+)	RI	.47	.31	.32	− .37	− .20	(.79)	
Energy/fatigue (+)	EF	.68	.37	.29	− .60	− .21	.38	(.88)

Note: Internal consistency reliability on the diagonal. All coefficients are significant ($p < .001$). N ranged from 2,910 to 3,023.
[a] A (+) high score indicates better health; a (−) high score indicates poorer health.

Table 8–11 Correlations between Health Perceptions, Health Distress, and Energy/Fatigue Scales and First Principal Factor

Scale	Correlation	h^2	Reliability
Current health (+)	.90	.81	.88
Health distress (−)	− .80	.64	.94
Energy/fatigue (+)	.77	.59	.88
Resistance to illness (+)	.62	.39	.79
Health outlook (+)	.62	.38	.87
Prior health (+)	.59	.35	.74
Health concern (−)	− .49	.24	.73

Note: h^2 = communality.
[a] A (+) high score indicates better health; a (−) high score indicates poorer health.

Resolution of Issues and Future Directions

The MOS developed six measures of health perceptions and one measure of energy/fatigue that correspond very closely to the hypothesized concepts. Four of the health perceptions measures are either very similar or identical to the original measures from the HIE (current health, prior health, health outlook, resistance to illness). The health concern and health distress measures are new. The energy/fatigue measure is derived from the HIE vitality measure.

The MOS successfully disaggregated the original HIE measure of health worry/concern into two measures: health concern and health distress. Health concern focuses on the extent to which people think about or are concerned about their health. The reliability of the health concern scale is fairly low and could still be improved. The health concern measure is the least related to all other measures of health status; thus, it may be the least useful as a measure of general health. Its pattern of correlations suggests that people with greater health concern tend to be less healthy, although the correlations are low. Health concern could be easily eliminated from the health perceptions battery because it is so difficult to define and measure and because of the ambiguity of its meaning.

The MOS developed a new measure of health distress, one which focuses on the psychological distress attributed to health problems. This measure taps feelings of frustration, despair, and other negative emotions resulting directly from health problems and is an offshoot of the health worry component of the HIE health worry/concern measure. Despite its skewed distribution, it is substantially related to all of the other health measures. It correlates almost as highly with other measures as current health. Its correlation with the mental health index is substantial, as expected, given that both measures assess psychological distress and use the same response scale. However, its correlation with many other health measures is as high as or higher than that with the mental health index, indicating that it is distinct from general psychological distress/well-being. Future studies will determine the validity of health distress.

Four potential aggregate health perceptions indexes were developed: three are based on combinations of different MOS subscales, and the fourth was intended to replicate as closely as possible the original HIE GHRI. One difference between the three MOS indexes and the original HIE GHRI is that the MOS indexes do not include prior health. Because of its very high stability, the prior health scale is not useful as an outcome measure in evaluating health care. It is, however, a very good baseline measure of case mix differences. Two of the MOS indexes do not include resistance to illness, and one does not include health outlook, because these components reflect beliefs and attitudes as well as health.

The results regarding which is the best index are inconclusive, because all did very well in the preliminary validity studies. The HIE GHRI did the poorest, while still doing well, and thus might be the least useful of the four. All three MOS indexes performed fairly well in all of the studies, although the most homogeneous of the three (GHP13) performed consistently better than the other two. It is necessary now to test the indexes in terms of their relative validity in other MOS studies.

The MOS refined and improved some of the psychometric characteristics of the HIE scales. Specifically, the reliability of the health outlook scale was increased from 0.73 to 0.87 by adding three new items and eliminating one old item. The reliability of the resistance to illness scale was increased from 0.70 to 0.79 by replacing one item. Finally, the number of items in the current health scale was reduced from nine to seven, but it retained its reliability of 0.88. Because of the high percentage of people responding "don't know" to the health outlook items (30–48%), further evaluation of the amount of useful information contained in this measure is warranted.

The MOS successfully constructed an energy/fatigue scale that is balanced in terms of positively and negatively worded items and is distinct from similar concepts such as sleep problems and psychological distress and well-being. This is the first time that a measure of energy/ fatigue has been included in a comprehensive set of health measures and constructed to be clearly distinct from concepts to which it is related. This inclusion is valuable because of the importance of fatigue in primary care.

9. Social Functioning: Social Activity Limitations Measure

Cathy D. Sherbourne

Definition and Issues

Social functioning is a broad and a general concept that can include all human behavior in social roles and contexts (Kane, Kane, and Arnold, 1985; Weissman, Sholomskas, and John, 1981). More specifically, social functioning can be viewed in terms of a person's adjustment or adaptation to the normative expectations regarding behavior or social roles within the community. To the extent that peoples' performance conforms to social expectations and responsibilities, they are seen as functioning well.

Social functioning is defined as the ability to develop, maintain, and nurture major social relationships. Although prior conceptualizations of social functioning have considered it one of three underlying health dimensions, we have taken a different approach. We do not consider social functioning per se as health (Donald and Ware, 1982; Ware, Johnston, Davies-Avery, et al., 1979). Instead, we view social functioning measures as being indicative of physical and mental health status; problems in social functioning can be caused by physical or mental health problems. Thus, measures of such problems serve to indicate the need for care and might be appropriate outcomes of health care (McDowell and Newell, 1987).

We differentiate functioning in interpersonal relationships from functioning in role and other daily activities, although both are commonly thought to be measures of social functioning. Role functioning refers to the performance of activities typical for a specified age and social role, such as work, housework, or schoolwork (chapter 12). Role functioning is defined separately because of the societal importance and economic implications of limitations in a person's usual role activities.

Social support is also differentiated from the more general category of social functioning (Donald and Ware, 1982; Sherbourne and Stewart, 1991). Social support refers to the context in which social interactions occur. It is defined in terms of the variety of resources provided by other persons (e.g., tangible or emotional support). A person may have good social functioning, yet have a small social support system (e.g., a person who has few friends available but who interacts well with those few). Similarly, a person might have some limitations in social functioning yet have a strong support system (e.g., a chronically ill person who cannot get out socially, yet who has a large number of supportive friends and relatives).

Lerner (1973) recommended that social functioning measures focus on such constructs as role-related coping, family functioning, and social participation. He hypothesized that persons functioning well socially would be better able to adjust to day-to-day challenges arising from their major social roles; would live in more stable and cohesive families; would be more likely to participate in community activities; and would be more apt to conform to the norms or moral codes of society. Because an individual's behavior occurs within multiple spheres of life, social functioning has often been defined in terms of the individual's behavior within a number of areas: marital (as a spouse or partner and as a parent), within an extended family (with parents, siblings, and close relatives), with friends and acquaintances, and in the community (e.g., participation in organizations) (Donald, Ware, Brook, et al., 1978; Kane, Kane, and Arnold, 1985). Functioning within each of these areas is often assessed separately, because adaptation can take place unevenly across them. For example, a chronically ill individual may be functioning well with close family members but may be unable to adapt with respect to acquaintances.

The MOS concentrated on three components of social functioning: health-related effects on social activities (such as visiting with family, friends, neighbors, and groups), family functioning (both marital and within the family in general) (chapter 10), and sexual functioning (chapter 11).

The common use of social activities as a component of social functioning assumes a consensus regarding the importance of social participation and interpersonal interactions to one's health and quality of life. However, there is some evidence that defining social functioning in these ways has not been useful as an indicator of health status (Sherbourne, 1988). For example, one study has shown that measures of social resources predict mental health better than do measures of social contacts (Donald and Ware, 1982) and that there is no relationship between frequency of social contacts and subsequent use of mental health services (Sherbourne, 1986) or between social contacts and measures of physical and mental health (Ware, Johnston, Davies-Avery, et al., 1979). Social activity can be a function of nonhealth factors external to the individual such as the environment, the community, and significant others. Levels of activity can also differ due to personal factors unrelated to health such as differences in personality, preferences, and opportunity for social interaction. We hypothesized that a more useful definition of social functioning for the purpose of measuring the health impact of disease and treatment would be one focusing on whether people's health problems limited their usual social activities. Such a definition would not only emphasize limitations in contacts due primarily to health-related reasons but would also leave it up to the individual to determine what his or her usual social activities were.

Two types of health effects on social activities are defined: the extent to which health problems limit an individual's ability to interact with or participate in activities with others, and the changes in usual levels of social activity (increases or decreases) due to changes in health. This definition represents a departure from most prior definitions of social activities, which focused on numbers of contacts (e.g., visits) and activities with family and friends (e.g., number of telephone calls, trips with friends) and frequency of participation in group activities (Donald, Ware, Brook, et al., 1978).

Measures of social contacts and activities have generally been identified under the domain of "social support" (i.e., specifically as measures of social integration or isolation). For MOS purposes, we conceptualized measures of social activity separately from the dimension of social support (Sherbourne and Stewart, 1991), although the two are logically interrelated (House and Kahn, 1985). For example, the frequency of contacts with others may partially determine the functional content (i.e., type of support) of those interactions.

In measuring social functioning in terms of health-related effects on social activities, the major issue was how to define and operationalize the concept. Because people differ in terms of their preferred level of social activities, we wanted to define health-related limitations in a general way so that people could respond according to their personal level of those activities. A variety of others developed measures of social activities (see review by Donald, Ware, Brook, et al., 1978), but most focused on the numbers of contacts and activities or the frequency of participation in different activities. These assessments are relatively objective and reliable measures of the existence and quantity of social relationships. However, they usually do not ask respondents to indicate whether their social activities have been affected by their own health problems. This approach to the measurement of social activities is appropriate for those interested in developing measures for general populations with few health problems or those interested in developing measures that are not confounded with other variables such as stress and health.

Social activities encompass interactions with or participation in activities with other people, including friends, relatives, neighbors, and groups, and health can affect these types of activities in a number of ways. Health problems can interfere with the person's usual activities. If the interference persists for a long time, then the person might come to define a new level of usual activity. Also, if a person has adjusted to a lower level of activity, then improvements in health can cause an increase in usual activity. Since the first case is probably more common, it was the focus for the development of our social activity items. However, we also decided to try to detect increases in the level of social activities that might occur because a person's health improved, wanting to define changes in activities due to both physical health and emotional problems. Finally, we thought it useful to define people's level of limitations due to health in comparison to others their own age.

A final issue we considered was how to deal with the fact that people had different usual levels of social activity, and given the respondent burden constraint, we needed to assess this using a relatively small number of items. The Sickness Impact Profile (SIP) addresses this issue by interviewing respondents about restrictions in specific activities due to health problems (Gilson, Gilson, Bergner, et al., 1975). The SIP asks respondents detailed questions about specific types of social activities that are limited due to health (e.g., going out to visit less often, cutting down the length of visits with friends, staying alone most of the time). Similarly, Jette, Davies, Cleary, et al. (1986) evaluated the amount of time patients had difficulty with various social activities but did not ask whether these difficulties were due to health problems. Ideally, it would be best to develop a series of questions that ask in detail about different types of social activities that are limited, as does the SIP. This would allow one to pursue hypotheses about how different types of social activities are more or less limited by health problems than others. Respondent burden kept us from this approach in favor of developing a few general questions that would cover a variety of unspecified social activities.

Content and Measurement Strategy

Pilot Study An MOS pilot study indicated that role functioning can be affected by purely emotional problems as well as or instead of physical health problems. We felt limitations in social functioning (i.e., contacts) might also be affected by either type of health problem specified. We therefore wrote the MOS items to detect limitations due to either physical health or emotional problems.

Final Items We developed our own set of questions that appeared, on the basis of face validity, to reflect the concept we were trying to assess. All four items ask about limitations in social activities as a result of either physical health or emotional problems. The actual items are shown on pages 375, 394, and 395 in the Appendix. The first two items assess limitations in social activities in terms of the extent of the limitation (with five response categories ranging from "not at all" to "extremely") and the amount of time the person feels limited (with five response categories ranging from "all of the time" to "none of the time"). The third item assesses limitations in social functioning in comparison to usual level (with five response categories ranging from "much less socially active than before" to "much more socially active than before"). This item was designed to tap potential increases in activity due to health care, especially mental health care. The fourth item assesses limitations in comparison to others of the same age (with five response categories ranging from "much more limited than others" to "much less limited than others").

Construction and Evaluation of Measure

Analysis Plan We first examined item frequency distributions to assure adequate variability for purposes of scale construction and to begin to estimate the prevalence of social activity limitations in our sample. We used multitrait scaling techniques, which are described in chapter 5 on methods, to make sure that items included in the hypothesized social activity scale were internally consistent and met our criteria for item convergence and item discrimination. Other scales included to test item discrimination are satisfaction with family life, marital functioning, overall happiness with family life, tangible support, affectionate support, emotional/informational support, positive social interaction, number of close friends and relatives, psychological distress/well-being, feelings of belonging, and current health perceptions. The social support scales are described in Sherbourne and Stewart (1991).

Item Variability The percentage distribution of responses to the four items are shown in Table 9–1. The means and standard deviation for the four items are shown in the multitrait analysis table (Table 9–2). The first two social activity items are skewed, with 52% and 59% of the patients reporting that physical or emotional problems interfered with their social activities "not at all" or "none of the time," respectively. However, the fact that at least 40% of the sample felt that their health was interfering at all with their social activities suggests that this concept is an important one to assess.

Sixty-six percent of the patients reported that they were about as socially active as before, 23% were less active, and only 11% were more active than before. Forty-six percent of the patients reported that their social activity was about the same as others their age, 25% said their activity was more limited, and 29% said their activity was less limited than others. Standard deviations for these four items ranged from 0.77 (activity compared to usual) to 1.10 (activity compared to others your age). The percentage missing on the four items ranged from 2 to 4.

Scale Construction Results of the multitrait scaling analysis are shown in Table 9–1. In this matrix, row entries represent correlations between each item and the sum of the items in each scale grouping. Footnote "a" indicates the hypothesized scale placement of each item and also indicates item-scale correlations that were corrected for overlap (i.e., each item is correlated with the sum of the other items in the scale).

The four social activity items met the stringent convergent validity criterion of 0.40—that is, they correlated at least 0.40 with their own scale, corrected for overlap. As shown in Table 9–2, all items also met the criterion of item discrimination (i.e., they correlated higher by two standard errors with their own scale than with other measures in the matrix).

Table 9–1 Percentage Distribution of Social Activity Limitations Items: P A Q
Baseline Sample ($N = 3,053$)

Abbreviated Item Content	Item Variable Name	Response Choice[a]	Item Response[b]					%of Total Missing
			1	2	3	4	5	
Extent interfered with social activities	SACT4	NE	52	27	12	7	2	4
Time interfered with social activities	SACT3	AT	2	6	13	20	59	2
Social activity compared to usual level	SACT2	ML	8	15	66	8	3	3
Social activity compared to others your age	SACT1	MM	8	17	46	14	15	3

[a]NE: 1–not at all; 2–slightly; 3–moderately; 4–quite a bit; 5–extremely. AT: 1–all of the time; 2–most of the time; 3–some of the time; 4–a little of the time; 5–none of the time. ML: 1–much less socially active than before; 2–somewhat less socially active than before; 3–about as socially active as before; 4–somewhat more socially active than before; 5–much more socially active than before. MM: 1–much more limited than others; 2–somewhat more limited than others; 3–about the same as others; 4–somewhat less limited than others; 5–much less limited than others.
[b]Percentage of those who responded to each item.

Scoring Rules In order to score a 4-item social activity scale, it was first necessary to rescore three of the raw items so that a high score indicated more limitations. Precoded responses for the item about extent of interference with social activities were not recorded. The other three items were reversed as follows: 1 = 5, 2 = 4, 4 = 2, 5 = 1. Scores were then averaged across items that were answered. We did not standardize or weight items before they were scored. Respondents missing more than two items received a missing scale score. The multi-item measure was subsequently transformed to a 0–100 scale.

Characteristics of Measure

Descriptive Statistics Table 9–3 presents descriptive statistics for the M O S Social Activity Limitations due to Health measure. The percentage missing the multi-item measure was 2%.

Variability For the multi-item measure, all possible scores were observed. The measure was skewed with more people having few limitations in social activity.

Table 9–2 Item-Scale Correlation Matrix, Social Activity Limitations Due to Health: PAQ Baseline Sample ($N = 2,181$)

Item	Mean	SD	SOCACT	FAMSAT	MARFUN	FAMHAP
SACT1	3.13	1.10	.50[a]	.26	.18	.26
SACT2	2.86	0.77	.46[a]	.18	.16	.20
SACT3	4.33	0.98	.70[a]	.34	.29	.38
SACT4	4.23	0.98	.67[a]	.28	.24	.33

Note: Standard error of correlation = 0.02. SOCACT = Social activity limitations due to health; FAMSAT = Satisfaction with family life; MARFUN = Marital functioning; FAMHAP = Overall happiness with family life; TANSUP = Tangible support; AFFSUP = Affectionate support; EMOSUP = Emotional/informational support; POSINT = Positive social interaction;

Reliability The internal-consistency reliability coefficient for the 4-item social activity limitations scale is 0.77. The homogeneity coefficient is 0.46.

Resolution of Issues and Future Directions

The social activity limitations measure can be used to assess health-related limitations in normal or usual social activities. The items are general in nature (e.g., they leave it up to the respondent to define his or her own social activities, although several examples of types of activities are given) and specifically ask about social activity that is affected by either physical health or emotional problems. Our items emphasize functioning in general rather than the impact of a specific condition on the patient or family because we feel that patients would have trouble isolating the effects of their illness on social activities. This strategy also allows for administration of the same battery of items to the entire sample.

We have several recommendations for future research studies using this measure. Given more space for additional items, we would suggest the evaluation of more specific types of social activity limitations. In other words, in addition to our approach of asking about social activities in general, we would include items that specify in more detail how specific activities might be limited as in the SIP (e.g., decreases in number of social activities, decreases in length of participation time spent in activities, changes to less physically taxing social activities,

TANSUP	AFFSUP	EMOSUP	POSINT	CLOSER	MHI5	BEL	CURR
.18	.18	.19	.22	.07	.40	− .30	.44
.09	.14	.15	.17	.03	.30	− .21	.34
.28	.30	.29	.35	.11	.60	− .43	.51
.22	.24	.22	.29	.09	.54	− .36	.51

CLOSER = Number of close friends and relatives; MHI5 = Mental health index; BEL = Feelings of belonging; CURR = Current health perceptions.
ª Denotes hypothesized item grouping and item-scale corrections corrected for overlap.

Table 9–3 Descriptive Statistics and Reliability Coefficient for Social Activity Limitations Due to Health Measure: PAQ Baseline Sample (N = 3,053)

Measureª	k	Mean	SD	Observed Range	% Missing	Reliability
Social activity limitations due to health (+)	4	− 34.8	19.2	0–100	2	0.77

ª A (+) high score indicates better health.

etc.). This would allow one to test more specific hypotheses about how illness impacts on social functioning. Furthermore, it would be useful to develop separate measures of limitations in social activity due to physical health problems and due to emotional problems, as we did for role functioning (chapter 7).

10. Social Functioning: Family and Marital Functioning Measures

Cathy D. Sherbourne and Caren J. Kamberg

Definition and Issues

Social functioning is a broad and a general concept defined in terms of limitations in social activities (chapter 9), sexual functioning (chapter 11), and family functioning, discussed in this chapter.

Family functioning refers to the quality of interactions among family members. Most frequently, it is conceptualized in terms of the degree of cohesion within the family. However, there are a wide variety of other, more specific, characteristics of families that have been measured in previous research, including adaptability, the amount of communication, conflict, acceptance, support, affection, expressiveness, time spent together, independence of family members, achievement orientation, morality/religiosity, locus of control, problem solving, family style, concern, and resentment.

Moos (1974) and Bloom (1985) have grouped these concepts into three broad dimensions: (1) a relationship dimension, which includes the extent to which family members feel that they belong to and are proud of their family, the extent to which there is open expression within the family, the degree to which conflictual interactions are characteristic of the family, family sociability, and disengagement; (2) a personal growth dimension, which includes a set of value orientations (intellectual-cultural, moral-religious, active recreational) as well as emphasis within the family on achievement and independence; and (3) a systems maintenance dimension, which refers to the structure or organization within the family (e.g., family style) and the degree of control exerted by various family members.

There is some consensus that cohesion and adaptability (both part of the relationship dimension) are two of the most fundamental aspects of family functioning (Bloom, 1985). Cohesion is defined as the emotional bonding members have with one another and the degree of individual autonomy a person experiences in the family system (Olson, Russell, and Sprenkle, 1983). Family adaptability is defined as the ability of a family system to change its power structure, role relationships, and relationship rules in response to situational and developmental stresses. In addition, family communication (e.g., empathy, reflective listening, supportive comments) is considered critical for the development of a cohesive and adaptable family system (Olson, Russell, and Sprenkle, 1983).

Two issues were addressed in developing measures of family functioning: the identification of the areas of family functioning most relevant to patients with chronic disease and that could potentially be affected by health care; and the development of family functioning measures that would be applicable to all types of family configurations (e.g., families with and without children).

In order to identify relevant areas of family functioning, the universe of family functioning concepts had to be identified. Six instruments selected from a review of literature appeared collectively to contain many of the most commonly measured components of family functioning: (1) the Family APGAR (Smilkstein, Ashworth, and Montano, 1982; Good, Smilkstein, Good, et al., 1979; McNabb, 1983; Smilkstein, 1978); (2) the Family Environment Scale or FES (Moos and Moos, 1981); (3) the Family Functioning Index or FFI (Pless and Satterwhite, 1973, 1975; Pless, Roghmann, and Haggerty, 1972); (4) the Family Life Questionnaire or FLQ (Guerney, 1977); (5) the Social Adjustment Scale Self-Report or SAS-SR (Weissman and Bothwell, 1976; Weissman, Sholomskas, and John, 1981); and (6) the Community Adaptation Schedule or CAS (Roen, Ottenstein, Copper, et al., 1966).

A variety of concepts related to the family were measured in each instrument: emotional (Family APGAR), communication/sharing (Family APGAR, FFI, FLQ, SAS, CAS), support (Family APGAR, FLQ, FES, SAS), acceptance (Family APGAR), affection (Family APGAR, SAS), time together (Family APGAR), expressiveness (FES), conflict (FES, FFI, FLQ, SAS, CAS), independence (FES), achievement orientation (FES), active/recreational orientation (FES), morality/religiosity (FES), organization (FES), control (FES), cohesion/closeness (FFI, FES, FLQ), problem solving (FFI), concern (FLQ), and resentment (FLQ).

Examination of the items themselves showed that many of these categories, although named differently, actually measured the same thing (e.g., affection and emotional).

To narrow the scope of this complex phenomenon, six aspects of general family functioning were chosen that were most likely to be affected by the chronic disease conditions of MOS patients: together-ness/cohesiveness, conflict, expressiveness, support/understanding, communication, and affection/emotional. These are aspects of family life that could easily be affected by the symptomatology of chronically ill family members. A set of items designed to measure aspects of the marital relationship were also developed.

In the many instruments designed to measure family functioning, the term "family" has been variously defined. In some cases, respondents are specifically told to answer questions in regard to their nuclear or traditional type family. In other cases, no specific definition of the term is given, leaving respondents to use their own interpretation of the word "family." Other methods used are to gear questions toward a specific population (i.e., families with chronically ill children) or to create different forms of the questionnaire for specific groups (e.g., one questionnaire for married persons and another for parents with chil-dren). Another method is to make questions so general that they are applicable to all types of respondents. The approach used depends on the specific goals of the investigators. The disadvantage of using questions focused on specific groups is that those persons not defined by the group do not answer those questions. The resulting reduction in sample size in analyses using these items affects the ability to detect differences or to measure change over time.

Content and Measurement Strategy

Pilot Study A pilot study was conducted before the beginning of the formal MOS to identify a set of family functioning items. For the measures related to family in general, items were constructed asking about the person's satisfaction with each of the six categories of functioning of interest (e.g., satisfaction with the amount of affection the family expresses). The interpretation of the term "family" was left to the respondent, and items were general enough to apply to everyone. All satisfaction items were expressed in a 6-point scale ranging from completely satisfied to completely dissatisfied. One overall measure of happiness with family life was also included. Responses for this item ranged from 1 ("extremely happy") to 6 ("very unhappy").

For the measures related to functioning within the context of the marital situation, relevant items (e.g., we had trouble sharing our personal feelings) were identified from reviewed instruments to assess each of the six categories (new items were written where necessary to fill out a particular category) and a subset of two to eight items was selected from each category, for a total of thirty items. For each item, subjects were asked to agree or disagree about their experiences during the prior thirty days using a 5-point scale (definitely true to definitely false). Only respondents with a spouse or partner were asked to answer these questions.

Item variability for the six general family functioning items was skewed in the direction of "satisfied." The most skewed distributions (i.e., 15% or less expressing any dissatisfaction) were seen for two items pertaining to satisfaction with the amount families expressed themselves and the amount of affection they expressed. The item about happiness with family life was similarly skewed, with 90% reporting that they were at least somewhat happy with their family life. These findings suggested that it would be difficult to construct a measure with good variability.

Thirty-seven of the sixty-eight pilot study respondents (54%) had a spouse or partner and thus completed the marital functioning items. Items pertaining to marital functioning were also skewed. Almost all respondents answered positively (definitely or mostly true) to these items. At least 85% expressed positive family functioning on fifteen of the thirty items. All but one of these was positively worded.

The two main hypothesized family functioning constructs (e.g., general family functioning and marital functioning) were analyzed using multitrait scaling techniques (chapter 5). A matrix of item-scale correlations was computed in order to evaluate the internal consistency of each hypothesized scale and the item convergence and discrimination. Other measures included in the matrix to test item discrimination were number of chronic disease conditions, number of medications taken, current health, mental health, loneliness, social support, physical functioning, and social contacts. The six items in the general family functioning scale had high item-scale correlations, and all discriminated well from the other scales in the matrix. Coefficient alpha for this 6-item scale was 0.95. To reduce the number of items, we eliminated two items (amount we express ourselves and amount of affection we express) that had highly skewed response distributions. The resulting 4-item scale had a reliability of 0.94.

To shorten the 30-item marital functioning scale, those items that showed poor item discrimination and/or low item-scale correlations were eliminated. Additional items were eliminated based on overlapping item content, direction of scoring (balance between negatively and positively worded items), and amount of skewness. The resulting 6-item marital functioning scale had a reliability of 0.86 in this pilot study sample. These items discriminated from the general family functioning scale, supporting their distinction as a separate measure.

Final Items The final MOS family functioning battery contains ten items, assessing the following hypothesized aspects of family functioning: satisfaction with family life (three items), overall happiness with family life (one item), and marital functioning (six items). The actual questionnaire items are given in the Appendix, pages 395 and 396.

The items concerning satisfaction with family life asked respondents to indicate their satisfaction with three specific aspects of their family life: the amount of togetherness and cohesion they had, the support and understanding they gave each other, and the amount they talked things over. Because of the extremely skewed responses in the pilot study, the response format was changed to one that did not refer to satisfaction. Respondents were asked: "In terms of your satisfaction with your family life, please rate the following." The response choices (poor, fair, good, very good, and excellent) have been found to reduce the tendency to report satisfaction (Ware and Hays, 1988). By presenting the "poor" response as the first choice, the tendency to report satisfaction was minimized. One item, taken from the pilot study, asked respondents to indicate how happy they were, overall, with their family life. Response choices were: extremely happy, very happy, somewhat happy, not too happy, somewhat unhappy, and very unhappy.

The six marital functioning items were those selected in the pilot study. The items asked respondents to tell how true or false was each of six statements about their relationship with their spouse or partner during the previous month: (1) "we said anything we wanted to say to each other," (2) "we often had trouble sharing our personal feelings," (3) "it was hard to blow off steam with each other," (4) "I felt close to my spouse/partner," (5) "my spouse/partner was supportive of me," and (6) "we tended to rely on other people for help rather than on each other." Response choices were: definitely true, mostly true, don't know, mostly false, and definitely false.

To increase responses to the marital functioning questions, we asked respondents without a spouse or partner to answer the questions about the person with whom they felt closest, but also asked people if they had a spouse or partner so that they could be identified, if necessary.

Construction and Evaluation of Measures

Analysis Plan The general goals were to confirm the dimensionality of the two family functioning concepts, to determine whether measures of family functioning were distinct from other measures of social functioning and mental health, and to develop a single-item measure for happiness with family life.

Item frequency distributions were examined to assure adequate variability for purposes of scale construction. The dimensionality of the family functioning concepts was evaluated using multitrait scaling techniques. The goal was to construct two multi-item measures of satisfaction with family life and marital functioning that were distinct from each other and from measures of mental health, feelings of belonging, social support, and social activity limitations. A limitation of the analysis is that people who are not close to anyone and therefore do not complete the marital functioning items are excluded from the analysis. Thus, the sample is slightly biased.

The validity of the item on overall happiness with family life was tested by evaluating the correlation between the item and each of the family functioning scales. A valid item should be substantially correlated with the scales. The mean family functioning and marital functioning scores were calculated for each response level of the item to evaluate the interval properties of the item. A valid single-item measure should show mean levels of family and marital functioning for those reporting that they were extremely happy with their family life that were substantially higher than mean levels for those reporting an extremely unhappy family life.

Item Variability Item frequency distributions are shown in Table 10–1. The three family satisfaction items were skewed in the direction of "satisfied." For example, for the item about satisfaction with support and understanding, only 19% rated their satisfaction as poor or fair; over 80% rated it as good to excellent. There was variability in the items, however, among the "satisfied" categories. For example, 25% rated their amount of togetherness as excellent, while 32% rated it as very good, and 22% rated it as good. Twenty-two percent rated their amount of togetherness as poor or fair. The variability of these items was improved slightly over that for the same pilot study items (which had used responses of "completely satisfied" to "completely dissatisfied"). Responses were also skewed for the item concerning happiness with family life.

Items pertaining to marital functioning were also skewed. Almost all respondents (greater than 82%) answered definitely or mostly true to the positively worded items (e.g., "said anything we wanted to each other"), while approximately 62% answered definitely false or mostly false to the negatively worded items (e.g., "had trouble sharing our feelings").

The percentage missing varied across items. At most, only 4%

Table 10–1 Percentage Distribution of Family Functioning Items: PAQ Baseline Sample (N = 3,053)

Abbreviated Item Content	Item Variable Name	Response Choice[a]	Item Response[b]						% of Total Missing
			1	2	3	4	5	6	
Amount of togetherness	FF01	EP	8	14	22	32	25	—	4
Support and understanding	FF02	EP	6	13	22	31	28	—	4
Amount you talk things over	FF03	EP	10	16	23	30	20	—	4
How happy with family life	FF04	EH	20	40	24	7	4	4	2
Said anything they wanted	FF06	DT	33	49	4	9	4	—	9
Trouble sharing feelings	FF07	DT	9	22	6	36	26	—	9
Hard to blow off steam	FF08	DT	9	22	8	35	26	—	10
Close to spouse/ partner	FF09	DT	47	34	5	8	4	—	10
Spouse/partner supportive	FF10	DT	49	34	6	6	5	—	10
Rely on other people	FF11	DT	6	11	6	27	50	—	10

[a]EP: 1–poor; 2–fair; 3–good; 4–very good; 5–excellent. EH: 1–extremely happy; 2–very happy; 3–somewhat happy; 4–not too happy; 5–somewhat unhappy; 6–very unhappy. DT: 1–definitely true; 2–mostly true; 3–don't know; 4–mostly false; 5–definitely false.
[b]Percentage of those who responded to each item.

missed any of the general family functioning items, while 10% missed the marital functioning items. The larger percentage missing the marital functioning items was most likely due to persons without a spouse, partner, or someone they felt close to skipping the battery. However, it is interesting to note that many people without a spouse or partner did answer the items (31% reported being without a spouse or partner). Item means and standard deviations are shown below in Table 10–2.

Scale Construction The two multi-item family functioning scales were analyzed using multitrait scaling techniques. The multitrait correlation matrix is presented in Table 10–2.

All items in the satisfaction with family life scale met the MOS criterion of item discrimination—that is, they correlated higher by two standard errors with their own scale than with the marital functioning scale or the other measures. Item-total correlations were substantial, ranging from 0.83 to 0.89. All items in the marital functioning scale also met the criterion of item discrimination and item-total correlations ranging from 0.43 to 0.71. The item with the lowest item-total correlation was that pertaining to "hard to blow off steam with each other."

The single-item satisfaction with family life measure was evaluated in terms of the strength of its relationship with the multi-item family functioning measures. The item correlated highly with the measure for satisfaction with family life ($r = 0.80$) and substantially with the marital functioning measure ($r = 0.59$). The higher correlation in the first case might be expected due to the fact that this multi-item measure asks about satisfaction with specific aspects of family life, while the marital functioning measure focuses more narrowly on the relationship with a spouse or partner. As anticipated, the mean scores for satisfaction with family life (results not shown here) were substantially lower for those reporting that they were very unhappy with their family life than for those reporting that they were extremely happy with their family life. However, differences between means for each level of the item were not of equal distance, with differences being fairly small at the unhappy end of the distribution. Thus, although the item does appear to reflect differences in functioning as expected, its inability to discriminate well at the dysfunctional end of the distribution leads one to question its value. Family functioning might be too multifaceted a phenomenon to capture well with a single item.

Scoring Rules Table 10–3 presents a summary of the final family functioning measures.

No rescoring of raw items was required for the three items in the

Table 10–2 Item-Scale Correlation Matrix, Family Functioning: PAQ Baseline Sample (*N* = 2,181)

Item	Mean	SD	FAMSAT	MARFUN	FAMHAP	TANSUP	AFFSUP
FF01	3.55	1.20	.87a	.58	0.78	0.43	0.55
FF02	3.61	1.19	.89a	.60	0.77	0.41	0.54
FF03	3.34	1.24	.83a	.61	0.71	0.37	0.52
FF06	3.98	1.04	.45	.61a	0.42	0.27	0.39
FF07	3.47	1.32	.49	.65a	0.41	0.24	0.38
FF08	3.48	1.32	.33	.43a	0.28	0.20	0.26
FF09	4.14	1.09	.58	.71a	0.58	0.39	0.56
FF10	4.09	1.06	.52	.67a	0.53	0.36	0.53
FF11	4.05	1.20	.49	.62a	0.45	0.31	0.43
FF04	4.56	1.22	.80	.59	n.a.	0.43	0.56

Note: Standard error of correlation = 0.02. FAMSAT = Satisfaction with family functioning; MARFUN = Marital functioning; FAMHAP = Overall happiness with family life; TANSUP = Tangible support; AFFSUP = Affectionate support; EMOSUP = Emotional/informational support; POSINT = Positive social interaction; CLOSER = Number of close friends and relations;

measure for satisfaction with family life (i.e., all items were in the direction of a higher score, indicating more satisfaction with family life). Scores for the nonmissing items were averaged to calculate the scale score. Because item variances for the family satisfaction items were generally comparable, it was not necessary to standardize or weight items before they were scored. Respondents missing more than one item received a missing scale score.

Precoded response categories for the single-item measure of overall happiness with family life were also reversed so that a high score would indicate more happiness with family life. Thus categories were reversed as follows: 1 = 6, 2 = 5, 3 = 4, 4 = 3, 5 = 2, 6 = 1.

To score the marital functioning measure, it was first necessary to rescore three of the raw items so that a high score would indicate a better relationship with one's spouse or partner. Precoded response categories for three items (we said anything we wanted to say to each other; I felt close to my spouse or partner; my spouse or partner was supportive of me) were reversed as follows: 1 = 5, 2 = 4, 4 = 2, 5 = 1. After reversal of these three items, all nonmissing items were averaged to calculate the marital functioning scale. Because item variances for the marital functioning items were generally comparable, it was not necessary to standardize or weight items before they were scored. Respondents missing more than three items received a missing scale score.

EMOSUP	POSINT	CLOSER	SOCACT	MHI5	BEL	CURR
0.46	0.51	0.15	0.34	0.49	−0.66	0.24
0.47	0.50	0.18	0.34	0.50	−0.66	0.23
0.48	0.47	0.16	0.30	0.45	−0.61	0.21
0.36	0.36	0.14	0.22	0.34	−0.43	0.15
0.37	0.38	0.16	0.22	0.35	−0.45	0.19
0.26	0.26	0.09	0.15	0.22	−0.29	0.13
0.47	0.50	0.14	0.27	0.43	−0.63	0.18
0.45	0.47	0.10	0.22	0.37	−0.56	0.14
0.34	0.37	0.12	0.21	0.35	−0.48	0.14
0.47	0.53	0.17	0.38	0.57	−0.70	0.26

SOCACT = Social activity limitations due to health; MHI5 = Mental health index; BEL = Feelings of belonging; CURR = Current health perceptions; ªDenotes hypothesized item grouping and item-scale correlations corrected for overlap.
N.a. = not applicable.

Table 10–3 Content and Scoring of Family Functioning Measures

Abbreviated Content	Item Variable Name	FAMSAT	FAMHAP	MARFUN
Number of items		3	1	6
Satisfaction with family life				
Amount of togetherness	FF01	NR		
Support and understanding	FF02	NR		
Amount you talk things over	FF03	NR		
Overall happiness with family life				
How happy with family life	FF04		R	
Marital functioning				
Said anything they wanted	FF06			R
Trouble sharing feelings	FF07			NR
Hard to blow off steam	FF08			NR
Close to spouse/partner	FF09			R
Spouse/partner supportive	FF10			R
Rely on other people	FF11			NR

Note: FAMSAT = Satisfaction with family functioning; FAMHAP = Overall happiness with family life; MARFUN = Marital functioning. R = Reversed before summing; NR = Not reversed before averaging.

The multi-item family functioning measures were subsequently transformed to a 0–100 scale.

Characteristics of Measures

Descriptive Statistics Table 10–4 presents descriptive statistics for the MOS family functioning measures. The percentage missing the general family functioning measure was 3.7 percent, while 9.0 percent had missing data for the marital functioning scale.

Variability For both scales, all possible scores were observed. Both measures were skewed with more people having better family functioning, although only 15% and 10% of patients reported perfect functioning on the satisfaction with family life and marital functioning scales, respectively.

Reliability Internal-consistency reliability coefficients for the two multi-item measures are shown in Table 10–4. As can be seen, reliability estimates are high for both measures (0.93 and 0.83). The homogeneity coefficient for the three satisfaction items is quite high (0.83), while that for the six marital functioning items is low (0.45). This suggests that the marital functioning items are less homogeneous and is probably due to the low correlation of the one item designed to measure conflict in the marital context.

Validity The measures for satisfaction with family life and marital functioning are substantially correlated ($r = 0.64$). The measure for overall happiness with family life correlates 0.79 with satisfaction with family life and 0.59 with marital functioning.

Resolution of Issues and Future Directions

The family functioning measures can be used to evaluate satisfaction with specific aspects of family life and to evaluate the degree of cohesion, communication, support, and understanding within the marital context. The family functioning items are deliberately general, allowing respondents to form their own interpretation of "family" and "spouse" or "partner" so that scores can be constructed for as many people as possible.

A disadvantage of the MOS family functioning measures is that they do not focus on specific aspects of family processes (e.g., cohesion only

Table 10–4 Descriptive Statistics and Reliability Coefficients for Family Functioning Measures: P A Q Baseline Sample (N = 3,053)

Scale[a]	k	Mean	SD	% Perfect	Observed Range	% Missing	Reliability
Satisfaction with family life (+)	3	62.2	28.7	15	0–100	3.7	.93
Overall happiness with family life (+)	1	4.5	1.2	20	1–6	2.0	.80[b]
Marital functioning (+)	6	71.8	22.0	10	0–100	9.0	.83

[a] A (+) high score means better functioning.
[b] Alternate forms reliability.

as opposed to the present combination of cohesion with communication, conflict, and support). In the future, a number of items designed to measure specific types of functioning could be included to see if a number of subscales could be developed that reflect the variety of aspects indicative of family life. Specifically, results seem to suggest that conflict might be a very distinct aspect of family functioning that should be developed further. The family functioning areas studied could be broadened to include family adaptability, which seems to be a particularly relevant area of functioning for families with a chronically ill family member. Finally, although the variability of the M O S general family functioning items improved slightly over pilot study findings with the use of an excellent- to poor-response format, responses were still skewed, indicating that further improvement could be made. Further empirical study of different response choice methods is needed to see if one is better than another at detecting differences.

11. Social Functioning: Sexual Problems Measures

Cathy D. Sherbourne

Definition and Issues

Social functioning is a broad and general concept. It is defined in terms of limitations in social activities (chapter 9) and family functioning (chapter 10) and in terms of sexual functioning, discussed in this chapter.

Sexual functioning is commonly defined by sexual problems and dysfunction. The MOS limited the definition to include any impairment of the capacity of an adult man or woman to achieve sexual arousal and orgasm (Conte, 1986). Types of dysfunctions are erectile dysfunction or retrograde ejaculation in the male, vaginal infections or dyspareunia (i.e., pain) in the female, and inadequate sexual interest or sexual pleasure in the male and the female. Erectile dysfunction involves some impairment of vasocongestion in the penis so that the male is unable to obtain a sufficiently firm erection or to maintain it during intercourse (Jehu, 1979). Retrograde ejaculation is the involuntary discharge of semen backwards into the bladder rather than forwards through the urethra. Dyspareunia is characterized by intercourse accompanied by pain. Inadequate sexual interest occurs when a person considers the level of interest to be lower than he or she would like it to be. A member of either sex may complain of an absence of feeling during intercourse or that it is insufficiently pleasurable or satisfying. The definition involves subjective judgments of inadequacy as well as a description of the actual behavior concerned (Jehu, 1979).

Two basic issues were addressed in developing a measure of sexual functioning for the MOS: the identification of specific sexual problems that could be caused by the five chronic conditions or that might result from interventions and treatments for these conditions, and practical issues related to how best to word the sexual problem items, the appropriate response format to use, and how to deal with persons who did not have a sexual partner or had not experienced a sexual encounter during the time frame of interest. The MOS was interested in assessing general sexual problems that could be due to one of the MOS chronic tracer conditions or that might result from interventions and treatments for these conditions. The MOS wanted to identify sexual problems that would be applicable across conditions, rather than those that were condition-specific, since the patient might not know that a sexual problem was due to a condition or treatment for a condition. The MOS also concentrated on current sexual problems rather than on changes in usual sexual functioning due to illness. The reason for this focus was that patients might be unable to recognize an association between sexual problems and their condition.

The literature revealed a variety of assessment methods and measures used by others to evaluate male, female, and couple sexual dysfunction. A wide variety of types of questions have been used, including questions related to sexual history or the extent of a person's sexual experience (e.g., types of sexual behaviors and frequency with which each behavior is experienced), subjective ratings of the intensity of sexual desire, ratings of the importance of sexual experiences, ratings of the preferred frequency of sexual intercourse, the occurrence of specific sexual dysfunctions, satisfaction with aspects of one's sex life, and attitudes toward sex. The methods used include interviews, self-report questionnaires, physiological techniques, and self-report behavioral records (Conte, 1986).

To narrow the focus, specific sexual problems considered to be either symptoms of one of the tracer conditions or side effects of treatment were defined based on the judgment of one of the study physicians (Table 11–1). General problems in sexual functioning were also defined that could result from some of these specific problems and side effects (e.g., fear of failure, less frequent intercourse than desired).

Three studies that had assessed sexual dysfunction in ways considered relevant to the MOS definition were identified, although only one focused on patients with a chronic condition. Snyder and Berg (1983) included a 15-item symptom checklist of sexual dysfunctions in their study of couples presenting with complaints of sexual dissatisfaction at a sexual dysfunction specialty clinic. The fifteen items ranged in content

Table 11–1 Sexual Functioning Problems Associated with MOS
Chronic Conditions

Chronic Condition	Symptom of Condition	Side Effect of Treatment
Hypertension	None	Impotence Retrograde ejaculation Decreased sexual desire Less feelings

Diabetes	Impotence
	Retrograde ejaculation
	Decreased ability to have
	  orgasms
	Low libido
	Painful intercourse
	  (women)
	Vaginal infections
	  (women)
		None

Myocardial infection
  and congestive
  heart failure
	None	Impotence
		Decreased sexual desire

Depression	Low libido Impotence Difficulty becoming aroused	Low libido Impotence Difficulty becoming aroused Retrograde ejaculation

from specific dysfunctions (e.g., erectile or orgasmic problems) to more general sexual difficulties (e.g., frequency of sex too high or too low, lack of affection for partner). Each item was rated on a 4-point Likert scale, ranging from "not at all a problem" to "very much a problem."

Frank, Anderson, and Rubinstein (1978) examined the frequency of sexual problems experienced by married couples. Each subject was asked to report on what sexual problems, if any, were currently occurring. The sexual problems were classified as either dysfunctions, which included erectile and ejaculatory problems in the husbands and arousal and orgasmic problems in the wives, or as difficulties, which included complaints about inability to relax, lack of interest, different sexual practices, or too little tenderness. This classification was based on the distinction between problems of performance and problems that are more related to the emotional tone of sexual relations.

Hogan, Wallin, and Baer (1980) measured sexual dysfunction in a hypertensive population receiving hypertensive medications by assessing loss of interest in sex, inability to achieve an erection, inability to maintain an erection, and inability to ejaculate. On subsequent visits to a hypertension clinic, the patients were asked whether any of the sexual problems had improved, worsened, stayed the same, or were no longer a problem. Croog, Levine, Testa, et al. (1986) adapted these four items to a 5-point response scale in which hypertensive patients rated how distressed they were due to each sexual problem from "not at all" to "extremely."

In these studies, three approaches were used to measure sexual problems. Respondents were asked to indicate whether or not different sexual problems were experienced, the extent of distress due to a given problem, and the degree to which each problem was bothersome. All response formats generate primarily subjective data about how subjects perceive their behavior. Which type of response format (i.e., yes/no, degree of distress, how much of a problem) to use depends on the purpose of the survey. For those interested in determining prevalence of problems, asking whether or not a sexual problem occurred would be sufficient. However, because the determination of a sexual problem is likely to depend on individual preferences and past experiences, it may be more important to ask about the degree to which sexual problems bother the subject or cause distress.

None of the studies discussed how to deal with people who did not have a partner or who did not have a sexual experience in a given interval.

Content and Measurement Strategy

Pilot Study The pilot study was designed to identify a small group of items (about five) that would best assess sexual problems among patients with the MOS chronic conditions. Other goals of the pilot study were to assess the variability of specific items and the degree to which items were internally consistent and exhibited adequate re-liability. The MOS was also interested in determining how patients without a spouse or partner or who had not had a sexual experience in a given interval would respond to these items (e.g., would they respond "not a problem" or "not applicable"?).

Included in the pilot study were questions about thirteen sexual problems: fear that sex may be harmful to your health; less frequent intercourse than you desire; pain during intercourse; lack of sexual interest; unable to relax and enjoy sex; less feeling in various parts of your body; fear of failure in sex; difficulty in becoming aroused and maintaining arousal; difficulty in obtaining an erection (men only); difficulty in maintaining an erection (men only); difficulty in ejaculating (men only); difficulty in having an orgasm (women only); and vaginal infection (women only).

The MOS response format used was similar to that used by Snyder and Berg (1983), requiring subjects to rate how frequently each item had been a problem for them during the past month. Because the MOS was unsure how a person would respond who had not experienced a sexual encounter during the past month, a "not applicable" column was added.

Two items were included that asked whether or not the subject was involved sexually with someone at present or had experienced sex with a partner in the last month. These two items were designed to help determine how subjects without a partner or who had not had a sexual experience would answer the items about sexual problems. The sample was sixty-eight people from an outpatient clinic.

Item variability and frequency were examined to determine the most commonly experienced types of sexual problems. For both men and women, the sexual problem with the highest incidence of any degree of problem was that of having "less frequent intercourse than you desire." For men, the item with the smallest variability (in other words, most people did not report it as a problem) was the item about "pain during intercourse." Among women, none reported a problem on the item "fear that sex is harmful to your health." Thus, this item was dropped from the analysis. For the remaining items, the percentage having any degree of problem ranged from 8% to 42% for men and from 9% to 55% for women.

Hypothesized sexual functioning measures were analyzed using multitrait scaling techniques. Because several of the items were gender-specific, item-scale correlations were computed separately for men and women. "Not applicable" responses for individual items were coded as missing. Item-scale correlations were evaluated only for those persons who were either involved in a sexual relationship at present or had had a sexual experience in the past month, to avoid artificially inflating the reliability of the items. For men, item-total correlations (not shown) were substantial for all but one item, ranging from a low of 0.44 (for the item "less frequent intercourse than you desire") to a high of 0.96 (for the items pertaining to difficulties in becoming aroused and obtaining an erection). The internal-consistency reliability of this 11-item measure was 0.95. For women, item-scale correlations were much lower, ranging from lows of 0.24 and 0.29 ("fear of failure" and "pain during intercourse") to a high of 0.84 ("difficulty in having an orgasm"). It should be noted that the "fear" and "pain" items exhibited low variability. In this case, it is difficult to know whether the low item-total correlations are due to the fact that these are poor items or to the low variability of the items themselves. The internal-consistency reliability of this 9-item measure was 0.84.

Responses for respondents without a partner or who had not experienced sexual intercourse were reviewed to determine which response category they were most likely to choose. Seventy-one percent of the pilot study sample reported being involved in a sexual relationship or having a sexual experience in the past month. Most of the men and women without a partner or who had not experienced sexual intercourse in the given interval responded "not a problem" to the sexual functioning items, rather than "not applicable." This indicated that a total score could be calculated that included those without a sexual experience.

Final Items To reach the MOS goal of five sexual problem items, the items with low variability and low item-total correlations—"less frequent intercourse than desired," "fear that sex is harmful to your health," "fear of failure," and "pain during intercourse"—were omitted. Two items that were symptoms primarily of diabetes and not the other tracer conditions, "less feeling in various parts of your body" and "vaginal infection," were also omitted. To reduce respondent burden, the two male-only questions about obtaining and maintaining an erection were combined into one item. The third gender-specific question about difficulty in ejaculation was deleted mainly due to space considerations and because this would allow construction of scales of equal length for both men and women.

The final battery thus contains three items that are appropriate for either men or women, one item appropriate for men only, and one for women only (see page 397 in the Appendix). These items are lack of sexual interest, inability to relax and enjoy sex, difficulty in becoming sexually aroused, difficulty getting or keeping an erection (men only), and difficulty in having an orgasm (women only). Respondents were asked to indicate how much of a problem each of the items was during the past four weeks, consistent with the pilot study items. Five response choices were given: not a problem, a little of a problem, somewhat of a problem, very much a problem, and not applicable. The "not applicable" response choice was retained for those respondents without a spouse or partner. This response choice was considered equivalent to the "not a problem" category, based on pilot study results.

Construction and Evaluation of Measure

Analysis Plan In addition to the usual analyses, some preliminary tests of the validity of our sexual functioning measure in terms of known groups validity were conducted (chapter 18). The mean sexual problems score was calculated for three groups: MOS patients who had a major medical condition (diabetes, hypertension, myocardial infarction, or congestive heart failure) and no major depression or dysthymia; patients who had both a major medical condition and major depression or dysthymia; and patients with major depression or dysthymia but no medical condition. Mean sexual problem scores were expected to be highest for patients with both depression and a major medical problem. The mean sexual problem scores were calculated for the separate tracer condition groups and were expected to be highest for depressed patients and lowest for patients with hypertension.

Item Variability Table 11–2 presents frequencies for the sexual problem items separately for men and women. Among men, the sexual problem with the highest incidence of any degree of problem was that of "difficulty in getting or keeping an erection." The percentage reporting any degree of problem ranged from 42% to 53% across items. Among women, the variability was the same across sexual problem items. From 36% to 40% of women reported that they had at least a little of a problem across items. Thus, more men reported problems than women. Eight to 14% of men responded "not applicable" to one or more sexual problem items. A greater proportion of women responded "not applicable" (24–29%). Interestingly, the percentage missing a sexual problem item was also higher for women, ranging from 15% to 20%, versus 6% to 7% for men. The variability of all items was considered sufficient to include in subsequent analyses.

Scale Construction The sexual functioning scale was analyzed separately for men and women. Item-total correlations (Table 11–3) were substantial, ranging from 0.70 to 0.85 for men and from 0.75 to 0.89 for women.

Table 11–2 Percentage with Sexual Functioning Problems: PAQ Baseline Sample of Men (N = 1,199) and Women (N = 1,852)

| | ITEM RESPONSE[a] | | | | | |
Abbreviated Item Content	Not a Problem 1	A Little of a Problem 2	Somewhat of a Problem 3	Very Much a Problem 4	Not Applicable 5	% of Total Missing
Men						
Lack of sexual interest	48	16	16	12	8	6
Unable to relax and enjoy sex	44	15	13	14	14	6
Difficulty in becoming sexually aroused	46	18	14	14	9	6
Difficulty getting or keeping an erection	40	17	14	22	8	7
Women						
Lack of sexual interest	35	14	12	14	24	15
Unable to relax and enjoy sex	34	15	10	12	29	16
Difficulty in becoming sexually aroused	36	15	10	13	27	16
Difficulty having an orgasm	36	14	10	12	28	20

[a] Percentage of those who responded to each item.

Scoring Rules The sexual problems scale was scored so that a high score indicated more problems. Raw items were first recoded so that the category "not applicable" was given the same value as the category "not a problem." Thus, raw item scores of 5 were recoded to 1. Scores for men and women were then calculated by averaging across the nonmissing items that had been administered to all patients (e.g., lack of interest in sex, unable to relax and enjoy sex, and difficulty becoming sexually aroused) as well as the one gender-specific item (e.g., men:

Table 11–3 Item-Scale Correlations for Sexual Problems Scale
Corrected for Overlap of Men (N = 1,074) and Women
(N = 1,234)

Item	Men	Women
Lack of sexual interest	.75	.81
Unable to relax and enjoy sex	.82	.86
Difficulty in becoming sexually aroused	.85	.89
Difficulty getting or keeping an erection	.70	N A
Difficulty having an orgasm	N A	.75

difficulty getting or keeping an erection; women: difficulty having an orgasm). Because item variances for the sexual problem items were generally comparable, it was not necessary to standardize or weight items before they were scored. The multi-item sexual problems measure was subsequently transformed to a 0–100 scale.

Characteristics of the Measure

Descriptive Statistics Table 11–4 presents descriptive statistics for the sexual functioning measure. Twelve percent received a missing scale score.

Variability The sexual problems measure is skewed toward the positive end of the distribution (i.e., more people reported the absence of sexual problems). However, more than 69% of men and 54% of women reported at least "a little of a problem" in one or more areas of their sexual functioning.

Reliability Internal-consistency reliability coefficients for the sexual problems measure were very high (0.90 for men and 0.92 for women).

Validity Mean sexual problem scores for three groups of patients are shown in Table 11–5. As expected, mean sexual problems scores were highest for patients with both depression and a major medical problem. Mean sexual problem scores were lowest for patients with a medical condition but no depression.

Mean sexual problem scores were evaluated separately for the four different medical conditions and depression. As expected, mean sexual problem scores were highest for depressed patients (41.76) and lowest for patients with hypertension (24.43). Means for the other medical

Table 11–4 Descriptive Statistics and Reliability Coefficients for MOS Sexual Problems Scales: PAQ Baseline Sample (N = 3,053)

Scale	k	Mean	SD	% with Problems	Observed Range	% Missing	Reliability
Sexual problems	5	27.2	32.0	59	0–100	12.0	
Men	5	30.3	31.9	69	0–100	—	.90
Women	5	24.9	32.1	54	0–100	—	.92

Note: A high score indicates more problems.

Table 11–5 Mean Sexual Problems Scores for Three Patient Groups

Group	Score
Major medical condition/no depression	24.48
Major medical condition/depression	43.50
Depression/no major medical condition	41.13

condition groups were 32.30 for congestive heart failure, 30.46 for myocardial infarction, and 26.75 for diabetes.

Resolution of Issues and Future Directions

The sexual problem measure can be used to assess sexual problems common among patients with MOS tracer conditions and can be administered to both men and women. The items focus on problems that respondents perceive in their capacity to achieve sexual arousal and orgasm. Sexual satisfaction is not assessed since there are so many other, non-health-related factors associated with the rating of sexual satisfaction. The MOS items are limited to only those problems most likely to occur in patients with the MOS tracer conditions (diabetes, hypertension, myocardial infarction, congestive heart failure, and depression).

For future measures of sexual problems, the MOS recommends including a number of other items. Specifically, in order to increase the ability to detect differences, the male-specific items related to difficulty obtaining and maintaining an erection could be separated. An item about difficulty in ejaculation could be included. The disadvantage to this approach, however, is that the scales would not be of equal length for both men and women.

How to deal with respondents who have had no sexual experiences in a given time interval deserves further study. Although the MOS solution of rescoring "not applicable" responses to "not a problem" is reasonable, confirmation of this approach is needed.

12. Role Functioning Measures

*Cathy D. Sherbourne, Anita L. Stewart,
and Kenneth B. Wells*

Definition and Issues

Role functioning refers to the degree to which an individual performs or has the capacity to perform activities typical for a specified age and social responsibility. Measurement of this construct presents several issues. Historically, the definition of role functioning has focused narrowly on job-related limitations, although many measures also included limitations in the performance of housework or schoolwork. For the MOS, role functioning was defined more broadly to include roles related to volunteer work, caring for children, being a spouse or partner, and being involved in community activities. Two other important issues were addressed: the appropriateness of distinguishing between role limitations due to physical and to mental health problems, and the way to improve sensitivity to various levels of role limitations.

Assessing functioning in a variety of roles is important. The three most commonly assessed roles are work for pay, whether for financial or for other reasons, which is considered a major component of quality of life (Levine and Croog, 1984); work as a housewife, which typically refers to the ability to perform household tasks; and being a student (Stewart, Ware, Brook, 1978). Curiously, none of the measures reviewed by Stewart et al. refers to child care as a major role, and only two refer to children (NCHS, 1974; Reynolds, Rushing, and Miles, 1974). None of the reviewed measures refers to volunteer or community work. Thus important roles held especially by women in our society have often not been assessed in the context of role functioning. To improve on the existing measures a variety of role activities had to be defined:

child care, community activities, and volunteer work, in addition to work, housework, and schoolwork. The MOS definition of role functioning excludes the role of spouse or partner because social functioning is separately assessed.

Most role functioning measures assume that one "major" role can be defined for each person—typically, either work, housework, or schoolwork—which causes two problems. One problem is that measures focusing on one major role cannot account for the fact that people might have more than one important role. At times, separate measures are developed for each of the three roles (workers, housewives, and students), and respondents are assigned a score on the measure only if they perform that role (Commission on Chronic Illness, 1957; Nagi, 1969). At other times, measures incorporate information regarding the one most appropriate role into an overall index (National Center for Health Statistics, 1974; Haber, 1970; Patrick, Bush, and Chen, 1973b; Nagi, 1976; Reynolds, Rushing, and Miles, 1974; Stewart, Ware, and Brook, 1978, 1981, 1982). A second problem with defining a single major role is that it does not consider the relative importance of various roles to the individual. For example, a working mother might consider her parent role more important than her worker role.

Although a good role functioning measure should be applicable to a range of roles, it is usually impractical to ask separate questions about peoples' various roles. For this reason, the MOS developed a measure sensitive to limitations in a variety of roles with only one set of questions, which was accomplished through instructions asking respondents to answer one set of questions regarding their regular daily activities, such as working at a job, keeping house, taking care of children, attending school, volunteer work, and taking part in community activities.

A variety of factors affect role functioning, such as the social environment (e.g., attitudes of coworkers), personality variables (e.g., motivation), and interest in or satisfaction with roles. To increase the validity of a role functioning measure as an indicator of the outcome of medical care, it is important to focus on those role limitations caused specifically by health problems. The most widely used role functioning measures in studies of health status focus specifically on limitations due to health problems.

Both physical and mental health problems can impact role functioning. However, the pros and cons about distinguishing between different causes of role limitations have not yet been evaluated. Many measures of role limitations ask the respondent about degree of limitations due to health problems in general or due to physical health problems specifically (Wells, Burnam, Leake, et al., 1988). People might be less likely to define personal and emotional problems as "health problems" when reporting role limitations. As a result, limitations due to emotional problems might go unreported in most existing measures.

In the MOS, we sought to improve the validity of role functioning measures by separately defining and assessing role limitations due to physical and emotional problems. Although our main interest in this approach was due to the focus of the MOS on patients with depression, psychological distress is common enough among patients with chronic medical conditions that limitations due to such distress should be captured and distinguished in studies of patients in general.

Another kind of problem with existing role functioning measures is their lack of sensitivity to the extent of limitation among those who are limited. Most previous measures have been coarse, having only three levels: no limitations, some limitations, and cannot perform role activities at all (e.g., Reynolds, Rushing, and Miles, 1974; National Center for Health Statistics, 1974; Stewart, Ware, and Brook, 1978). Such coarseness limits the ability to detect important differences in role functioning that might occur among individuals within a given category.

Other role functioning measures are insensitive because they assess only certain types of limitations. Of the measures reviewed (Stewart, Ware, and Brook, 1978), most focus only on limitations in the amount of work or the kind of work that can be done. Some measures are more specific about the kinds of limitations and do ask about reductions in hours worked, reductions in work efficiency, and changes in kinds of work, conditions of work, or location of work (Commission on Chronic Illness, 1957; Nagi, 1969; Haber, 1970; Gilson, Bergner, Bobbitt, et al., 1975). A measure based on a broader definition can be more sensitive.

Two strategies for improving the sensitivity of MOS role measures were including questions about a broad range of possible types of limitations and selecting a scaling method that captures as much of that information as possible. For the first strategy, we assessed a broader range of limitations due to poor health (e.g., the need for frequent rests, doing work less carefully than usual); for the second, we used a simple summated-rating scaling method. We abandoned the Guttman cumulative scale approach because it forced a small number of scale levels

(Stewart, Ware, and Brook, 1978). By simply counting limitations, we constructed a continuous measure with more scale levels, which should increase the ability to detect true differences and true changes in levels of functioning over time.

Content and Measurement Strategy

Pilot Study A pilot study was designed to help determine the content of the final role functioning battery and to address practical issues, such as the battery length, the specific types of prevalent role limitations, and the rate of missing data for different types of items. Another reason for the pilot study was to conduct formal empirical tests of any gains in precision of a longer role functioning measure over a short-form measure in order to determine if any gains justified the additional respondent burden of administering a longer version. The pilot study was administered to a sample of patients and other people waiting to see physicians in a typical ambulatory clinic.

To determine the need for any additions to the content of a role functioning battery, previous work was reviewed to compile a list of types of limitations people might experience in the performance of daily activities (Patrick, Bush and Chen, 1973b; Gilson, Bergner, Bobbitt, et al., 1975; National Center for Health Statistics, 1974; Stewart, Ware, and Brook, 1978). Ten types of limitations were identified: limiting the kind of activities; limiting the amount of time spent on activities; accomplishing less than desired; working less carefully than usual; having to take frequent rests; having to take breaks to deal with health problems; acting irritably toward others; performing activities with difficulty; experiencing pain or discomfort; and needing special assistance performing activities.

Respondents in the pilot study were asked to report if any of these problems occurred with their work or other regular daily activities due to health. A subset of four of the limitations were repeated, but respondents were asked specifically whether these limitations were due to emotional problems. Open-ended questions, asking respondents to identify other possible problems not included in the sample of items from published questionnaires, were included in the questionnaire. To assess limitations across multiple roles, the instructions named a variety of different roles: working at a job, keeping house, taking care of children, attending school, working as a volunteer, and taking part in community activities. The best two out of three items from the Health Insurance Experiment measure of role limitations (Stewart, Ware, and Brook, 1981) were included as a benchmark for estimating any gains in precision due to a longer role functioning measure.

Item variability and frequency were examined to determine the most commonly experienced types of limitations. Of the fifteen specific types of limitations piloted, all but one (changing jobs due to emotional problems) were prevalent enough to warrant inclusion in a final scale. Written responses to the open-ended items were reviewed to determine if important types of limitations were omitted. Few people listed other problems in the open-ended items. All other problems mentioned (e.g., family or sexual functioning) were covered by items in other MOS scales.

Factor analyses and multitrait scaling tests were used to evaluate the internal consistency of hypothesized scales and the item discrimination of the role items in relation to other MOS health scales. The results supported the construction of an overall scale of role limitations "due to health" based on all ten items. Correlations of items with the first unrotated principal component ranged from 0.59 to 0.88, suggesting an internally consistent total scale. The internal-consistency reliability of this scale was 0.89. Multitrait scaling results indicated that all but one item—acting irritably towards others—met the established criterion of item discrimination.

Based on the factor analytic and multitrait scaling results, a 4-item measure of limitations due to emotional problems was constructed. Item-scale correlations ranged from 0.41 to 0.58, and the internal-consistency reliability of the scale was 0.70. Although items correlated highest with their own scale, considerable overlap between these items and measures of anxiety and depression was observed. To compare the sensitivity of measures of role limitations due to health problems with measures of limitations due to emotional problems, a series of cross-tabulations between comparable items was performed. A substantial percentage, 27% or more, of people who reported a limitation due to emotional problems did not report the same limitation as being "due to health." We estimated that an additional 11% to 14% of the total sample would be added to the "limited" category of role functioning by asking about limitations due to emotional problems over and above the percentage limited due to health. Thus, it seems important to ask specifically whether role functioning has been affected by emotional problems in addition to asking about the effects of health problems in general. We concluded that this method of distinguishing between the two types of health problems improves the sensitivity of role limitations measures.

We compared the ability of the 2-item short form with the long-form role functioning measure to predict a number of conceptually related variables. We regressed measures of current health, mental health, and an item about not doing things as well as you should because of illness separately on the physical functioning scale and short-form role functioning scale and the longer MOS pilot role functioning scale. Results showed that the longer MOS pilot role functioning scale added significantly more information over and above that due to the physical functioning and the short-form role functioning measures in the prediction of the dependent variables. These tests of the incremental validity of the MOS pilot role functioning scale showed that the increased precision gained with additional levels (eleven levels for the pilot measure and three levels for the short-form measure) was valid in terms of some increment in predictive efficiency over the information obtained from the shorter 2-item role functioning measure.

In addition, substantially more people were detected as limited using the longer pilot measures. Twenty-four percent reported having one or more limitations on the basis of the 2-item measure. Sixty-five percent reported having one or more limitations on the basis of the 10-item measure.

Final Items Because the pilot results indicated that people often do not equate emotional problems with health problems, we adopted two role functioning inventories for the formal MOS: one 7-item inventory that asks about various limitations due to physical health problems, and a second 4-item inventory that asks about limitations due to emotional problems. (See the Appendix for questionnaire items, page 380.) We eliminated four pretest items: (1) "acting irritable," because it did not discriminate well between role limitations and psychological distress; (2) having to take breaks, because it was redundant with the item pertaining to taking frequent rests; (3) experiencing pain or discomfort, because this item is measured more comprehensively in the pain scales; and (4) "some other problem." Respondents were asked to respond yes or no to an item about whether they had each limitation during the past four weeks. We also included a set of two items about the inability to work or do housework because of health (Appendix page 381). These items were included because we felt that the inability to do housework or to work because of health were extreme limitations that might not be adequately represented by the other role limitation items.

Construction and Evaluation of Measures

Analysis Plan We first examined item frequency distributions to assure adequate variability for purposes of scale construction and to estimate the prevalence of various types of role limitations. The goal in the multitrait scaling analysis was to make sure that items included in each role functioning scale were internally consistent and distinct from each other as well as from other health concepts. To provide stringent tests of the discriminant validity of the role items, we included in our multitrait matrix both physical and emotional role functioning scales and nine other measures: anxiety, depression/behavioral-emotional control, positive affect, feelings of belonging, cognitive functioning, physical functioning, energy/fatigue, current health, and social activity limitations due to health. Scales were included for different reasons: the psychological distress/well-being measures because of their similarity to role limitations due to emotional problems, the physical functioning measure because role and physical functioning tend to be highly related (Stewart, Ware, and Brook, 1981), and the social functioning, current health, and energy/fatigue measures to assure a good representation of competing health concepts.

As preliminary tests of the validity of the measures, we examined the correlations among the role functioning measures, expecting that they would be moderately correlated. We also evaluated correlations between the two role functioning scales and selected validity variables to see if they differed as hypothesized. Our hypotheses are summarized in Table 12–1. The role functioning scale due to physical health problems was expected to correlate higher with measures related to physical health than the role functioning scale due to emotional problems. Similarly, we predicted that the role functioning scale due to emotional problems would correlate higher with measures related to mental health than would the role functioning scale due to physical health. The study also compared average role functioning scores for groups of patients known to differ in their physical and mental health problems. The following MOS groups were compared: patients with a major medical condition (hypertension, diabetes, congestive heart failure,

Table 12–1 Hypothesized Results for Two Role Functioning Scales

	EXPECT HIGHEST CORRELATION WITH	
Validity Variables	Role/Physical Scale	Role/Emotional Scale
Physical demands of daily activities	x	
Emotional stress associated with daily activity		x
Physical functioning	x	
Mental health index I		x
Energy/fatigue	x	x

myocardial infarction) and no major depression and/or dysthymia; patients with major depression and/or dysthymia but no major medical condition; and patients with both a major medical condition and major depression and/or dysthymia. We expected mean levels of role limitations due to physical health to be higher for the first and third groups than the second group, while mean levels of role limitations due to emotional problems would be higher for the second and third groups than the first group.

Item Variability Table 12–2 shows the prevalence of role limitations, i.e., the percentage of those reporting a limitation during the past four weeks. The percentage limited ranged from a low of 11 (requiring special assistance) to a high of 54 (accomplishing less than they would like). The variability of all items was sufficient to include in subsequent analyses.

Scale Construction The multitrait matrix for ten physical and emotional role functioning items used to define two scales is presented in Table 12–3. One item, "acting irritable toward people," was deleted because it did not discriminate between role limitations and other mental health measures. The physical and emotional role functioning scales are labeled ROLPHY and ROLEMO, respectively. The other measures included in the matrix are presented in the order given previously.

All ten role items correlated substantially with their hypothesized scales and exceeded the standard for convergence or internal consistency as well as the criterion of item discrimination. These findings

Table 12–2 Percentage Limited on Role Functioning Items: PAQ Baseline Sample (N = 3,053)

Abbreviated Item Content	Item Variable Name	Percent Limited[a]	% of Total Sample Missing
Limitations due to physical health[b]			
Took frequent rests when doing work or activities	RPHY5	34	3.7
Cut down amount of time spent on work or activities	RPHY2	39	3.7
Accomplished less than you would like	RPHY3	54	4.3
Didn't do activities as carefully as usual	RPHY4	31	4.2
Were limited in kind of work or activities	RPHY1	38	3.9
Had difficulty performing the work or activities	RPHY6	44	3.4
Required special assistance to perform activities	RPHY7	11	3.6
Limitations due to emotional problems[b]			
Cut down amount of time spent on work or activities	REM1	26	3.6
Accomplished less than you would like	REM2	39	3.5
Didn't do activities as carefully as usual	REM3	26	3.7
Acted irritable toward people	REM4	39	3.4

[a] Percentage of those who responded to each item.
[b] Defined as a "yes" response to any item.

constitute strong empirical support for the hypothesized physical and emotional role functioning scales and the distinction between these role measures and other health measures.

Scoring Rules Table 12–4 presents the item content of the MOS role functioning scales. The two scales were scored by counting across "yes" responses for each activity limitation. Respondents missing more than two items or one item for the role limitations due to physical health and emotional problems scales, respectively, were assigned a missing value on the scale. Each multi-item measure was subsequently transformed to a 0–100 scale. All measures were scored negatively, with a high score indicating more limitations. Two other dichotomous role functioning measures were also computed: inability to work because of health scored "limited" if unable to work, and inability to do housework because of health scored "limited" if unable to do housework.

Table 12–3 Item-Scale Correlation Matrix, Role Functioning: P A Q Baseline Sample (N = 2,678)

Item	Mean	S D	ROLPHY	ROLEMO	ANX	DEPBC
RPHY1	1.62	.48	.70[a]	.28	.19	.20
RPHY2	1.61	.48	.72[a]	.39	.24	.26
RPHY3	1.46	.49	.65[a]	.41	.27	.27
RPHY4	1.69	.46	.58[a]	.46	.30	.28
RPHY5	1.66	.47	.66[a]	.31	.21	.23
RPHY6	1.56	.49	.69[a]	.38	.31	.32
RPHY7	1.88	.31	.43[a]	.29	.20	.19
REM1	1.73	.43	.42	.69[a]	.48	.58
REM2	1.60	.48	.42	.73[a]	.50	.58
REM3	1.74	.43	.42	.64[a]	.46	.51

Note: Standard error of correlation = 0.02. R O L P H Y = Role limitations due to physical health; R O L E M O = Role limitations due to emotional problems; A N X = Anxiety; D E P B C = Depression/behavioral-emotional control; P O S = Positive affect; B E L = Feelings of belonging;

Characteristics of Measures

Descriptive Statistics Table 12–5 presents a summary of information, including descriptive statistics, for all measures of role functioning. The percentage missing a role functioning measure ranged from a low of 3.3% to a high of 5.6%.

Variability For all scales, all possible scores were observed. For the two multi-item scales, although the largest percentage was observed to be in the "no limitations" category, the frequencies were fairly evenly distributed over the remaining levels. The percentage with any limitations on these measures ranged from 67 for the role limitations due to physical health scale to 16 for unable to do housework.

Reliability Summarized in Table 12–5 are the internal-consistency reliability coefficients for the multi-item scales. Reliability estimates are high for both measures (0.86 and 0.83 for limitations due to physical health and emotional problems, respectively).

Validity Correlations relevant to the construct validity of the role functioning measures are shown in Table 12–6. The magnitude of the correlations conformed to the hypotheses that the role functioning scale due to physical health problems would correlate higher with measures related to physical health than would the role functioning scale due to

POS	BEL	COG	PHYS	CURR	ENERGY	SOC
.21	.11	.26	.59	.48	.46	.43
.27	.17	.30	.52	.48	.49	.45
.31	.20	.32	.44	.45	.54	.40
.29	.19	.36	.40	.39	.43	.39
.23	.12	.29	.56	.48	.50	.43
.34	.21	.33	.48	.48	.52	.45
.17	.08	.23	.39	.33	.30	.37
.49	.39	.50	.21	.36	.42	.50
.53	.41	.50	.22	.37	.45	.47
.46	.35	.50	.23	.34	.40	.43

COG = Cognitive functioning; PHYS = Physical functioning; CURR = Current health perceptions; ENERGY = Energy/fatigue; SOC = Social activity limitations due to health.
[a] Denotes hypothesized item groupings and item-scale correlation corrected for overlap.

Table 12–4 Content of Final Role Functioning Scales

Abbreviated Item Content	Item Name	ROLE LIMITATIONS DUE TO	
		Physical	Emotional
Number of items		6	3
Role limitations due to physical health			
Took frequent rests	RPHY5	x	
Cut down amount of time	RPHY2	x	
Accomplished less	RPHY3	x	
Didn't do activities as carefully	RPHY4	x	
Were limited in kind of activities	RPHY1	x	
Had difficulty performing activities	RPHY6	x	
Required special assistance	RPHY7	x	
Role limitations due to emotional problems			
Cut down amount of time	REM1		x
Accomplished less	REM2		x
Didn't do activities as carefully	REM3		x
Acted irritable[a]			

[a] Not included in any measure.

Table 12–5 Descriptive Statistics and Reliability Coefficients for Role Functioning Measures: PAQ Baseline Sample ($N = 3,049$)

Scale[a]	k	Mean	SD	% Limited	Observed Range	% Missing	Reliability
Role limitations due to physical health	7	35.80	34.40	67	0–100	3.4	.86
Role limitations due to emotional problems	3	30.00	39.20	43	0–100	3.3	.83
Unable to do housework due to health	1	0.16	0.36	16	0–1	3.7	—
Unable to work due to health	1	0.17	0.38	17	0–1	5.6	—

[a] High score indicates more limitations on all measures.

Table 12–6 Correlations between Role Functioning Measures and Validity Variables

	ROLE LIMITATIONS DUE TO	
Validity Variables	Physical	Emotional
Physical demands of daily activities	−.11	−.09
Emotional stress associated with daily activities	.00	−.23
Physical functioning	−.65	−.25
Mental health	−.36	−.63
Energy/fatigue	−.63	−.49

emotional problems, and vice versa. These results provide support for the validity of the two scales. The correlation between the two scales is 0.48.

As a further test of the validity of the measures for use in clinical applications, we calculated the mean role scale scores for three clinical groups of patients which were defined above. Results are presented in Table 12–7. The pattern of results conforms partially to what would be expected if the two scales discriminate between physical health and

Table 12–7 Mean Role Functioning Scores for Three Clinical Groups

Clinical Conditions	Role/Physical Subscale	Role/Emotional Subscale
Major medical condition/no depression	33.73	22.55
Depression/no major medical condition	43.45	62.83
Major medical condition and depression	59.39	62.42

emotional problems. Mean levels of role limitations due to emotional problems are significantly higher for the two groups including depressed patients relative to the group with a medical condition and no depression. Contrary to our hypothesis, the mean level of role limitations due to physical problems was not higher in the group with a medical condition and no depression than in the group with depression only.

Resolution of Issues and Future Directions

We improved upon existing measures in three respects. First, we defined a broader variety of roles (e.g., volunteer work, caring for children, and being involved in community activities) and not just common roles related to work, housework, or being a student. Second, we demonstrated the usefulness of distinguishing between role limitations attributed to physical and mental health problems. Third, we improved the sensitivity of the measures to various levels of role limitations (i.e., decreased the coarseness of scales) by asking about a broad range of types of limitations and by selecting a scaling method that would reflect as much of that information as possible.

The MOS role functioning scales represent a noteworthy departure from how role functioning has traditionally been measured. In the past, most measures of role functioning focused on only three types of roles: workers, housewives, and students. The one originally used in the Health Insurance Experiment distinguished only three levels of limitations: no limitations, some limitations, and inability to perform role activity at all. The MOS role functioning scales take into account multiple roles. By including a variety of types of problems that people can have in their role functioning and by using a simple sum as our scoring method, we have increased the number of possible scale levels to eight for the role functioning due to physical health scale and four for the role functioning due to emotional problems scale. All possible scores were observed in these analyses.

MOS role functioning scales are also unique in that they allow for distinctions between limitations due to physical health problems and limitations due to emotional problems. The latter are sometimes missed in surveys that do not ask explicitly about limitations due to personal and emotional problems. Further work is needed to study the validity of these measures including studies of whether the two scales are more or less sensitive to change in health over time.

The internal-consistency reliabilities of the two scales are high (0.83 and 0.86); this level of reliability was achieved while enumerating a larger number of scale levels. Finally, incremental validity results (from the pilot study) suggest that these gains will translate into more precise tests of hypotheses.

In the future, we would further expand the sensitivity of our measures by using three or four response choices per limitation item rather than a yes/no format. For example, we could ask about the extent to which people experience each limitation (a lot, a little, not at all) or the proportion of time each was experienced.

By specifically asking about limitations "due to health," we may be missing some important limitations caused by treatments. It would be useful to determine if patients are experiencing additional limitations due to inconveniences of treatments or side effects of medications. However, patients commonly may not know if they are experiencing side effects or how to attribute limitations to an underlying illness or to side effects of treatment. To the extent that side effects are manifested in physical symptoms, we are probably detecting those limitations. However, it would be helpful to address this question empirically.

A tremendous amount of role dysfunction in the baseline sample of patients (who have either hypertension, diabetes, heart disease, or depression) was observed. Sixty-seven percent experienced at least some limitations due to physical health problems and 43% experienced at least some limitations due to emotional problems. The finding that 17% were completely unable to work due to health underscores the importance of better understanding the nature of these limitations and how to help patients with these conditions improve their functioning in these areas. An even stronger statement is made by the finding that 37%

of those who are presently not working are not working because of health. Are these patients unable to work because their health problems are very severe, their jobs demanding, or for other reasons? These are questions for future studies.

13. Pain Measures

Cathy D. Sherbourne

Definitions and Issues

Pain refers to subjective feelings of distress or discomfort experienced in various parts of the body and includes headaches, backaches, muscle pains, and joint pains. Pain has been defined by the International Association for the Study of Pain (IASP) as "an unpleasant sensory and emotional experience associated with actual or potential tissue damage or described in terms of such damage" (IASP, 1979). Pain is one of the most common complaints seen by physicians (Keefe, 1982). In many cases, pain is the result of an injury or a specific disease; however, some patients do complain of pain that has no obvious cause or that seems disproportionate to a disease or injury (Institute of Medicine, 1987). Psychosocial factors, which include social and cultural variables and physiologic conditions, all appear to play an important role in the experience of pain (Institute of Medicine, 1987).

Two basic issues in developing measures of pain—the most important dimensions of the pain experience to assess and the best way to measure selected dimensions of pain—were examined for the MOS. The important dimensions of pain were identified. Pain, a multidimensional concept, can be assessed in general or in terms of specific areas of the body that might be involved in a particular condition. Pain can be described in terms of location, intensity or severity, duration or persistence, frequency of occurrence, precipitating and aggravating factors, quality, and the amount of pain relief that can be obtained from various treatments and behaviors. Pain is often categorized as acute, meaning of recent onset or short duration, or chronic, meaning of at least several months' duration (Sternbach, 1978). Of all the dimensions of pain, intensity or severity is probably the most important and the most commonly assessed (McDowell and Newell, 1987).

In recent years, attention has focused on the assessment of the effects of pain. This more indirect approach asks how pain affects various activities (e.g., physical activities, work, sleep) and how pain affects emotions (e.g., distress, worry). This indirect approach has the advantage of eliminating an evaluation of a sensation by the subject. A disadvantage of this approach is that it may be difficult to specify pain reduction or other factors as the cause of a change in activities.

Theoretically, pain severity and functional impairment might be independent constructs. Some patients can function with pain; they do not allow the pain to interfere with their daily activities. Other patients evidence some degree of limitation due to pain. No clear relationship between the amount of tissue damage and the degree of pain or functional disability has been identified (Institute of Medicine, 1987). For those concerned with the return of the patient to normal functioning and the assessment of pain relief, it seems important to measure not only the intensity of the pain experience but the effects of pain on normal functional abilities.

Because pain is an internal sensation that cannot be directly observed or measured, its measurement depends on the subjective response of the person experiencing it (McDowell and Newell, 1987). No direct, objective way to measure pain exists at present (Institute of Medicine, 1987). No completely adequate measures of pain are available due to the difficulties of quantifying a complex, perceptual experience such as pain. Pain is measured by using subjective evaluations (self-reports) of the pain experience and through direct observation of the subject's nonverbal behaviors (e.g., observation of facial expressions, limitations in mobility). The accuracy and reliability of the latter approach is not well understood (Bradley, Prokop, Gentry, et al., 1981). Detailed overviews of pain measurement are numerous (Bradley, Prokop, Gentry, et al., 1981; Chapman, Casey, Dubner, et al., 1985; McDowell and Newell, 1987).

Two widely known instruments designed to measure pain, representative of the different approaches, are the McGill Pain Questionnaire (Melzack, 1975) and The Wisconsin Brief Pain Questionnaire (WBPQ) (Daut, Cleeland, and Flanery, 1983). The McGill Pain Questionnaire, an interviewer-assisted questionnaire, consists of three major classes of word descriptions: sensory, affective, and evaluative. The seventy-eight descriptors are used by patients to specify their own pain experience. Subjects are asked to circle one word in each of twenty classes that describes their present pain. One advantage of this approach is that patients appear grateful when provided words to describe their pain. Several problems include: the meaning of selected word descriptors might be misunderstood by respondents and the instructions can be difficult, especially when the items are self-administered.

The McGill Pain Questionnaire also contains items asking about things that relieve the pain, the overall intensity of the present pain, and descriptions of the intensity of pain at its worst and at its least. The questionnaire requires fifteen to twenty minutes to complete. A separate, revised pain assessment questionnaire for use in a pain clinic and a home recording card to record pain levels at home are also available. Both include questions regarding treatment for the pain, pain patterns, accompanying symptoms, and the effects of pain on various activities. There is support for the reliability and validity of the McGill Pain Questionnaire (Chapman, Casey, Dubner, et al., 1985).

The Wisconsin Brief Pain Questionnaire, a self-report instrument for assessing pain in cancer and other diseases, contains approximately nineteen pain-related questions which focus on pain frequency, severity, and the effects of pain. Patients who report pain during the past month are asked to rate their pain at its worst, usual pain, and present pain; to report medications received and percentage of relief provided by the medications; and to rate the degree to which pain interferes with mood, relations with other people, and other aspects of daily activities. The reliability of selected items in the questionnaire ranges from moderate to high based on test-retest studies. Validity studies showed that the percentage of patients taking medications increased with higher pain ratings. The correlation between pain ratings and ratings of interference with activities was moderately high. It appeared that ratings of pain at their worst rather than ratings of usual level of pain were more highly correlated with activity interference.

Aspects of the pain experience have been measured by a variety of other researchers. Although intensity is one of the most frequently measured aspects of pain, studies differ in terms of the way they measure it. Several basic methods have been used to assess intensity. A visual analogue scale asks respondents to mark the point along a straight line at which their experience of pain is represented. The ends of the line are anchored by extremes (e.g., no pain versus the worst pain imaginable). A numeric rating scale is similar, but places numbers (e.g., from 1 to 10) along the line. A graphic rating scale places descriptive terms (e.g., severe, mild) at selected intervals along the line. A verbal rating scale asks respondents to select one of four or five response categories that best describes the pain (mild, moderate, severe). Some claim that the visual analogue, numeric rating scales, and graphic rating scales might be more sensitive to changes in pain than are simple verbal rating scales. Experience suggests, however, that patients need to be shown how to use these kinds of scales. The advantage of the verbal rating scale is that it is simple for the patient to understand; however, it might not be as sensitive to change as a more continuous rating scale with more levels. Other disadvantages are that response scale descriptors mean different things to different people, and controversy exists about whether the intensity descriptors in verbal rating scales reflect equal intervals—that is, the difference between mild pain and moderate pain may not be the same as the difference between moderate pain and severe pain (Melzack and Torgerson, 1971; Ohnhaus and Adler, 1975).

One measurement issue is how to deal with the fact that patients might experience more than one pain during a given interval (e.g., back pain, headache, joint pain). Most studies deal with this issue by focusing on one type of pain (e.g., back pain) and asking respondents to describe their experience with regard to that particular pain. Other studies ask the same items for each different type of pain experienced. The difficulty with both approaches is that they do not deal well with patients with multiple chronic conditions, who are likely to experience a number of different types of pain. Asking questions about each type of pain is cumbersome and unrealistic in terms of questionnaire space constraints. One solution is to ask respondents who experience more than one pain to describe their feelings of pain in general.

Content and Measurement Strategy

The MOS focused on two basic dimensions of pain: severity in terms of intensity, frequency, and duration, and behavioral/mood effects. These dimensions of pain were chosen because they reflect both the sensory and the performance aspects of the pain experience.

A 12-item battery of pain items was constructed (see pages 374, 378, and 379 in the Appendix). Eight of the twelve items were adaptations from the WBPQ: the ratings of effects of pain and two intensity numeric rating scales about pain on average and pain at its worst. Three of the twelve items, verbal ratings of the frequency and duration of pain and a report about the number of days in which pain interfered with activities, were adapted from the Health Information Study Questionnaire (S. Kaplan and S. Greenfield, personal communication). Both numeric rating and verbal rating scales of the intensity pain dimension were used to provide different approaches to the measurement of this important pain component.

Table 13–1 presents a summary of the pain items grouped by hypothesized pain dimension (i.e., intensity, frequency, duration, and effects).

The verbal rating scale asked all respondents to indicate how much (none, very mild, mild, moderate, severe, very severe) bodily pain they generally experienced. This overall pain item was administered on the second page of the questionnaire. The remaining questions were asked later in the questionnaire only of those who reported experiencing some pain during the prior four weeks. A skip question, "Did you experience

Table 13–1 MOS Pain Items

Abbreviated Item Content	Item Variable Name	All Patients	Patients with Pain
Intensity			
Overall pain	PGLOB	x	
Pain on average	PINT2		x
Pain at its worst	PINT3		x
Frequency			
How often had pain	PFREQ		x
Duration			
How long pain lasted	PDUR		x
Effects			
Mood	PBEH1		x
Ability to walk about	PBEH2		x
Sleep	PBEH3		x
Normal work	PBEH4		x
Recreational activities	PBEH5		x
Life enjoyment	PBEH6		x
Days pain interfered	PDAYS		x

Note: All items referred to pain in the last 4 weeks. Only the overall pain item was asked of all respondents. The remaining items were completed only by respondents who reported that they had experienced some pain during the preceding 4-week interval, as assessed by a skip question (see text).

any bodily pain during the past 4 weeks?" reduced respondent burden by having patients experiencing no pain during the given time interval omit the remaining pain items. The numeric rating scales asked respondents to circle one number from 0 to 20 that best described their pain on the average and at its worst. The frequency item asked respondents how often (once or twice, a few times, fairly often, very often, every day or almost every day) they had pain or discomfort. The duration item asked how long (a few minutes, several minutes to an hour, several hours, a day or two, more than two days) pain that was experienced lasted. Respondents were asked to write in the number of days that pain interfered with things they usually did. The behavioral/mood effects items asked respondents to indicate how much (not at all, a little bit, moderately, quite a bit, and extremely) pain interfered with their mood, ability to walk or move about, sleep, normal work, recreational activities, and enjoyment of life. The focus was on current pain, defined as during the past four weeks, in order to be consistent with the recall period for other items in the questionnaire. This focus avoided problems associated with forgetfulness in longer recall periods. A disadvantage to the assessment of pain during only a four-week period, however, is that it does not allow for differentiation between chronic and acute pain. Respondents who experienced more than one pain in the last month were asked to describe their feelings of pain in general.

Construction and Evaluation of Measures

Analysis Plan Item frequency distributions were examined to assure adequate variability for purposes of scale construction and to begin to estimate the prevalence of pain in the MOS sample. By comparing the percentage missing on the numeric rating items and the verbal rating items, we could gain a sense of whether people had trouble with the numeric rating method. If people provided responses across all twenty levels of the numeric rating items, it was inferred that they basically understood the method. The correlation between the verbal rating scale and the two numeric rating items was examined to determine similarity.

Pearson product-moment correlations between pain measures and selected health measures were computed as a preliminary test of construct validity. Because pain measures have not typically been included as a component of large health batteries, little is known about the meaning of the scores in terms of their relationship with other aspects of health. Pain was expected to be related to a variety of health constructs symptomatic of underlying physical health problems, such as general symptoms, physical functioning, role limitations caused by physical health problems, and mental health problems, although the strength of the relationship with mental health problems was expected to be weaker than with physical health problems. Pain was expected to be least correlated with less immediate health problems such as perceptions of prior health, health outlook, resistance to illness, health concern, and sexual problems.

Because the respondents who experienced no pain were asked to skip the pain items, their missing scores for these items were recoded to a "no pain" response before constructing scales and performing correlational analyses. Scaling analyses, however, were conducted only on those patients who had experienced some pain during the prior four weeks.

Item Variability Item variability, summarized in Table 13–2, was adequate for purposes of scaling analyses. There is a substantial amount of pain experienced by these patients, as indicated by the item responses. On the overall pain item, approximately 78% of the PAQ baseline sample reported they experienced some pain during the preceding four-week period. Thirty-one percent reported moderate to very severe pain.

For items in the pain battery, 71% of the sample reported experiencing some pain in the preceding four-week period based on the skip item and thus responded to the remaining items in the battery. Of those persons with pain, 16% had had pain or discomfort once or twice, 34% a few times, 22% fairly often, 8% very often, and 20% every day or almost every day. For the majority of people, pain interfered at least a little bit with their mood, sleep, normal work, recreational activities, enjoyment of life, and ability to walk or move about. Pain interfered with activities on one or more days for 60% of the sample. Frequency distributions for the two numeric rating scales were fairly evenly distributed across the scales, which ranged from 0 to 20. A slight tendency for respondents to round off to the middle category (10) occurred. The mean score of average pain was 6.59 (SD = 4.83), while the mean score of pain at its worst was 9.03 (SD = 5.87).

The percentage missing for those who should have responded to the items ranged from 2% to 5% across items. The percentage missing the verbal rating item as opposed to the two numeric rating items was comparable, 4% versus 5% and 5% respectively.

Table 13–2 Percentage Distribution of Pain Items: PAQ Baseline Sample ($N = 3,053$)

Abbreviated Item Content	Item Variable Name	Response Choice[a]	ITEM RESPONSE[b]						% of Total Missing
			1	2	3	4	5	6	
Overall Pain	PGLOB	NV	22	26	20	24	6	1	4.0
How often had pain	PFREQ	OE	16	34	22	8	20	—	1.5
How long pain lasts	PDUR	AM	20	23	19	13	24	—	2.6
Interferes with mood	PBEH1	NE	33	38	16	11	2	—	4.6
Interferes ability walk	PBEH2	NE	40	29	26	11	4	—	3.7
Interferes sleep	PBEH3	NE	42	28	15	11	4	—	4.1
Interferes normal work	PBEH4	NE	38	31	15	12	4	—	4.0
Interferes recreation	PBEH5	NE	37	29	14	13	7	—	4.1
Interferes life enjoyment	PBEH6	NE	38	32	14	11	4	—	3.6

Days Pain Interfered		%	Pain on Average		%	Pain at its Worst		%
None	0	40	No Pain	0	6	No Pain	0	6
	1	3		1	7		1	4
	2	7		2	9		2	5
	3	5		3	10		3	6
	4	4		4	8		4	6
	5	5		5	12		5	8
	6	2		6	5		6	4
	7	2		7	6		7	4
	8	2		8	5		8	5
	9	<1		9	3		9	2
	10	6		10	10		10	13
	11	<1		11	2		11	2
	12	1		12	4		12	5
	13	<1		13	1		13	2
	14	3		14	2		14	3
	15	3		15	4		15	7
	16	<1		16	1		16	3
	17	<1		17	1		17	2

Table 13–2 *(Cont.)*

Days Pain Interfered			Pain on Average			Pain at its Worst		
	%			%			%	
None	18	<1	No Pain	18	1	No Pain	18	3
	19	<1		19	<1		19	1
	20+	14		20	2		20	6

ᵃNV: 1–none; 2–very mild; 3–mild; 4–moderate; 5–severe; 6–very severe. OE: 1–once or twice; 2–a few times; 3–fairly often; 4–very often; 5–every day or almost every day. AM: 1–a few minutes; 2–several minutes to an hour; 3–several hours; 4–a day or two; 5–more than two days. NE: 1–not at all; 2–a little bit; 3–moderately; 4–quite a bit; 5–extremely.
ᵇPercentage of those who responded to each item.

Scale Construction A principal components factor analysis was undertaken to see whether subscales could be scored. Two factors were rotated to orthogonal structure to facilitate their interpretation. The first factor contained high loadings for the six behavioral/mood effects items, while the second factor contained high loadings for the pain severity items, which reflected intensity, duration, and frequency. The item pertaining to number of days in which pain interfered loaded equally on both factors. Results suggest that three independent pain measures could be constructed: the effects of pain, the overall severity of pain, and the number of days pain interfered.

These three hypothesized measures were then evaluated using multi-trait scaling techniques. The multitrait correlation matrix for the twelve items, grouped according to the three hypothesized subscales, is presented in Table 13–3. In this matrix, row entries represent correlations between each item and the sum of the items in each scale grouping. The items hypothesized to measure severity were first standardized due to the different number of response levels in each item.

For the two multi-item subscales, effects of pain (PBEH) and pain severity (PINT), all of the items correlated 0.57 or greater with their hypothesized scale, thus exceeding our stringent criterion of 0.40. All items met the MOS criterion of item discrimination, that is, they correlated higher by two standard errors with their own scale than with the other pain scales.

To determine if an overall index could be scored, the MOS evaluated whether a general underlying factor could be identified using factor analysis. All twelve pain items showed high loadings on the first

Table 13–3 Item-Scale Correlation Matrix, Pain: PAQ Baseline Sample (N = 2,190)

Item	Mean	SD	PBEH	PINT	DAYS
PBEH1	2.11	1.04	.70[a]	.53	.48
PBEH2	2.10	1.16	.69[a]	.56	.52
PBEH3	2.06	1.16	.66[a]	.54	.48
PBEH4	2.11	1.17	.84[a]	.64	.63
PBEH5	2.24	1.25	.81[a]	.60	.61
PBEH6	2.13	1.17	.78[a]	.56	.57
PGLOB	−0.00	1.00	.57	.61[a]	.49
PINT2	0.00	1.00	.68	.77[a]	.60
PINT3	−0.00	1.00	.64	.74[a]	.53
PFREQ	−0.00	1.00	.47	.67[a]	.51
PDUR	−0.00	1.00	.40	.57[a]	.36
PDAYS	7.61	8.80	.66	.63	n.a.

Note: Standard error of correlation = 0.02. PBEH = Effects of pain; PINT = Pain severity; DAYS = Days pain interfered. N.a. = not applicable.
[a] Denotes hypothesized item groupings and item-scale correlations corrected for overlap.

unrotated component, supporting the construction of an overall pain index. Loadings ranged from 0.53 to 0.84. Multitrait scaling analyses confirmed these findings.

Scoring Rules A summary of the final pain measures is presented in Table 13–4, including item groupings and item names. In scoring the pain measures, a high score indicates more pain or more negative effects of pain. No reversing of raw items is required (i.e., all original items were in the direction of a higher score indicating more pain). A behavioral/mood effects of pain measure was scored by averaging across the six effects items. Because item variances for these six items were generally comparable, it was not necessary to standardize or weight items before they were summed. The resulting raw score ranged from 1 to 5. All persons who skipped the pain battery because they had experienced no pain during the past four weeks were given a score of 1 (no interference) on the effects of pain measure. For those who should not have skipped the battery, a missing value was assigned if more than three items were missing. The score was transformed to a 0–100 scale.

A pain severity scale was constructed by averaging the ratings of five items: pain on average, pain at its worst, pain frequency, pain duration, and the overall pain item. Because these five items had different

Table 13–4 Content and Scoring of Pain Measures

Scale/Item Grouping	Item Variable Name	SCALES PBEH	SCALES PINT	SCALES DAYS	Index
Number of Items		6	5	1	12
Effects of Pain					
Mood	PBEH1	NR			NR
Ability to walk about	PBEH2	NR			NR
Sleep	PBEH3	NR			NR
Normal work	PBEH4	NR			NR
Recreational activities	PBEH5	NR			NR
Life enjoyment	PBEH6	NR			NR
Pain Severity					
Global pain	PGLOB		NR		NR
Pain on average	PINT2		NR		NR
Pain at its worst	PINT3		NR		NR
How often had pain	PFREQ		NR		NR
How long pain lasted	PDUR		NR		NR
Days Pain Interfered	PDAYS			NR	NR

Note: NR = Not reversed before combining.

numbers of response choices, items were first standardized to a mean of zero and a standard deviation of one. Before items were standardized, all persons who skipped the pain battery because they had experienced no pain during the past four weeks were given a score of zero for the four items included in the main battery. The overall pain item, which was also included in this scale, was answered by everyone; therefore, no adjustments were made to this item. For those who should not have skipped the battery, a missing value was assigned if more than two of the remaining four items were missing.

An overall pain index was constructed by averaging all twelve pain items with scores of zero or one added as indicated above for people who skipped the battery. Because items had different numbers of response choices, and hence item variances differed across these items, it was necessary to standardize each item to a mean of zero and a standard deviation of one before computing the average score. For those who should not have skipped the battery, a missing value was assigned if more than six items were missing.

The number of days on which pain interfered with the patient's activities was scored as a single-item continuous measure that ranged from 0 to 28.

Characteristics of Measures

Descriptive Statistics Table 13–5 presents descriptive statistics for the measures of pain. The percentage missing a pain measure ranged from a low of 1.9 to a high of 4.7. The percentage receiving a nonperfect score in the total sample, meaning the presence of pain or effects of pain, ranged from 85% for the pain index and pain severity to 45% for the scale for the days pain interfered. For only those patients reporting some pain, the percentage receiving a nonperfect score ranged from 100% to 64% for the same measures respectively.

Variability The effects of pain and pain severity measures were both skewed, with people tending to report less severe interference of pain with their behavior and mood and less severe pain intensity. The measure of days pain interfered was also skewed with people tending to report fewer days on which pain was experienced.

Reliability Internal-consistency reliability coefficients for the two multi-item pain scales and the pain index are shown in Table 13–5. Internal-consistency reliability estimates are high for all three measures. Examination of the consistency of responses to the skip question (yes

Table 13–5 Descriptive Statistics and Reliability Coefficients for Pain Measures: PAQ Baseline Sample (N = 3,053)

Scale[a]	k	Mean	SD	Total Sample	With Pain	Observed Range	% Missing	Reli- ability
				% WITH NONPERFECT SCORE				
Effects of pain	6	22.0	24.3	68	92	0–100	3.4	.91
Pain severity	5	0.0	0.9	85	100	−1.17–2.26	1.9	.86
Days pain interfered	1	5.1	8.2	45	64	0–28	4.7	.78[b]
Pain index	12	0.0	0.8	85	100	−0.93–2.52	2.9	.93

[a] A high score indicates more pain or more effects of pain.
[b] Alternate forms reliability.

or no, pain was experienced) and the overall pain item (the degree of bodily pain experienced during the past four weeks) showed that 85% of the respondents answered consistently, indicating yes or some degree of pain to both questions or no, no pain to both questions. Fifteen percent had inconsistent responses (i.e., they answered yes to one and no to the other).

Validity Correlations relevant to the construct validity of the pain measures are presented below. Table 13–6 presents correlations among the pain measures. Correlations for nonoverlapping measures are strong, ranging from 0.68 to 0.79. Correlations are strongest ($r > 0.95$) between the subscales and the index, as expected due to overlapping items. The verbal rating item correlated 0.66 with the numeric rating item pertaining to average pain and 0.62 with the numeric rating item pertaining to pain at its worst (results not shown).

Table 13–7 presents correlations between the pain measures and selected validity variables. As expected, the pain measures are highly related to many of the health measures. Pain measures are most highly related to physical/psychophysiologic symptoms, physical functioning, role limitations due to physical problems, current health, and health distress and least related to measures of prior health, health outlook, health concern, and sexual problems.

Resolution of Issues and Future Directions

Using only twelve items, the MOS empirically developed measures of three fairly independent aspects of pain: severity, behavioral/mood effects of pain, and the number of days pain interfered with activities. An overall index can be scored that summarizes all three components. This battery of pain items appears to be simple to use and requires no

Table 13–6 Correlations among Pain Measures

	PBEH	PINT	INDEX	DAYS
Effects of pain (PBEH)	(.91)			
Pain severity (PINT)	.79	(.86)		
Pain index (INDEX)	.95[a]	.93[a]	(.93)	
Days pain interfered (DAYS)	.71	.68	.78	—

[a] Coefficients are inflated due to item overlap. Internal consistency reliability on the diagonal.

Table 13-7 Correlations between Pain Measures and Selected Validity Variables

Validity Variables[a]	Effects of Pain (−)	Pain Severity (−)	Days Pain Interfered (−)	Pain Index (−)
Physical/ psychophysiologic symptoms (−)	.63	.66	.52	.68
Physical functioning (+)	−.54	−.47	−.48	−.54
Role limitations/ physical (−)	.66	.56	.54	.65
Role limitations/ emotional (−)	.39	.28	.30	.36
Sleep disturbance (−)	.44	.36	.34	.43
Cognitive functioning (+)	−.40	−.29	−.28	−.37
Psychological distress (−)	.45	.33	.30	.41
Psychological well-being (+)	−.40	−.29	−.27	−.37
Current health (+)	−.58	−.51	−.46	−.58
Health distress (−)	.57	.43	.44	.54
Prior health (+)	−.29	−.27	−.21	−.29
Health outlook (+)	−.28	−.22	−.20	−.27
Resistance to illness (+)	−.33	−.30	−.23	−.33
Health concern (−)	.23	.17	.18	.22
Sexual problems (−)	.20	.15	.14	.19

Note: N ranged from 2,577 to 2,997 due to missing data. All coefficients are significant at $p < .001$.
[a] A (−) high score indicates poorer health; a (+) high score indicates better health.

special instructions other than asking subjects to generalize their pain experiences across all types of pain that they experienced during a four-week period.

Generally, results were very encouraging. The multi-item scales exhibited excellent reliability (internal-consistency reliabilities of 0.83 and greater). The items in the MOS severity and behavioral/mood effects subscales discriminated well from one another, supporting the distinction of these two pain constructs, as hypothesized. Preliminary tests of the construct validity of these pain measures confirm hypotheses about their relationship with other measures of health.

Two methods—numeric rating scales and verbal rating scales—were used to measure pain intensity with the goal of increasing the sensitivity of the severity measure (to facilitate detection of change in the sensation of pain over time). Patients appeared to have no difficulty using the numeric rating scales, as evidenced by the spread of responses across scale levels and by the low percentage of missing values on these items. The correlation between the verbal rating scale and each of the numeric rating scales was substantial ($r = 0.68$ and 0.64 with pain on average and pain at worst respectively) but not extremely high. The predictive validity of one method over another remains to be studied.

More study is needed on what respondents mean when describing pain in general and how these more general ratings compare to measures of specific types of pain (e.g., chest pain or headaches). Given additional resources (i.e., more questionnaire space), an attempt should be made to characterize the pain experience more fully by focusing on specific types of pain. Pain relief (e.g., how much relief pain treatments provide) might also be measured to see how reliably the respondent can evaluate the effectiveness of specific treatments for pain and to see how pain relief relates to more general measures of pain severity and behavioral/mood effects.

14. Sleep Measures

Ron D. Hays and Anita L. Stewart

Definition and Issues

Sleep is defined as a suspension of normal waking consciousness that involves a diminished capacity for interaction with one's environment (Birrell, 1983). A person spends nearly one-third of life asleep or trying to sleep. Sleep is critical to homeostasis and is an important element of functioning and well-being.

Sleep has been excluded from most health status batteries. Of seven health status batteries that are somewhat comprehensive in their definition of health (Bergner, Bobbitt, Carter, and Gilson, 1981; Brook, Ware, Davies-Avery, et al., 1979; Chambers, MacDonald, Tugwell, et al., 1982; Hunt, McKenna, McEwen, et al., 1981; Jette, Davies, Cleary, et al., 1986; Parkerson, Gehlbach, Wagner, et al., 1981; Patrick, Bush, and Chen, 1973a), only one included sleep problems as a component (Bergner, Bobbitt, Carter, and Gilson, 1981).

Sleep is in part a health practice or risk factor and in part an indicator of health status. The extent to which people make an effort to get enough sleep and regulate their sleep schedule reflects sleep as a health practice. For this reason, the quantity of sleep has often been considered a health-related behavior. For example, in the Alameda County Study, the number of hours of sleep was combined with six other health practices to predict subsequent health and mortality (Belloc, 1973; Berkman and Breslow, 1983). However, the disruption of sleep, which can affect the quantity of sleep, might be outside of a person's control and indicative of physical and mental health problems.

The theoretical dimensions of sleep have been defined by others. The

American Psychiatric Association's *Diagnostic and Statistical Manual of Mental Disorders* DSM-III (American Psychiatric Association, 1980), identifies four sleep disorders: (1) disorders of initiating and maintaining sleep, (2) disorders of excessive somnolence or drowsiness, (3) disorders of the sleep-wake schedule, and (4) disorders related to sleep stages or partial arousals like sleepwalking and nightmares. Nine components of sleep are reflected in existing measures (Bergner, Bobbitt, Carter, and Gilson, 1981; Cernovsky, 1984; Ellis, Johns, Lancaster, et al., 1981; Eisenstadt and Schoenborn, 1980; Simonds and Parraga, 1982, 1984; Snyder-Halpern and Verran, 1987) and in various clinical studies (e.g., Morewitz, 1988). These dimensions are summarized in Table 14–1.

Although different dimensions of sleep were hypothesized in these studies, little information existed about whether these dimensions were empirically distinct and could be scored and interpreted separately. Two studies attempted to evaluate the dimensionality, but neither included the full range of dimensions (Johns, 1975a, 1975b; Snyder-Halpern and Verran, 1987). Evidence of commonality between sleep initiation and sleep maintenance is shown in some samples (Johns, 1975a; Johns, Egan, et al., 1970), but notable distinctiveness in these aspects of sleep is shown in other samples (Johns, 1975a, 1975b; Johns, Egan, et al., 1971). It is also possible that measures of quantity of sleep and perceived adequacy assess the same underlying concept and do not warrant different interpretations. One important goal of the MOS, therefore, was to develop measures of important dimensions of sleep and to test empirically whether the concepts were sufficiently distinct so that they could be scored separately.

Sleep is associated with clinical status and other health indicators. Sleep problems are prevalent, even in general populations (Bixler, Kales, Soldatos, et al., 1979; Kales, Soldatos, and Kales, 1987; Karacan, Thornby, Anch, et al., 1976; Lamberg, 1985; Mellinger, Balter, and Uhlenhuth, 1985), and they are significantly related to self-rated health status (Urponen, Vuori, Hasan, et al., 1988). Sleep problems have been linked with depression (Bixler, Kales, Soldatos, et al., 1979; Mellinger, Balter, and Uhlenhuth, 1985), distress (Mellinger, Balter, and Uhlenhuth, 1985), impaired social/role functioning (Kales, Caldwell, Cadieux, et al., 1985), hospitalizations (Kales, Caldwell, Cadieux, et al., 1985), chronic conditions (Kales, Bixler, Cadieux, et al., 1984; Mellinger, Balter, and Uhlenhuth, 1985), and mortality (Kripke, Simons, Garfinkle, et al., 1979; Wingard and Berkman, 1983).

Table 14–1 Dimensions of Sleep Identified in Literature Review

Initiation	Time required to fall asleep; problems with initiation identify sleep onset insomnia
Maintenance	Ability to stay asleep; restlessness, movement, tenseness, and associated awakenings, and having trouble getting back to sleep are commonly used as indicators of inability to maintain sleep and therefore serve to identify sleep maintenance insomnia
Quantity	The number of hours of sleep per night
Perceived adequacy	Subjective evaluation of sufficiency of sleep in terms of amount and restoration; perception of getting enough sleep
Somnolence	Daytime drowsiness or excessive daytime sleepiness
Respiratory impairments	Breathing difficulties during sleep such as shortness of breath and snoring; sleep apnea[a] is a common respiratory problem
Regularity	Extent to which sleep onset and arising are consistent from day to day; regularity of onset probably reflects sleep as a health-related behavior more than as a health indicator per se; regularity of arising may reflect the external demands of the person's life situation as well
Sleep stage disorders	Sleepwalking, nightmares, enuresis (bedwetting), bruxism (teeth grinding while asleep)
Use of sleep medications	Use of tranquilizers or other medications intended to facilitate sleep

[a] Sleep apnea is defined clinically as the cessation of breathing for 10 seconds or more for a total of 30 or more times during 7 hours of sleep (Kales, Vela-Bueno, and Kales, 1987).

Problems with sleep initiation and sleep maintenance, which are symptomatic of a variety of medical and mental conditions, are the most commonly encountered sleep disorders in medical practice (Kales, Soldatos, and Kales, 1987). Sleep maintenance insomnia can impair daytime functioning (Coates and Thoresen, 1984) and is also a classic symptom of depression (Mead, 1974). Data from the 1979 National Survey of Psychotherapeutic Drug Use revealed that insomnia, defined as sleep onset or maintenance problems, was associated with distress, somatic anxiety, symptoms of major depression, and multiple health problems (Mellinger, Balter, and Uhlenhuth, 1985). Johns, Bruce, and Masterton (1974) reported that sleep onset delay was significantly correlated with MMPI-measured depression ($r = 0.25$) in a sample of medical students. Recent observations on new cases of overt ischemic heart disease during a three-year period showed that subjects who reported severe sleep disturbances during their last interview were at higher risk of developing a first lethal or nonlethal acute myocardial infarction within two subsequent years than were those with normal sleep (Siegrist, 1987).

The quantity of sleep is related to health status in a nonlinear way, with seven or eight hours per night appearing optimal. In one study, individuals reporting eight hours of sleep were healthier in terms of a summary measure of disability, symptoms, and chronic conditions than those sleeping more or less than eight hours (Reed, 1983). In the Alameda County study, those reporting seven or eight hours of sleep per night in 1965 had a lower mortality risk in 1974 than those reporting more or fewer hours of sleep (Wiley and Camacho, 1980). The relative mortality risk associated with those sleeping less than or more than seven or eight hours per night was 1.3 times or 30% higher than that for those sleeping seven or eight hours per night, after controlling for age, gender, race, socioeconomic status, physical health status, smoking history, physical inactivity, alcohol consumption, weight, use of health services, social networks, and life satisfaction (Wingard and Berkman, 1983). Data from a prospective American Cancer Society study indicated that self-reported sleep of less than five hours or more than nine hours was about as predictive of six-year mortality as were reports of having diabetes, hypertension, heart disease, or stroke (Kripke, Simons, Garfinkle, et al., 1979). Thus, hours of sleep and health outcomes are related quadratically, with better outcomes found for intermediate amounts of sleep. Sleep deprivation has substantial negative effects on mood and performance (Angus, Heslegrave, and Myles, 1985; Knab and Engel-Sittenfeld, 1983). The effects of sleep deprivation differ by age, health, and neuropsychiatric disease, with recovery from such deprivation more prolonged among the elderly and less healthy than among younger, healthier persons (Reynolds, Kupfer, Hoch, et al., 1987). In the National Health Interview survey, an association between hours of sleep and health care utilization has been established; those sleeping seven or eight hours per night made fewer doctors visits and spent fewer days in the hospital than those sleeping a lesser or greater number of hours (Wetzler and Cruess, 1975).

Perceived adequacy of sleep was significantly related to depression, hypochondriasis, paranoia, and schizophrenia (Johns, Bruce, and Masterton, 1974). Somnolence, or excessive daytime sleepiness, has been linked with a variety of underlying conditions in the elderly, including endocrine or metabolic disorders, neurological disorders, and others (Morewitz, 1988).

Patients with severe sleep apnea, defined by the investigators as a history of snoring, excessive daytime sleepiness, sleep attacks, nocturnal snoring and gasping sounds, and nocturnal breath cessations were somatic-depressive, according to the MMPI and SCL-90-R (Kales, Caldwell, Cadieux, et al., 1985). Most of the depression involved feelings of physical vulnerability. A significant relationship between depressive symptoms, measured by the Geriatric Depression Scale, and sleep-related respiratory disturbance, defined by the number of apneic and hypopneic events per hour of sleep, has been observed among elderly males but not among elderly females (Bliwise, Yesavage, Sink, et al., 1986). Other studies have shown that sleep apnea and hypertension are related (Kales, Vela-Bueno, and Kales, 1987; Lavie, Ben-Yosef, and Rubin, 1984), and that habitual snoring is associated with cerebral infarction (Partinen and Palomaki, 1985), hypertension (Koskenvuo, Kaprio, Partinen, et al., 1985; Lugaresi, Cirignotta, Coccagna, et al., 1980), and angina pectoris in men (Koskenvuo, Kaprio, Partinen, et al., 1985). In another study, sleep apnea was more common among patients with Alzheimer's dementia (42.9%) than among patients with unipolar, nondelusional major depression (17.6%) and healthy elderly control subjects (4.3%) (Reynolds, Kupfer, Taska, et al., 1985).

Use of sleep medications is rarely assessed (Carskadon, Dement, Mitler, et al., 1976). Information about medication usage is important because "well over half of any large population of individuals who complain of insomnia are likely to be using one or more sedative drugs on a daily basis" (Carskadon, Dement, Mitler, et al., 1976). Propanolol, a beta-blocker, has been linked with positive results in treating narcolepsy, but has detrimental effects with respect to sleep apnea and is a cause of restlessness during sleep and increased wakefulness (Rosen and Kostis, 1985).

Many challenges confront those measuring sleep, but one of the more important concerns is the source of information used to assess sleep. Self-reports and laboratory or objective measures have served as the primary sources of sleep information. But consistent differences between self-reports and laboratory observations have been observed (Birrell, 1983; Carskadon, Dement, Mitler, et al., 1976; Coates, Killen, George, et al., 1982; Lewis, 1969). Self-reports are generally faulted for this lack of convergence; failure of memory is cited as a major limitation of self-reported information. Despite these criticisms, disturbed sleep as reported by the individual is the basis upon which millions of prescriptions for hypnotic drugs are written each year (Johns, 1975a).

Significant correlations between indicators of the same aspect of sleep measured by different methods have been reported (e.g., $r = 0.56$ between subjective and objective estimates of sleep onset delay; Johns, 1975b), and subjective reports may be accurate to within a few minutes for information such as sleep onset and quantity of sleep (Johns, 1971). Self-reports can provide "more reliable information about certain aspects of sleep at home than do detailed EEG studies in the sleep laboratory, which tend to make sleep more disturbed than usual" (Johns, 1971). Responses to a sleep questionnaire provide information which electronic monitoring methods cannot easily provide, such as the usual time a person goes to bed at night and gets up the next morning, the number of times a person dozes during the day, the frequency of taking sleeping pills, and the adequacy of sleep (Johns, 1975b; Johns, Gay, et al., 1971).

The sleep battery developed by Simonds and Parraga (1982, 1984), consisting of questions about the frequency from "daily" to "less than once a month" of twenty-six sleep-related behaviors, is the most comprehensive self-report measure, assessing eight of the nine concepts identified in Table 14–1. However, the Simonds and Parraga questionnaire consists of over forty items and is constructed to enable parents to report on their children's sleep. Because of its length and its focus on proxy reports of the sleep problems of children and not adults, it could not be adopted for the MOS but was helpful in structuring MOS measures.

No other comprehensive battery is available. The St. Mary's Hospital sleep questionnaire is limited to quantity, adequacy, and disturbance (Ellis, Johns, Lancaster, et al., 1981). The RAND Health Insurance Experiment (HIE) included single items to measure quantity of sleep, sleep onset, and use of sleeping pills. The National Survey of Personal Health Practices and Consequences (Eisenstadt and Schoenborn, 1980) included a quantity of sleep item similar to the HIE. The Sickness Impact Profile (SIP) developed by Bergner, Bobbitt, Carter, and Gilson (1981) has a 7-item sleep and rest scale that includes items pertaining to somnolence and maintenance. Cernovsky (1984) asked respondents about their nightmare frequency, dream frequency, and several questions about dreams and nightmare content. In addition, four questions about the incidence of insomnia and related disorders are included. The

Verran and Snyder-Halpern (vsh) Sleep Scale (Snyder-Halpern and Verran, 1987) is a visual analogue instrument consisting of ten analogue lines for each of eight items: midsleep awakenings, movement during sleep, total sleep period, sleep latency, soundness of sleep, rest upon awakening, method of awakening, and subjective quality of sleep.

Most studies present results for their sleep measures without providing information about reliability and validity. Two studies provide reliability estimates. Test-retest correlations for the items in the St. Mary's Hospital questionnaire were found to be acceptable in a sample of medical inpatients, psychiatric inpatients, surgical inpatients, and normal volunteers (Ellis, Johns, Lancaster, et al., 1981). An estimate of scale reliability was also given for the vsh. Because the vsh items are hypothesized to be indicators of sleep adequacy, Snyder-Halpern and Verran computed theta reliability for the items. They found the reliability of the vsh to be acceptable (theta = 0.82), supporting the existence of a large general factor of sleep adequacy (Armor, 1974).

Content and Measurement Strategy

Pilot Studies The basic strategy in developing the mos measures of sleep was to build a set of measures conforming to eight of the theoretical dimensions. Sleep stage disorders (e.g., nightmares) were excluded because such measures are expected to be less reflective of health status than the other concepts in the sleep battery.

Two pilot studies were conducted, which consisted primarily of adults visiting physicians in a medical clinic in an academic setting and in a rural health clinic. Seven dimensions of sleep were represented in the first pilot study battery. Respiratory impairments were included only in the second pilot study. The purposes of the pilot studies were to assess the hypothesized item groupings, especially in terms of whether sleep initiation and maintenance could be scored separately, and to identify the smallest number of items necessary to assess the independent dimensions.

A battery of sleep items was compiled that represented a synthesis of previous measures and the addition of some new items. The mos selected items for the initial item pool from existing measures to the extent possible, primarily from the sleep measures used in research reported by Simonds and Parraga (1982, 1984), Cernovsky (1984), and the HIE (Brook, Ware, Davies-Avery, et al., 1979).

Eight conclusions resulted from the pilot study regarding each sleep construct. Two items, sleep initiation and sleep maintenance, could not be distinguished as independent constructs in either pilot study, even though prior research suggested they were independent (Johns, 1975a, 1975b; Johns, Gay, et al., 1971). It appears that a single construct of sleep disturbance will prevail. However, because of their theoretical distinction, two items for initiation and two for maintenance, which allows an adequate representation of each construct, were retained. The MOS evaluated their distinctiveness again in the main study sample. Two perceived adequacy items, "enough sleep to feel rested" and "got amount of sleep you need," were tested in both pilot studies. These two items had an internal-consistency reliability of 0.84 and 0.71 in the two studies.

Three somnolence items were tested in the first pilot and four in the second. The addition of the fourth item proved not useful; thus, the best measure is the three original items, which have an internal-consistency reliability of 0.65 in both pilots. It is of special importance that the somnolence items define a cluster distinct from the energy/fatigue measure because of their conceptual similarity. In the first pilot, all items met the criterion of item discrimination with the energy/fatigue scale. In the second pilot, however, the somnolence items correlated almost as high with energy/fatigue as they did with the somnolence scale, corrected for item overlap. Because of the success of this scale in the first pilot and because the standard error of the correlation is very high in the second pilot study, due to a small sample size, the MOS decided to retain these items in the final somnolence scale, pending evaluation in the main MOS sample. Respiratory problems, defined in terms of snoring and shortness of breath, were assessed only in the second pilot study. Those results indicate that these might need to be scored separately. Both items were retained.

Sleep-wake schedules were fairly regular for respondents in both studies. Sleep onset was somewhat less regular than wake-up, which can be attributed to the fact that many people use an alarm clock to wake up in the morning or wake in response to external demands (e.g., children). The percentage reporting regularity was greater when items were worded to ask whether they went to sleep "within one hour of the same time." The two regularity items had an internal-consistency reliability of 0.72 and 0.82 in the first and second pilot studies.

In the first pilot, the MOS asked separately about use of sleeping pills and use of tranquilizers, sedatives, or nerve pills. These items were empirically indistinguishable and had a high internal-consistency reliability (alpha = 0.83). Because of the high correlations between these two sleep medications items in the first pilot, the MOS asked about the use of prescribed as well as over-the-counter medications in the second pilot study. Separate scores for these could be constructed in the second pilot study.

Correlational and factor analyses indicated that quantity and perceived adequacy are highly interrelated. However, multitrait scaling analyses indicated that the two concepts can be scored separately if extremely stringent criteria are not applied.

Because the two concepts are theoretically distinct—quantity is relatively objective and adequacy reflects personal values—it is preferable to maintain their separation. Empirical evidence that the two concepts could be distinguished was provided by the fact that these two measures manifested different patterns of correlations with the validity variables in both pilot studies. Based on all of these considerations, we decided to maintain them as distinct concepts and further test their independence in the main study.

Final Items The final sleep battery consists of twelve items which assess the following constructs: initiation (2 items), maintenance (2 items), respiratory problems (2 items), quantity (1 item), perceived adequacy (2 items), and somnolence (3 items). Actual questionnaire items are shown on pages 399 and 400 in the Appendix.

Sleep regularity and use of sleep medications were determined empirically to be additional independent dimensions of sleep in the pilot studies and demonstrated adequate reliability. Respondent burden considerations, however, led us to eliminate these two concepts from the final battery. We eliminated the sleep regularity measure because we considered it to be less subject to change due to health care than some of the other sleep constructs. We eliminated the items concerning sleep medications because their use is indicative of other factors besides sleep problems (e.g., willingness to take medications) and because we assessed these during the health examination.

Respondents were asked to report the actual number of hours of sleep obtained each night during the past four weeks. Response choices for the remaining items were framed in terms of the amount of time during the past four weeks the particular item was true. Six choices were offered ranging from all of the time to none of the time. For one item, "how long did it usually take to fall asleep?" five response choices were offered ranging from 0–15 minutes to more than 60 minutes.

Construction and Evaluation of Measures

Analysis Plan The goals of the analysis were (1) to construct measures of the six hypothesized sleep constructs (subscales); (2) to determine whether or not a dichotomous measure of "optimal" sleep could be justifiably scored from the quantity of sleep measure; (3) to construct an overall sleep index that summarized information across all of the constructs; (4) to construct a short-form sleep index that could be used in more constrained surveys; and (5) to perform preliminary validity studies of the measures.

In constructing measures of the separate constructs, several issues were of interest: (1) whether sleep initiation and sleep maintenance could be distinguished as independent constructs (although they have been hypothesized by some as independent, the two pilot studies indicated they are not); (2) whether the two respiratory symptoms items could be combined into a single scale (in the pilots, they could not); (3) whether sleep quantity and sleep adequacy could be scored and interpreted separately (in the pilot studies, they were highly intercorrelated); and (4) whether a measure of somnolence could be constructed that was independent from energy/fatigue.

A series of multitrait analyses was performed to evaluate the hypothesized sleep constructs. The first analysis included six hypothesized sleep constructs: five multi-item scales, including separate scoring of initiation and maintenance, and one single-item measure. Because we wanted to construct the measures of sleep to be independent of other health concepts that might conceivably be related, several validity variables were included: energy/fatigue, anxiety, depression, positive affect, and socially desirable response set. The first four of these measures were included because of their conceptual similarity to sleep. Their inclusion provided a rigorous assessment of the discriminant validity of the sleep items. The measure of socially desirable response set (Hays, Hayashi, and Stewart, 1989) was included to evaluate possible self-report bias in the measures.

Because the relationship of quantity of sleep to other health outcomes was not always linear (Berkman and Breslow, 1983), an additional measure of "optimal" sleep was derived from the question about quantity of sleep. "Optimal" was defined as seven or eight hours based on the literature review. To confirm this cutpoint and test for alternates, mean current health perceptions and perceived adequacy scores were plotted for each category of hours of sleep.

For purposes of constructing an overall sleep index, the MOS considered including all twelve of the sleep items. Because it was thought that the quantity item might not be linearly related to the other items, we included the optimal sleep quantity measure instead. The items were standardized using a mean of 0 and a standard deviation of 1 because two of the items had a different number of response choices than the other ten. Multitrait scaling techniques and factor analysis were used to construct the index. The criterion for inclusion in the overall index was that items should correlate at least 0.30 with the index. We also wanted to represent each of the sleep constructs.

The goal in constructing a short-form index was to arrive at the best compromise between good scaling properties and representativeness of the universe of sleep content. Six items were selected from those in the long-form index. The MOS criteria were to include items with the highest item-scale correlations and to represent all constructs as evenly as possible, with a focus on sleep disturbance and sleep adequacy as representing the heart of the sleep problems concept. The selection was limited to the ten items with the same response format to facilitate short-form administration, using a grid-type format. Thus, the optimal sleep measure and one of the sleep initiation items were excluded from consideration. To select the six items for the short-form index, the content of the sleep items and the magnitude of their item-total correlations were examined simultaneously.

As a preliminary test of the validity of all of the sleep measures, the correlations among the sleep measures as well as correlations between the sleep measures and the other health measures were evaluated.

Item Variability Table 14-2 presents a summary of the sleep items, grouped by hypothesized constructs, and shows the frequency distributions for each item. The sleep items have fairly good distributions, in general, in the MOS sample. One item, awakening short of breath or with a headache, was notably skewed (skewness $= -1.8$), but this fact accurately reflects that this is relatively rare.

The modal respondent reported never having trouble falling asleep and being able to fall asleep within fifteen minutes, but the majority of respondents reported having some difficulty with sleep initiation. The sleep maintenance items displayed similar distributions to the sleep

Table 14–2 Percentage Distribution of Sleep Items: PAQ Baseline Sample (N = 3,053)

Abbreviated Item Content	Item Variable Name	Response Choice[a]	ITEM RESPONSE[b]						% of Total Missing
			1	2	3	4	5	6	
Initiation									
Trouble falling asleep	SLEEP1	AT	4.9	7.0	7.3	17.2	27.9	33.3	2.4
How long to fall asleep	SLEEP2	U	42.5	31.4	10.8	5.0	7.2	—	2.6
Maintenance									
Sleep was not quiet	SLEEP3	AT	3.3	9.7	11.4	18.9	30.6	23.1	3.0
Trouble falling asleep again	SLEEP4	AT	2.8	7.1	11.3	21.1	32.9	22.0	2.8
Respiratory									
Snore	SLEEP5	AT	5.5	8.0	6.7	20.2	21.6	28.3	9.6
Awaken short of breath or w/headache	SLEEP6	AT	1.0	2.6	4.2	10.1	17.0	62.5	2.8
Adequacy									
Feel rested in morning	SLEEP8	AT	8.9	37.8	14.5	18.6	12.0	5.6	2.6
Amount of sleep needed	SLEEP9	AT	10.9	42.3	12.1	16.1	9.7	6.0	3.0
Somnolence									
Drowsy during day	SLEEP10	AT	2.0	7.7	12.2	30.3	32.0	13.3	2.5
Trouble staying awake	SLEEP11	AT	0.9	2.2	5.0	16.0	31.6	41.2	3.1
Take naps	SLEEP12	AT	2.8	6.1	6.8	19.7	26.6	33.1	3.0
Quantity									
Hours sleep each night	SLEEP7	HR	10.8	24.4	30.2	22.4	5.6	2.8	3.0

[a] AT: 1–all of the time, 2–most of the time, 3–a good bit of the time, 4–some of the time, 5–a little of the time, 6–none of the time. U: 1-0–15 minutes, 2-16–30 minutes, 3-31–45 minutes, 4-46–60 minutes, 5-more than 60 minutes. HR: Open-ended response options recoded for this table to 1-5 or less hours, 2-6 hours, 3-7 hours, 4-8 hours, 5-9 hours, 6-10 or more hours.
[b] Percentage of those who responded to each item.

initiation items, although more people reported some maintenance problems.

Scale Construction In the first analysis, item-scale correlations provided support for scoring adequacy and somnolence. The scoring of sleep respiratory problems was not supported. The two sleep respiratory items correlated $r = 0.11$ with one another. This result is not surprising given the pilot study findings for similar items. Snoring and waking up with a headache appear to tap fairly independent aspects of sleep respiratory problems. The "how long it takes to fall asleep" item was analyzed with the sleep initiation scale as is rather than standardizing the items because its mean and standard deviation were comparable to the other item in the scale. Sleep initiation and maintenance items were not empirically distinguishable from one another, consistent with the pilot study results.

Based on these findings, the respiratory items were scored separately and the initiation and maintenance items were combined. A second multitrait analysis was performed with this respecification. Item-scale correlations for this second analysis are given in Table 14–3. The results in Table 14–3 are quite good, with the two sleep adequacy items intercorrelating 0.60. The sleep quantity item correlated only 0.36 with the sleep adequacy scale, indicating that these two constructs can be scored and interpreted separately. Item-scale correlations ranged from 0.60 to 0.79 for sleep disturbance and 0.50 to 0.69 for sleep somnolence. Correlations of the sleep items with their hypothesized scales were significantly higher than their correlations with scales measuring energy/fatigue, anxiety, depression/behavioral-emotional control, positive affect, and SDRS.

Table 14–4 presents the item-total correlations of the twelve sleep items after standardization. The quantity of sleep item, SLEEP7, was first scored dichotomously as optimal sleep (1 = 7 or 8 hours, 0 = all others). Mean scores on sleep adequacy, health distress, and current health perceptions by hours of sleep supported this dichotomous scoring scheme. Based on these results, we selected nine items for the overall sleep problems index: 1, 2, 3, 4, 6, 8, 9, 10, 11. The optimal sleep item correlated so weakly with the scale that it was eliminated and the analysis rerun. The conclusions reached in this additional analysis were identical to those of the original analysis. These nine items represent all sleep concepts except quantity and emphasize sleep disturbance.

Using the criteria outlined in the analysis plan, the six items listed in Table 14–5 were selected for the shorter index. SLEEP11 was selected

Table 14–3 Item-Scale Correlations, Sleep: Analysis #2 (N = 2,607)

Item	Mean	SD	SLPD	SLPSNR	SLPSOB	SLPQ
SLEEP1	2.36	1.43	.79a	.01	.34	−.32
SLEEP2	1.97	1.18	.66a	−.04	.29	−.32
SLEEP3	2.61	1.39	.60a	.11	.35	−.23
SLEEP4	2.52	1.28	.66a	.08	.36	−.31
SLEEP5	2.57	1.51	.05	n.a.	.07	−.07
SLEEP6	1.65	1.07	.41	.07	n.a.	−.17
SLEEP7	7.95	1.31	−.36	−.07	−.17	n.a.
SLEEP8	3.96	1.40	−.40	−.03	−.26	.24
SLEEP9	4.13	1.39	−.51	−.05	−.30	.41
SLEEP10	2.73	1.19	.39	.16	.35	−.13
SLEEP11	1.94	1.07	.34	.18	.31	−.11
SLEEP12	2.28	1.34	.16	.16	.15	−.04

Note: Standard error of correlation = 0.02. SLPD = Sleep disturbance (initiation and maintenance); SLPSNR = Snoring; SLPSOB = Awaken short of breath or with headache; SLPQ = Quantity of sleep; SLPA = Sleep adequacy; SLPS = Somnolence; ENERGY = Energy/fatigue; ANX = Anxiety; DEPBC = Depression/behavioral-emotional control; POS = Positive affect; SDRS = Socially desirable response set. N.a. = not applicable.

Table 14–4 Item-Total Correlations of Twelve Sleep Items Corrected for Overlap (N = 2,607)

Itema	Item Total
SLEEP1	.64
SLEEP2	.49
SLEEP3	.59
SLEEP4	.61
SLEEP5	.12
SLEEP6	.44
OPTIMAL SLEEP	−.03
SLEEP8	.47
SLEEP9	.57
SLEEP10	.60
SLEEP11	.55
SLEEP12	.28

a See Table 14–2 for item content.

SLPA	SLPS	ENERGY	ANX	DEPBC	POS	SDRS
−.46	.29	−.37	.43	.41	−.39	−.08
−.37	.19	−.30	.33	.33	−.31	−.01
−.43	.33	−.39	.47	.43	−.41	−.19
−.40	.35	−.38	.38	.36	−.34	−.09
−.04	.20	−.10	.08	.04	−.02	−.05
−.31	.33	−.40	.35	.32	−.31	−.04
.36	−.11	.09	−.14	−.13	.16	.02
.60a	−.27	.41	−.40	−.40	.45	.18
.60a	−.29	.41	−.43	−.43	.46	.17
−.42	.61a	−.53	.41	.40	−.37	−.16
−.34	.69a	−.46	.33	.33	−.29	−.13
−.05	.50a	−.27	.09	.10	−.07	−.03

a Denotes hypothesized item groupings and item-scale correlation corrected for overlap.

Table 14–5 Items Used to Score the 6-item Overall Sleep Problems Index

Item	Abbreviated Item Content	Construct
SLEEP1	Have trouble falling asleep	(Disturbance-initiation)
SLEEP4	Awaken during your sleep time and have trouble falling asleep again	(Disturbance-maintenance)
SLEEP6	Awaken short of breath or with a headache	(Respiratory problems)
SLEEP8	Get enough sleep to feel rested upon waking in the morning	(Adequacy)
SLEEP9	Get the amount of sleep needed	(Adequacy)
SLEEP11	Have trouble staying awake during the day	(Somnolence)

over SLEEP10, despite its slightly smaller item-scale correlation in Table 14–4, because SLEEP11 was judged to indicate a definite sleep-related problem (trouble staying awake during the day), whereas SLEEP10 could easily represent a normal state of affairs for the average person (i.e., "feel drowsy or sleepy during the day"). All six items in this short-form index are also part of the 9-item overall index. These two indices intercorrelated $r = 0.97$ with one another.

Scoring Rules Based on the above analyses, seven subscales and two overall indexes were scored as shown in Table 14–6.

A summary of the items included in each of these measures and an indication of whether the item is to be reversed in the measure is presented in Table 14–7. The multi-item sleep scales were constructed by averaging nonmissing item responses. Because of differing numbers of response options for items comprising them, the sleep disturbance and overall sleep index items were standardized prior to averaging. The quantity of sleep scale was scored as the number of hours of sleep; the optimal sleep measure was a dichotomized version of sleep quantity, with "1" representing optimal sleep. Sleep scales other than the standardized scales and the quantity measures were transformed linearly to range from 0 to 100. All measures were scored so that a high score reflects more of the attribute implied by the scale name (e.g., greater sleep disturbance, greater sleep adequacy).

Characteristics of Measures

Descriptive Statistics A summary of descriptive statistics for the nine sleep measures is shown in Table 14–8. The percentage of missing data was 4% or below for all measures except the snoring item. Ten percent of the respondents did not provide an answer to this item. The snoring item did not display the same degree of problems in the second pilot study sample.

Variability The full range of possible scores was observed for the sleep measures. The distributions of scores also tended to be fairly normal, with skewness ranging from −0.55 (adequacy) to 1.81 ("awaken short of breath or with a headache").

Reliability Internal-consistency reliabilities are summarized in Table 14–8 for the three multi-item subscales and the two indexes. Reliabilities ranged from 0.75 to 0.86, which are all well above the minimum level of 0.50 necessary for purposes of group comparisons.

Table 14–6 Summary of Sleep Subscales and Overall Indexes

Subscale/Index	# of Items
Sleep disturbance (initiation and maintenance)	4
Snoring	1
Sleep shortness of breath or headache	1
Sleep adequacy	2
Sleep somnolence	3
Sleep quantity	1
Optimal sleep	1
Sleep problems index I	6
Sleep problems index II	9

Validity A summary of the correlations among the sleep subscales and indexes is presented in Table 14–9. Perceptions of adequacy were moderately correlated with all subscales except snoring, indicating that such perceptions do in fact reflect an integration of other sleep dimensions. Sleep disturbance was most highly associated with adequacy, followed by shortness of breath. Snoring was most highly correlated with somnolence. Shortness of breath was moderately correlated with adequacy and somnolence and was somewhat related to quantity and optimal sleep. Quantity of sleep and optimal sleep were associated with adequacy. Adequacy and somnolence were moderately intercorrelated. Snoring was the most distinct of all the sleep items. The sleep indexes were both most correlated with disturbance, sleep adequacy, somnolence, and the awaken short of breath or with a headache item.

Correlations between the measures of sleep and eighteen of the MOS health measures are presented in Table 14–10. Snoring (SLPSNR) was the least correlated with the other health measures (range from 0.02 to 0.14, absolute magnitude). The correlations of the quantity of sleep (SLPQ) and optimal sleep (SLPOP) with other health measures were also fairly low (range was from 0.07 to 0.20, absolute magnitude). In all cases, the optimal sleep measure correlated as high or higher with the other measures than did the quantity of sleep measure. The measures of sleep disturbance (SLPD), sleep shortness of breath (SOB), and sleep adequacy (SLPA) correlated with other measures in parallel ways. Among the sleep measures, the sleep problem indices (SLP6, SLP9) displayed the strongest correlations with the health measures. The correlations of SLP6 and SLP9 with other measures were virtually

Table 14–7 Content and Scoring of Final Sleep Measures

Item Content	Item Variable Name	SLPD	SLPSNR
# of items		4	1
Trouble falling asleep	SLEEP1	R	
Time to fall asleep	SLEEP2	NR	
Sleep restlessness	SLEEP3	R	
Awaken during sleep	SLEEP4	R	
Snore during sleep	SLEEP5		R
Awaken SOB or with a headache	SLEEP6		
Quantity of sleep	SLEEP7		
Enough sleep, feel rested	SLEEP8		
Amount sleep needed	SLEEP9		
Feel drowsy	SLEEP10		
Trouble staying awake	SLEEP11		
Take naps	SLEEP12		

Note: NR = not reversed; R = reverse scored; C = scored as 7, 8 hours = 1, otherwise = 0. All of the SLP9 and SLPD items were standardized before they were combined. SLPD = Sleep disturbance (initiation and maintenance); SLPSNR = Snoring; SLPSOB = Awaken short of

identical. This similar pattern of correlations and the large correlation between SLP6 and SLP9 (r = 0.97) suggests that the short version is nearly equivalent to the long version.

Resolution of Issues and Future Direction

A relatively short (twelve items) yet comprehensive battery of sleep is provided whose dimensions have been empirically verified. The twelve items were identified based on two pilot studies that tested seventeen items each. Both a short- and a long-form overall sleep problems index have been constructed. Each index summarizes information across most or all sleep dimensions. The construction of a comprehensive sleep battery fills an important gap in health status assessment.

The MOS has taken a first step in identifying the independent dimensions of sleep based on empirical studies. We can be confident that the measures are not redundant and that each separate measure contributes unique information about sleep. Because this is the first

| | SCALES | | | | INDEXES | |
SLPSOB	SLPQ	SLPOP	SLPA	SLPS	SLP6	SLP9
1	1	1	2	3	6	9
					R	R
						NR
						R
					R	R
R					R	R
	NR	C				
			R		NR	NR
			R		NR	NR
				R		R
				R	R	R
				R		

breath or with headache; SLPQ = Quantity of sleep; SLPOP = Optimal sleep; SLPA = Sleep adequacy; SLPS = Somnolence; SLP6 = Sleep problems index I; SLP9 = Sleep problems index II.

study in which the dimensions were studied empirically, using a comprehensive set of items, it is important to replicate these findings in other samples and populations.

An issue that warrants more attention is whether sleep initiation and sleep maintenance should continue to be combined into a sleep disturbance measure as we have done. If sleep initiation and sleep maintenance have different clinical or therapeutic meanings, it may be important to try harder to develop separate measures. There is evidence that sleep-maintenance insomnia is more difficult to treat than sleep-initiation insomnia (Hoelscher and Edinger, 1988). The use of more items per concept would facilitate their discrimination. Evidence that initiation and maintenance are conceptually similar will increase confidence in the decision to score them together rather than separately.

The fact that the two respiratory items did not correlate with one another suggests that some thought needs to be given to the meaning of sleep respiratory problems in relation to other sleep problems and to health problems. Although few people reported awakening short of breath or with a headache, this item was highly correlated with the

Table 14–8 Descriptive Statistics and Reliability Coefficients for Sleep Measures: PAQ Baseline Sample ($N = 3,053$)

Scale	k	Mean	SD	% with Problems[a]	Observed Range	% Missing	Reliability[b]
Subscales							
Sleep disturbance	4	0.0	0.8	—	−1.0–2.5	2	.84
Snoring	1	31.4	30.2	68.6	0–100	10	—
Sleep shortness of breath or head-ache	1	13.3	21.8	35.8	0–100	3	—
Sleep quantity	1	6.9	1.4	—	1–23	4	—
Optimal sleep	1	0.6	0.5	45.9	0–1	4	—
Sleep adequacy	2	60.8	25.3	—	0–100	1	.75
Sleep somnolence	3	26.5	19.8	—	0–100	3	.76
Indexes							
Sleep problems index I	6	28.3	18.2	—	0–100	1	.78
Sleep problems index II	9	0.0	0.7	—	−1.1–2.9	2	.86

Note: High scores indicate more of the concept (e.g., high scores on sleep disturbance indicate greater disturbance). High scores on the indexes indicate more sleep problems.
[a] Calculated only for single-item measures.
[b] Calculated only for multi-item measures.

Table 14–9 Intercorrelations among Sleep Measures

Scale	Name	SLPD	SLPSNR
Sleep disturbance	SLPD	—	
Snoring	SLPSNR	.06	—
Sleep shortness of breath or headache	SLSOB	.41	.07
Sleep quantity	SLPQ	−.36	−.06
Optimal sleep	SLPOP	−.32	−.07
Sleep adequacy	SLPA	−.51	−.05
Sleep somnolence	SLPS	.35	.19
Sleep problems index I	SLP6	.82[a]	.10[a]
Sleep problems index II	SLP9	.88[a]	.11[a]

Note: High scores indicate more of the concept (e.g., high score on sleep disturbance indicates greater disturbance). High scores on the indexes indicate more problems. N ranged from 2,676 to 3,025. All correlations are statistically significant ($p < 0.01$).

other sleep items. The more common respiratory problem of snoring was not associated with other sleep problems. Snoring by itself is thus not a good indicator of sleep problems. Awakening short of breath or with a headache is a better indicator of sleep problems than snoring is because it defines a severe form of apnea with significant clinical effects.

Because quantity of sleep is one of the most commonly used measures, it is important to understand better how it relates to other health measures relative to the other sleep concepts. By scoring quantity in its original scale as well as in the form of an optimal quantity measure, such studies can be performed.

The sleep problems index provides a useful summary measure of the different types of sleep problems and will be helpful when a single score is desired. For those who cannot administer all the items, a short-form version is provided. In the MOS sample, the two indices were virtually indistinguishable, having 94% shared or common variance. Until more is known about the sensitivity of the short version relative to the long in other samples, the authors recommend using the full battery and index whenever possible. Because the short-form index is a subset of the long-form index, any studies including the long-form index can evaluate the validity of the short-form index as well.

Although there is much information on the relationship of sleep problems to other indicators of health, a unique contribution of the MOS is to allow a comparison of how the different aspects of sleep

SLSOB	SLPQ	SLPOP	SLPA	SLPS	SLP6
—					
−.16	—				
−.14	.39	—			
−.33	.34	.33	—		
.32	−.10	−.16	−.30	—	
.60[a]	−.37[a]	−.36[a]	−.82[a]	.54[a]	—
.59[a]	−.35[a]	−.35[a]	−.75[a]	.61[a]	.97

[a] Coefficient inflated due to overlapping items.

Table 14–10 Correlations between Sleep Measures and Eighteen Other Health Measures

	SLPD	SLPSNR	SLPSOB
Effects of pain (−)	.44	.08	.39
Pain severity (−)	.38	.09	.37
Physical/psychophysiologic symptoms (−)	.45	.11	.51
Energy/fatigue (+)	−.44	−.10	−.40
Physical functioning (+)	−.30	−.12	−.30
Satisfaction with physical abilities (+)	−.34	−.12	−.31
Mobility (+)	−.27	−.09	−.31
Role limitations due to physical health (−)	.38	.10	.33
Role limitations due to emotional problems (−)	.36	.05	.28
Unable to work due to health (−)	.22	.06	.22
Social activity limitations due to health (−)	.44	.07	.36
Cognitive functioning (+)	−.42	−.10	−.34
Depression/behavioral-emotional control (−)	.47	.03	.35
Anxiety (−)	.48	.07	.35
Feelings of belonging (+)	−.32	.03	−.24
Positive affect (+)	−.44	−.02	−.32
Current health (+)	−.41	−.14	−.37
Health distress (−)	.42	.12	.36

Note: SLPD = Sleep disturbance; SLPSNR = Snoring; SLPSOB = Awaken short of breath or with headache; SLPQ = Quantity of sleep; SLPOP = Optimal sleep; SLPA = Sleep adequacy; SLPS = Somnolence; SLP6 = Sleep index I; SLP9 = Sleep index II.

relate to a comprehensive set of health measures in the same sample. The MOS results reveal generally high associations of many of the sleep measures to other health measures. Thus, sleep measures appear to be useful indicators of health and should not be ignored.

The finding that sleep problems are so highly correlated with the MOS indicators of mental health, in addition to their correlations with physical health indicators, suggests that sleep problems might be especially important outcomes in studies of mental health care.

The direction of effect between sleep problems and other health measures can go either way. Sleep can be adversely affected by physical health problems and by psychological distress. Poor sleep can also adversely affect physical and mental well-being and disrupt daily functioning. Longitudinal studies are essential to estimate and interpret properly the nature of the association between sleep and physical and

SLPQ	SLPOP	SLPA	SLPS	SLP6	SLP9
−.17	−.19	−.36	.38	.50	.53
−.15	−.17	−.31	.33	.44	.44
−.19	−.20	−.39	.40	.55	.57
.09	.18	.46	−.49	−.57	−.60
.11	.12	.15	−.36	−.33	−.35
.11	.18	.32	−.35	−.42	−.44
.10	.11	.18	−.34	−.33	−.34
−.11	−.16	−.27	.46	.44	.47
−.10	−.16	−.34	.30	.43	.44
−.07	−.07	−.17	.24	.27	.27
−.11	−.19	−.39	.37	.52	.54
.08	.16	.38	−.38	−.51	−.53
−.11	−.20	−.47	.33	.56	.57
−.12	−.19	−.45	.31	.56	.57
.10	.16	.36	−.18	−.39	−.39
.14	.18	.51	−.28	−.55	−.55
.11	.17	.37	−.42	−.51	−.52
−.12	−.17	−.36	.42	.50	.53

mental well-being. The MOS will evaluate this question in the future with longitudinal data.

The quantity of sleep and optimal sleep were the least related to other health measure, indicating that these may be among the least useful measures of health status per se. Sleep disturbance and sleep adequacy were the most highly related to other health measures; thus, they appear to represent the core of sleep as a health concept.

Some aspects of sleep, such as going to bed on time, are under the control of the individual; others are not. It will be of interest to understand better the extent to which changes in the behavioral aspects of sleep can affect sleep quantity and adequacy. For example, if people are experiencing substantial psychological distress and are at risk for poor sleep, can efforts to get enough sleep make a difference or must the psychological distress be reduced before a beneficial change is apparent? To minimize respondent burden, the measure of sleep regularity was not included in the MOS battery, although such a measure would be an important addition in studies focusing on the behavioral aspects of sleep in relation to health.

A fairly high prevalence of sleep problems was observed in this sample of patients with chronic disease and depression, not a surprising finding. To determine if sleep problems are generally common or are more prevalent in patient groups, these sleep measures need to be administered to a general population sample. Previous research in general populations has found about one-third of those studied to have some sleep problems (Kales, Soldatos, and Kales, 1987).

Little is known about the side effects of different treatments on sleep patterns. If, for example, certain treatments or medications cause sleep disturbances, which in turn cause other health problems, then understanding the effects of treatments on sleep would be an important step in achieving better long-term health outcomes. There have been some reports of the effects of medications on sleep. For example, sleepiness was one of the most common complaints of patients on methyldopa, an antihypertension medication (Bulpitt and Dollery, 1973; Rosen and Kostis, 1985). Clonidine use is associated with longer time asleep (Rosen and Kostis, 1985). The use of a multidimensional sleep battery would add much more information on the distinct effects of these types of medications. As sleep measures are increasingly incorporated into studies of health care, more can be learned about how various treatments affect sleep.

The correlations of the sleep measures with the other health measures were low enough to suggest that these measures tap distinct aspects of health and thus provide a useful complement to a set of generic health measures. The content and face validity of these measures also supports their distinctiveness from other measures. It would be useful if future studies could focus on the incremental validity of these measures or the extent to which the increased burden warrants their inclusion. For example, do the sleep measures increase the prediction of subsequent health or utilization over and above the other measures of functioning and well-being? Do treatments affect sleep when no adverse effects on other functioning or well-being concepts are observed? Are some of the adverse effects of medical treatments on functioning and well-being mediated by sleep problems?

One potential value of these sleep measures is in facilitating a better understanding of the nature of problems in other areas of functioning and well-being. For example, if a person is experiencing a great deal of fatigue but is sleeping well, the problem could be considered to be quite different from one in which the fatigue could be attributed to poor sleep. Similarly, if a person is not sleeping well and is depressed, the treatment for the depression might be different than if the person were sleeping well. The health problems can be interpreted differently depending on whether a sleep problem was occurring in conjunction with other problems in functioning and well-being.

Subsequent studies might show that many problems in functioning and well-being can be attributed to sleep problems, suggesting sleep-related avenues by which physicians can intervene indirectly to improve functioning and well-being. For example, poor job performance might be due to difficulty concentrating as a result of inadequate sleep. A patient might exhibit functional limitations in day-to-day life that are attributable to sleep deprivation arising out of marital problems rather than due to a physical illness. In contrast, inability to sleep because of occupational stress might make a person irritable at home, resulting in impaired family relationships and functioning. A final argument in favor of including sleep measures as part of a generic sleep battery is that sleep is a basic human attribute and an important measure in its own right.

15. Physical/Psychophysiologic Symptoms Measure

Cathy D. Sherbourne, Harris M. Allen, Caren J. Kamberg, and Kenneth B. Wells

Definition and Issues

A physical symptom is defined as a perception, feeling, or belief about the internal state of one's body (Pennebaker, 1982). Symptoms may or may not be disease-specific. Physical symptoms refer to problems encountered in the body's various functional systems. They range from relatively minor, frequently self-limiting conditions (e.g., an upset stomach for less than twenty-four hours) to more serious conditions (e.g., chest pain when exercising) for which medical care is often indicated. Physical symptoms reflect complaints specific to a particular body site (e.g., nasal congestion) as well as complaints of a vague, nonspecific nature (e.g., aches all over). Some symptoms can be observed by others (e.g., skin rash, vomiting), but most are not. Information about symptoms is usually obtained by asking the person directly experiencing the symptoms.

Symptom reports can be simple (e.g., a checklist asking whether or not different symptoms have been experienced) or more complex (e.g., asking further details about the severity of the symptom, frequency of occurrence, cause of the symptom, or actions taken in response to the symptom). A response relating to a given time period can be asked for (e.g., within the last six months), or more detailed information can be obtained about the onset and duration of the symptom, the timing of actions taken to deal with the symptom, or the character of repeated episodes (Verbrugge and Ascione, 1987).

Symptoms, the common pathway for a variety of physical and psychological conditions and disorders, are influenced by beliefs about the nature of illness, beliefs learned from others, past experiences, and specific situations (Pennebaker and Epstein, 1983). The probability that a symptom will be reported varies according to demographic and cultural factors. For example, women seem to report more symptoms than do men (Pennebaker, 1982).

A number of types of symptoms were included in the MOS: general physical symptoms, focusing especially on psychophysiologic sensations that can have a physical and/or psychological component; access symptoms designed to explore the patient's care-seeking behaviors when experiencing minor or serious physical symptoms; and tracer-specific symptoms or indicators directly associated with physical and/or mental problems stemming from one or more of the tracer conditions assessed in the MOS. In addition, other symptomatic problems were measured: pain, sleep disorders, sexual functioning, and energy/fatigue.

The focus in this chapter is on the development of a measure of general physical and psychophysiologic symptoms and not on measures of access or the MOS tracer-specific symptoms. Symptoms used to evaluate the accessibility of treatment when needed have been discussed (Shapiro, Ware, and Sherbourne, 1986). Tracer-specific symptoms, used in the MOS to develop measures of severity and comorbidity for case-mix analyses, are described elsewhere.

The MOS goal was to develop a brief, general measure indicative of general distress or lack of well-being associated with physical and psychological problems and, therefore, appropriate for patients with either physical or emotional problems. The MOS focused on both psychophysiologic symptoms and general physical health symptoms because a large proportion of patients presenting to physicians suffer from complaints for which no organic cause can be found on routine investigation (Kellner, 1985).

Psychophysiologic symptoms are those associated primarily with mental health status, with or without an association with physical health status. These types of symptoms cannot be assigned either a purely physiological or purely psychological etiology, but instead reflect a linkage between mind and body. The measure is referred to as general because a given symptom can result from a variety of physical or psychosocial disorders and the number and frequency of symptoms provide an indication of more severe disorder or poorer health status (Parkerson, Gehlbach, Wagner, et al., 1981).

Another reason for focusing on psychophysiologic symptoms was that other MOS measures of mental health status focus exclusively on emotional and cognitive states. However, many mental health measures developed by others contain psychophysiologic symptoms as indicators of mental distress. A complete picture of mental health requires examination of body states that are linked correlationally, if not causally, to purely psychological phenomena.

Many measures of physical/psychophysiologic symptoms already exist: the Health Insurance Experiment (HIE) Symptoms List (Shapiro, Ware, and Sherbourne, 1986), the Hopkins Symptom Checklist (Derogatis, Lipman, and Covi, 1973; Derogatis, Lipman, Rickels, et al., 1974), the Psychosomatic Symptom Checklist (Attanasio, Andrasik, Blanchard, et al., 1984), the Symptom Response Ratio (Aday and Andersen, 1975; Aday, Andersen, and Fleming, 1980), the Center for Epidemiologic Studies Depression Scale (CES-D) (Radloff, 1977), and the Cornell Medical Index (Brodman, Erdmann, Lorge, et al., 1949; Levav, Arnon, and Portnoy, 1977). Most of these measures contain items assessing affect, cognitive functioning and general and/or physiologic health. None was appropriate in its entirety for MOS purposes either because of length or because the measure was not scored to discriminate between affective and physical states. A subset of symptoms was selected from existing measures.

Content and Measurement Strategy

Pilot Study The MOS goal was to identify approximately eight symptom items, half primarily physical and half primarily psychophysiologic, that could be combined into a single general symptom scale.

A potential item pool of both physical and psychophysiologic symptoms was developed from the HIE symptoms list, the Hopkins Symptom Checklist (HSCL), the Symptom Response Ratio, and the Cornell Medical Index, and an additional list of psychophysiologic symptoms used on health status measures (e.g., the Beck Depression Inventory [Beck, 1967b] the HSCL, and the CES-D). The psychophysiologic symptoms proposed were restricted to symptoms of the physiologic effects of anxiety and depression defined by the *Diagnostic and Statistical Manual of the American Psychiatric Association,* third edition (DSM-III). The MOS focused on anxiety and depression because they are the commonest forms of psychological distress in general and primary care populations. The MOS specifically focused on a sample of patients with unipolar affective (i.e., depressive) disorder. Items were chosen that were not disease-specific, were common in a population of adult patients, sampled a variety of organ systems, and reflected a balance of physical and psychophysiologic symptoms. Forty-six self-reported symptom items were written.

The various existing measures from which symptom items were drawn differed considerably in response format and in the time frame over which symptoms were assessed. Three common response choice formats for symptom items were whether the patient has had a symptom (yes/no), whether the patient has talked to the doctor about the symptom, and the severity of the symptom. Severity can be assessed in terms of intensity or frequency of occurrence. Measures of symptom intensity and frequency are highly correlated (the Psychosomatic Checklist in Attanasio, Adrasik, Blanchard, et al., 1984). For the MOS, a time frame and an intensity format for symptom items was needed to assess current symptoms at periodic intervals.

To be consistent with other MOS health and functioning measures, patients were asked about symptoms experienced during the past four weeks. The severity of each symptom was assessed (Attanasio, Adrasik, Blanchard, et al., 1984). To reduce administration time and respondent burden, only one type of severity measure, frequency, was used. The response categories were "never," "once or twice," "a few times," "fairly often," and "very often" to the question of how often the patient had any of the symptoms during the four-week interval.

The pilot study sample was eighty-six patients who were visiting a doctor's office. Each subject completed a self-administered questionnaire. For each symptom, we hypothesized whether it measured purely physical health problems or could instead be considered psychophysiologic. Two types of analyses were performed: factor analysis and correlations with a measure of psychological distress.

A series of factor analyses was conducted on the pilot study symptom data to determine whether items appeared to be psychophysiologic or were purely physical. The analyses were intended to determine which symptom items loaded reasonably highly on mental health factors, with or without loading on physical health factors. The mental health factor was defined by measures of anxiety, depression, and general positive affect. The physical health factor was defined by measures of physical functioning, chronic medical conditions, and ratings of perceived future health.

Pearson product-moment correlations were calculated between each of the symptoms and a measure of psychological distress (scored 1 if in the upper 29% of the distribution of a scale combining anxiety and depression and 0 otherwise). Since these statistics are bivariate, the use of pairwise deletion is not problematic and the number of subjects in the sample was adequate.

Because of limitations in both approaches, items were chosen based on a synthesis of the two. The three criteria for selection of symptoms as physical health symptoms were: (1) symptom was hypothesized to be physical only; (2) symptom did not have a high loading (above 0.23 following the "five percent" rule) on the mental health factor; and (3) symptom did not correlate above 0.23 with the measure of psychological distress. The three criteria for the selection of psychophysiologic symptoms were: (1) symptom was hypothesized to be psychophysiologic; (2) symptom had a high loading (above 0.23) on the mental health factor regardless of its loading on the physical health factor; and (3) symptom correlated above 0.23 with the measure of psychological distress. Not all final items met all criteria.

According to these criteria, the MOS identified the primarily physical symptoms: weight loss; stiffness, pain, swelling in joints; backaches; skin rash; shortness of breath; toothache; chest pain; bleeding (nonaccidental); noises in ears; leg cramps; pains in arms and legs; itching; constipation; diarrhea; and urination (> 2/night). Of the remaining twenty-eight symptoms, the a priori classifications were not particularly well supported. Of the eighteen symptom items classified a priori as psychophysiologic (i.e., reflecting mental health status), ten yielded loadings greater than the 0.23 criterion on the mental health component: headache, early morning waking, lump in throat, poor appetite, heart (chest) pain, dizziness, heavy feeling in arms/legs, heart pounding, getting up exhausted, and acid indigestion. Nine of the ten symptoms initially classified as reflecting only physical health status: trouble falling asleep, sore throat, stomach flu, cough without fever, nose stopped up, nausea, heavy chest cold, being bloated, and swollen ankles, yielded loadings greater than 0.23 on the mental health component. The coughing symptom was the only a priori physical item that did not correlate greater than 0.23 on the mental health component.

In the case of the correlations of the items with psychological distress, the a priori classifications were better supported. Fourteen of the symptoms classified a priori as psychophysiologic (the ten listed above as well as low energy, soreness in muscles, trembling, lower back pains, and numbness) met or exceeded the 0.23 criterion. Four of the symptoms classified a priori as physical (cough without a fever, nose stopped up, swollen ankles, and coughing) did not correlate more than 0.23 with psychological distress.

Final Items We chose two symptoms reflecting primarily physical health from the list of physical symptoms meeting all three criteria: stiffness, pain, swelling in joints; and backaches. (See Appendix for actual questionnaire items, page 377.) The M O S expanded each of these item stems to include other similar symptoms shown in the factor analysis to be primarily physical indicators: stiffness, pain, swelling, or soreness of muscles or joints; and backaches or lower back pains. A third physical item, coughing, was chosen that loaded highest with the physical health factor in step two of the analyses and did not correlate with psychological distress. The symptom stem was expanded to "coughing that produced sputum" to more clearly indicate a physical symptom.

The psychophysiological symptoms included headache, nausea, feeling bloated, and heavy feelings in arms and legs, which met the "five percent rule" criterion in both sets of analyses. Two of these, nausea and feeling bloated, had been classified a priori as physical; however, both correlated above 0.23 on the mental health factor and above 0.23 with psychological distress. The headache stem was expanded to read "headaches or head pains," the nausea stem to read "nausea (upset stomach)," and the feeling bloated stem to include acid indigestion, a symptom that loaded highly on the mental health component in the factor analyses. A fifth symptom classified a priori as psychophysiological, "lump in throat," thought to be symptomatic of a generalized anxiety disorder, that met the five percent rule criterion in the factor analyses only was chosen.

The eight final symptom items were: *physical*—stiffness, pain, swelling, or soreness of muscles or joints; coughing that produced sputum; backaches or lower back pains; *psychophysiologic*—nausea or upset stomach; acid indigestion, heartburn, or feeling bloated after meals; heavy feelings in arms and legs; headaches or head pains; and lump in throat.

Construction and Evaluation of Measure

Data were used to confirm the internal consistency reliability of the 8-item symptom scale, to see whether the eight items defined a global symptom construct, and to examine whether the results regarding the classification of the symptom items as reflecting strictly physical or both mental and physical health status could be replicated.

Analysis Plan The item frequency distributions were examined to assure adequate variability for purposes of scale construction and to estimate the prevalence of the eight symptoms in the sample. Multitrait scaling techniques were used to assure that items included in the hypothesized symptom scale were internally consistent and that symptoms items were distinct from other health concepts. The matrix included measures of physical and role functioning, psychological distress/well-being, cognitive functioning, current health, pain, sleep problems, and energy/fatigue to assess the item discrimination of the symptom measure.

Unlike other multitrait analyses, the correlation of the symptom items with other measures was not used as a criterion for exclusion of an item from the symptom scale. The symptom items were expected to be highly correlated with other symptomatic measures. Thus a high correlation between a symptom item and other symptomatic measures supports the construct validity of the symptom measure itself. The analysis was intended to identify only the grossest problems of discriminant validity. The reliability of the multi-item scale was evaluated using Cronbach's alpha coefficient. Correlations among items were inspected to judge their homogeneity. The expectation was a weak correlation, given that items were selected to represent a variety of different types of complaints.

A factor analysis of the eight items was conducted to see whether results of the pilot study regarding the classification of symptoms as primarily physical or psychophysiologic could be replicated. As in the pilot study, the analyses focused on the relationship between the eight symptom items and factors defined by mental health and physical health "validity" measures. Measures to define physical health included role limitations due to physical health, unable to work due to health, physical functioning, satisfaction with physical ability, and mobility. Measures to define mental health included depression/behavioral-emotional control, positive affect, anxiety, and cognitive functioning.

Measures of health distress and current health were also included and hypothesized to load equally on both factors. Factors were rotated using the promax rotation. As in the pilot study analyses, a correlation of less than 0.23 with the mental health factor and a correlation of greater than or equal to 0.23 with the physical health factor was used to confirm symptoms classified a priori as physical. A correlation of 0.23 or greater with the mental health factor, regardless of the strength of the correlation with the physical health factor, was used to confirm symptoms classified a priori as psychophysiologic.

Item Variability Table 15–1 presents frequencies for the symptom items. The four most frequently occurring symptom items are: (1) stiffness, pain, swelling, or soreness of muscles or joints; (2) backaches or lower back pains; (3) acid indigestion, heartburn, or feeling bloated after meals; and (4) headaches or head pains. The least frequently occurring symptom is lump in throat. The percentage missing a symptom item ranged from 5% to 6%.

Scale Construction Multitrait scaling results are shown in Table 15–2. In this matrix, row entries represent correlations between each item and the sum of the items in each scale grouping. Footnote "a" indicates hypothesized correlations that were corrected for overlap. The symptom scale is identified across the top of the table by the acronym SYMP.

Item-total correlations for the symptom scale ranged from a low of 0.31 for the symptom of coughing that produced sputum, to a high of 0.50 for the symptoms of nausea and heavy feelings in arms and legs. In general, the symptom items discriminated well from other scales in the

Table 15–1 Percentage Distribution of General Physical and Psychophysiologic Symptoms: PAQ Baseline Sample (*N* = 3,053)

Symptom	Item Variable Name	ITEM RESPONSE[a]				
		Never	Once or Twice	A Few Times	Fairly Often	Very Often
Stiffness, pain, swelling, or soreness of muscles or joints	SYM1	26	18	25	17	14
Coughing that produced sputum	SYM2	62	14	13	8	4
Backaches or lower back pains	SYM3	34	23	22	12	10
Nausea (upset stomach)	SYM4	60	23	11	4	2
Acid indigestion, heartburn, or feeling bloated after meals	SYM5	37	27	21	10	8
Heavy feelings in arms and legs	SYM6	62	16	12	6	4
Headaches or head pains	SYM7	37	29	19	9	5
Lump in throat	SYM8	83	9	5	2	1

[a] Percentage of those who responded to each item.

Table 15-2 Item-Scale Correlation Matrix, Physical/Psychophysiologic Symptoms: PAQ Baseline Sample (N = 1,999)

Item	Mean	SD	SYMP	ROLE	ANX	DEPBC
SYM1	3.05	1.32	.44a	−.43	−.18	−.15
SYM2	1.87	1.19	.31a	−.25	−.20	−.17
SYM3	2.68	1.33	.47a	−.38	−.24	−.23
SYM4	1.75	1.01	.49a	−.32	−.38	−.38
SYM5	2.34	1.21	.48a	−.28	−.34	−.32
SYM6	1.86	1.18	.50a	−.44	−.29	−.27
SYM7	2.32	1.20	.45a	−.26	−.39	−.37
SYM8	1.35	0.81	.41a	−.24	−.24	−.25

Note: SYMP = Physical/psychophysiologic symptoms; ROLE = Role limitations index (Role limitations due to physical health plus three other items); ANX = Anxiety; DEPBC = Depression/behavioral-emotional control; POS = Positive affect; PHYS = Physical functioning; CURR =

matrix, specifically from the mental health and energy scales. As expected, there was some overlap between symptom items and scales that are symptomatic (e.g., the pain scales). The stiffness, pain, swelling, or soreness of muscles or joints symptom correlated significantly higher with the measure of pain severity and overlapped with measures of physical functioning, role functioning, and the effects of pain. The symptom "coughing that produces sputum" correlated higher with the current health scale, while the symptom "backaches or lower back pains" correlated higher with the two pain scales. The symptom "headaches or head pains" correlated higher with the sleep measure. Table 15-3 shows that correlations among the eight symptom items were relatively low, as expected, ranging from 0.18 to 0.51.

The factor analysis revealed that symptoms one through three were primarily associated with physical health status, while symptoms four through eight were associated with both physical and mental health status, i.e., they are psychophysiologic symptoms. Table 15-4 presents correlations (reference structure) from the promax rotated results. Coefficients for the validity variables are not given. As in the pilot study, symptoms one through three—stiffness of muscles, coughing, and backaches or lower back pains—loaded on the physical health component more than 0.23 and on the mental health component less than or equal to 0.23 (the five percent rule) supporting their a priori classification as primarily physical symptoms. Symptoms four, five, and seven loaded more than 0.23 on the mental health component, sup-

POS	PHYS	CURR	ENERGY	PBEH	PINT	SLEEP
−.19	−.47	−.38	−.38	.45	.58	.30
−.16	−.21	−.27	−.26	.24	.22	.24
−.20	−.36	−.34	−.35	.43	.48	.34
−.35	−.19	−.34	−.37	.37	.31	.40
−.30	−.21	−.32	−.34	.31	.27	.35
−.25	−.44	−.46	−.43	.43	.39	.39
−.37	−.14	−.31	−.38	.33	.34	.44
−.21	−.18	−.23	−.23	.23	.20	.27

Current health perceptions; ENERGY = Energy/fatigue; PBEH = Effects of pain; PINT = Pain severity; SLEEP = Sleep Problems Index II.
[a] Denotes hypothesized item groupings and scale correlation corrected for overlap.

porting their a priori definition as definitely psychophysiologic. One item, "heavy feelings in arms/legs," classified a priori as psychophysiologic, appeared to be primarily physical. The symptom "lump in throat" appears to reflect neither, but this could be due to its low occurrence.

Scoring Rules No rescoring of raw items was required for the eight items in the general symptom measure. All items were precoded in the direction of a higher score indicating more frequent experience of specific symptoms. Scores for the eight items were averaged to calculate the scale score. Because item variances for the symptom items were generally comparable, it was not necessary to standardize or weight items before they were scored. Respondents missing more than four items received a missing scale score. The scale was subsequently transformed to a 0–100 scale.

Characteristics of Measure

Descriptive Statistics Table 15–5 presents descriptive statistics for the physical/psychophysiologic symptoms scale. Four percent were missing a scale score. A high score indicates poorer health (more symptoms).

Variability The symptom measure was skewed in the direction of less frequent experience of symptoms, although only 4% reported that

Table 15-3 Correlations among Physical/Psychophysiologic Symptom Items

Symptom		SYM1	SYM2	SYM3	SYM4	SYM5	SYM6	SYM7	SYM8
SYM1	Stiffness, pain of muscles	—							
SYM2	Coughing	.18	—						
SYM3	Backaches	.51	.19	—					
SYM4	Nausea	.21	.18	.26	—				
SYM5	Acid indigestion	.26	.20	.26	.46	—			
SYM6	Heavy feeling arms/legs	.45	.21	.35	.29	.33	—		
SYM7	Headaches	.29	.19	.34	.40	.36	.29	—	
SYM8	Lump in throat	.20	.20	.22	.29	.26	.28	.28	—

Table 15-4 Correlations of Symptoms Items with Physical and Mental Health Factors

Symptoms		Physical Health (+)	Mental Health (−)
SYM1	Stiffness, pain, or soreness of muscles (P)	− .57	− .02
SYM2	Coughing producing sputum (P)	− .25	.10
SYM2	Backaches or lower back pains (P)	− .46	.07
SYM4	Nausea (PSY)	− .18	.37
SYM5	Acid indigestion (PSY)	− .21	.30
SYM6	Heavy feelings in arms/ legs (PSY)	− .47	.13
SYM7	Headaches or head pains (PSY)	− .17	.35
SYM8	Lump in throat (PSY)	− .19	.20

Note: P = Hypothesized as primarily physical; PSY = Hypothesized as psychophysiological. A (+) high score indicates better health; a (−) high score indicates poorer health.

Table 15–5 Descriptive Statistics and Reliability Coefficient for Physical/ Psychophysiologic Symptom Measure

Scale	k	Mean	SD	% without Symptoms	Observed Range	% Missing	Reliability
Physical/Psychophysiologic Symptoms (−)	8	25.0	17.6	4	0–93.8	4.3	.74

Note: A high score indicates poorer health (more symptoms).

during the last four weeks they had not experienced any of the eight symptoms.

Reliability The internal-consistency reliability, coefficient alpha, for the 8-item symptom scale was 0.74. The homogeneity coefficient was low (0.27), suggesting a fairly heterogeneous group of symptoms.

Issue Resolution and Future Directions

A brief 8-item measure of general physical and psychophysiologic symptoms was designed to reflect nondisease-specific problems experienced by the MOS patient sample. Three of the eight symptoms primarily reflected physical health status, and three were shown to be primarily psychophysiologic. One item, "heavy feeling in arms or legs," was hypothesized to be psychophysiologic but appeared to be primarily physical. This item was included in the physical symptom scale but with no specification as to its nature. Further tests of this item in more homogeneous samples (i.e., depressed patients only or hypertensive patients only) are needed to classify accurately this item as primarily physical or psychophysiologic. The nature of the eighth item, "lump in throat," is also unclear, due primarily to the low variability of this type of symptom in our sample. The eight items were fairly heterogeneous, a finding that might be expected due to the fact that the items were chosen to represent a variety of types of complaints within a variety of organ systems.

All eight items were designed to indicate severity of the symptom, with a high score indicating more frequent experience of symptoms within the four-week interval. The measure is reliable and is distinct from more affective mental health measures. As expected, some of the symptom items were highly related to other MOS symptomatic measures such as pain, supporting the construct validity of the scale.

The MOS symptom measure was designed specifically to assess physical symptoms commonly experienced by persons seeking health care, especially persons with chronic medical problems and/or depression. The measure was designed to complement our psychological distress/well-being measures that ask directly about positive and negative feelings and to complement the general physical health measures, which focus on functioning rather than symptoms. It may be less appropriate for assessing physical symptoms in persons without psychological or medical problems, sensitive in identifying adverse health states than longer, more comprehensive symptom checklists. A low score on the measure indicates not the absence of sickness but less severe symptomatology. Information from this scale combined with other indicators such as affective mental health, perceived current health, physical functioning, and chronic conditions gives an idea of the patient's overall level of well-being and general health status.

IV

Short-Form Measures

Part IV describes the MOS 20-Item Short-Form General Health Survey and the MOS 6-Item General Health Survey. The MOS 20-Item Short-Form General Health Survey, which is also referred to as the SF-20, was based on an 18-item survey originally developed and tested in a general population by Ware, Sherbourne, and Davies. Chapter 16 describes its development and the reliability and validity findings in the general population. The MOS 6-Item General Health Survey (chapter 17) represents an approach that is also comprehensive but is based on six single-item measures instead of multi-item scales. These items, which can be administered in less than two minutes, provide an option for those limited to extremely short health surveys.

The 20-item Short-Form General Health Survey was administered to the MOS screening sample, which allowed a test of its reliability in a patient population and further tests of its validity. The results of this administration are presented in an article, "The MOS Short-Form General Health Survey: Reliability and Validity in a Patient Population," published in *Medical Care* ([1988]26:724–35) and summarized here. To the original 18-item General Health Survey, two items, pain and limitations in usual social activities due to health, were added to increase its comprehensiveness before administering to the MOS screening sample. Six health concepts were represented: physical, role, and social functioning, health perceptions, pain, and mental health. (See Appendix pages 401–403).

The survey was administered to a random half of the total screening sample, consisting of 11,186 adult, English-speaking patients. Ages ranged from 18 to 103 years with a mean age of 47, which is slightly older than the general population sample. Thirty-eight percent of the sample were male, with women overrepresented relative to the general population sample. Eighty-seven percent had completed high school, with an average of 13.7 years of education. Seventy-nine percent were white, 11% black, 5% Latino, and 3% Asian or Pacific Islander. Fifty percent of the sample had a total household income of at least $20,000 in 1985.

The full range of possible scores was observed for all measures. The distributions of mental health and current health perceptions were roughly symmetric as desired. The distributions of physical and role functioning scores were skewed, with more people scoring along the positive end of the scale, but to a lesser degree than in the general population. The role functioning scale had a bimodal distribution, with the least prevalent category being the middle one, indicating some limitations. The distribution of the social functioning item was skewed in the direction of more people being healthy. The pain item was well distributed even though the modal score was no pain.

Internal-consistency reliabilities ranged from 0.81 to 0.88, nearly identical to those in the general population (0.76 to 0.88). Reliabilities were similar for depressed patients (0.82 to 0.87) and for other subgroups analyzed: patients with congestive heart failure (0.77 to 0.87), diabetes (0.83 to 0.87), myocardial infarction (0.77 to 0.88), less than a high school education (0.86 to 0.88), and who are over age 75 (0.84 to 0.89).

Preliminary validity studies were of four types. First, in the multitrait scaling analyses, excellent item-scale discrimination was observed for all items, supporting the six hypothesized scales. Second, correlations among the measures in the patient sample were all statistically significant ($p < .01$), and most were substantial in magnitude. Third, known-groups validity studies compared the percent limited and mean scores on the four comparable measures between the patient sample and the general population sample, hypothesizing that the scores should be lower in the patient sample. All hypotheses were confirmed. For example, 45% of patients were in the poor health range on physical functioning compared to only 22% in the general population. Fourth, correlations between the health measures and age, sex, education, income, and race were consistent with results obtained using comparable long-form measures. Although the validity of a health survey cannot be established in a single study, these findings support the validity of the measures. Additional studies of the validity of the 20-item Short-Form General Health Survey have been published that tested the measures in relation to several chronic medical conditions (Stewart, Greenfield, Hays, et al., 1989) and to depression (Wells, Stewart, Hays, et al., 1989). In support of the validity of the short-form measures in relation to clinical criteria, each medical condition studied had a unique profile of scores across the six scales. Hypertension had the least overall impact, as expected, and heart disease had the greatest impact. Patients with multiple conditions showed greater decrements in functioning and well-being than those with only one condition.

Other short-form health surveys based on the MOS measures described here are currently being evaluated, including a 36-item short form referred to as the SF-36 (Ware and Sherbourne, 1992). Tests of its validity and precision relative to long-form MOS measures have yielded some encouraging results (McHorney, Ware, Rogers, et al., 1992).

16. Developing and Testing the MOS 20-Item Short-Form Health Survey: A General Population Application

John E. Ware, Jr., Cathy D. Sherbourne, and Allyson R. Davies

Applications of standard scaling techniques have produced noteworthy improvements in the precision of health measures. Advances include more refined multi-item scales for measuring physical and role functioning, psychological distress and well-being, and current health perceptions. The superiority of multi-item health scales over the best single-item measures has also been demonstrated (Manning, Newhouse, and Ware, 1982; Davies and Ware, 1981). Single-item health measures are more likely than multi-item measures to fall short of the minimum level of precision necessary for statistical power in testing hypotheses because they are more coarse and less reliable (Manning, Newhouse, and Ware, 1982; Ware and Karmos, 1976; McHorney, Ware, Rogers, et al., 1992).

Investigators often choose not to use multi-item scales, however, because they are too long. When questionnaire length must be limited, as in most studies, investigators must choose between breadth and depth of measurement. Because there are good arguments for maintaining breadth, many health surveys have compromised by using single-item measures of health. The MOS tested an alternative strategy, which is to use a new, multidimensional, short instrument. The new instrument represents only the most important health concepts. Each concept is measured by a small number of questionnaire items, selected because they have good psychometric properties. The resulting short-form survey instrument provides a solution to the problem faced by many investigators who must restrict survey length. The instrument is designed to reduce respondent burden while achieving minimum standards of precision for purposes of group comparisons involving multiple health dimensions.

Description of the Short-Form Survey

The short-form survey included seventeen items adapted from longer surveys used successfully in the Health Insurance Experiment (HIE). Selected items represent four of the five health concepts recommended as a minimum set for comprehensive health surveys (Ware, 1987). The number of items included: physical functioning (6), limitations in role performance due to poor health (2), general mental health (5), and current health perceptions (4). Social functioning was not included.

Physical Functioning Six items were selected to assess physical functioning, a dimension measured in the HIE by aggregating twenty items measuring physical limitations and capacities, mobility, and self-care (Stewart, Ware, and Brook, 1978; Stewart, Ware, and Brook, 1982). The goal was to approximate as closely as possible the 6-level scale constructed in the HIE. Response choices and item wording were modified from the HIE version to capture better specific limitations of interest, to describe more accurately the scale level defined by each item, and to facilitate oral administration. One new item (moderate level of limitation in physical functioning) was added to fill a gap in the HIE scale.

Role Functioning Two items were selected to measure limitations in role functioning due to poor health. These are the two best items from the 3-item HIE role functioning scale (Stewart, Ware, and Brook, 1978, 1981, 1982).

Mental Health General mental health was assessed using five items derived empirically from the HIE Mental Health Inventory (MHI). This set is the best 5-item predictor of the summary score based on the full 38-item MHI (Davies, Sherbourne, Peterson, and Ware, 1988). The set represents the four major mental health dimensions (anxiety, depression, loss of behavioral-emotional control, and psychological well-being) as confirmed in factor-analytic studies of the MHI (Veit and Ware, 1983). These five items correlated 0.95 with the MHI total score in the HIE sample used to derive the short-form scale. On cross-validation using another HIE sample, the scale correlated 0.92 with the MHI total score (Davies, Sherbourne, Peterson, and Ware, 1988).

Current Health Perceptions The 22-item Health Perceptions Questionnaire (HPQ) (Davies and Ware, 1981; Ware and Karmos, 1976; Ware, 1976) includes six subscales that are substantially intercorrelated. The Current Health subscale is the most reliable and empirically valid of these (Davies and Ware, 1981). That subscale also best represents the overall HPQ concept, accounting for the largest amount of variance common to the HPQ subscales. For these reasons, four items are selected from the Current Health subscale, as recommended elsewhere (Davies and Ware, 1981). These items have high correlations with the Current Health subscale, have substantial and roughly equal correlations with other physical and mental health measures, and achieve the balance between favorably and unfavorably worded items necessary to control for acquiescent and opposition response sets.

Validity Variables Two other health measures are included in the survey as part of a preliminary evaluation of validity: a single-item rating of health in terms of excellent, good, fair or poor; and a report of days spent in bed due to illness during the past year. Sociodemographic variables included age, sex, education, and income.

Methods: Data Collection and Sample Characteristics

Louis Harris and Associates included the 17-item short form in a 100-item telephone interview. The short-form health items, which were administered toward the end of the interview, required about three or four minutes to complete. Respondents included 2,008 persons aged eighteen years and older. Half of those sampled represented United States households enrolled in health maintenance organizations (HMOs) and half represented those enrolled in the fee-for-service (FFS) system. The FFS sample was identified using the random-digit-dialing method and a sampling frame stratified by region and by the Census Bureau's "size of place" designations. The same procedure was used for the HMO sample: households were first screened to identify those falling into known HMO market areas, and sampling from 195 Standard Metropolitan Statistical Areas known to include HMOs yielded additional HMO enrollees. Additional details regarding study design are reported elsewhere (Montgomery and Paranjpe, 1985).

The mean age of the combined respondent sample was thirty-six years, and twenty-seven percent (unweighted) were fifty-five years or older. The median household income was approximately $25,000. High school graduation was reported by eighty-four percent of respondents; ninety-one percent were white, and forty-four percent were male.

Plan of Analysis

Scale Construction Item-scale correlations are examined to evaluate the internal consistency of each scale and the discriminant validity of each item. For these tests, scores for items in each scale are summed and item-scale correlations are adjusted downward to correct for the inflation caused by including the item in the scale total (Howard and Forehand, 1962). The M O S required adjusted item-scale correlations of 0.40 or greater to satisfy the Likert-type criterion of internal consistency.

The validity of each item in discriminating its hypothesized scale from other health scales is evaluated by examining each item's pattern of correlations across the four scales. The M O S required that each item discriminate well by correlating significantly higher with its hypothesized scale than with each of the other three scales.

Items in the physical and role functioning scales are further evaluated using Scalogram analysis (Guttman, 1944), as in previous studies (Stewart, Ware, and Brook, 1978, 1981, 1982; Davies, Sherbourne, et al., 1988). This analysis tests whether the items are ordered by severity of limitation and whether a single pattern of responses across items is associated with each scale score. The coefficient of reproducibility (C R) indicates the extent to which these ideals have been achieved. Very high C R values can be obtained by chance when item responses are highly skewed, as in most general population studies. Therefore, the M O S estimated whether the observed C R for each scale represented an improvement over the minimum possible C R value, which is indicated by the coefficient of scalability (C S). C R and C S estimates are based only on data from respondents who completed all items. To achieve more conservative tests, respondents with no limitations are excluded.

Tests of hypothesized scales are performed independently for the H M O and F F S samples as well as for the combined sample. Because the results are similar, the M O S reports results for the combined samples.

Reliability The reliability of each scale is estimated using Cronbach's alpha coefficient (Cronbach, 1951), an internal-consistency estimate. The coefficient of reproducibility (C R) is also estimated for the physical and role functioning scales. C R values of 0.90 or greater are usually accepted for cumulative scales when C S also exceeds 0.70 (Guttman, 1944; Edwards, 1957). Internal-consistency reliability estimates above

0.70 are considered satisfactory for group comparisons (Nunnally, 1978).

Validity Correlations among the four health scales and between these scales and the two validity variables are evaluated to see if they reveal the same direction and magnitude of correlations that have consistently been observed for longer versions of the scales. The MOS hypothesized a substantial positive association between the two scales measuring physical and role functioning. Both have correlated higher with each other than with mental health (Ware, Davies-Avery, and Brook, 1980). The measure of current health perceptions was expected to be significantly and substantially correlated with both mental and physical health and most highly correlated with the single-item rating of health as excellent, good, fair, or poor (Ware, Davies-Avery, and Brook, 1980; Davies and Ware, 1981). The MOS expected measures of all four concepts (favorably scored) to correlate negatively with days in bed due to illness (Ware, Davies-Avery, and Brook, 1980).

Correlations between the health scales and demographic variables are also evaluated. Prior research suggests that, if the new short-form measures are valid: (1) older persons should report poorer physical and role functioning and perceive their health less favorably, but should rate their mental health more positively; (2) men should rate their current health more favorably and report better mental health than women; and (3) education and income should be positively correlated with all four scale scores.

Results: Construction of Short-Form Scales

The MOS first tested the physical and role functioning items to see whether they defined cumulative scales. The two role functioning items defined a reproducible scale with three levels. CR was 0.97 for the combined sample, and CS was 0.90 ($N = 459$). Both coefficients well exceeded minimum scaling criteria.

The six physical functioning items are combined to define a 7-level scale of physical functioning with CR = 0.89 and CS = 0.57. The MOS uses two items (difficulty in bending, lifting, or stooping, and difficulty walking uphill or climbing a few flights of stairs) to define one level. People who indicated that they were limited on one or both of these items are classified at that particular level. This pattern differed from that found for the HIE scale, in which items about limitations in vigorous activities and difficulty in bending, lifting, or stooping are combined. However, the short-form items are worded slightly differently, which might account for this discrepancy in scaling results.

Item-Scale Correlations Items in the physical functioning, role functioning, mental health, and current health scales correlate substantially with their respective total scale scores (Table 16–1). Item-scale correlations (adjusted for overlap) ranged from 0.41 to 0.74 for the physical functioning scale. These correlations ranged from 0.54 to 0.65 for mental health and from 0.57 to 0.72 for the current health scale. Because the role functioning scale contains only two items, the item-scale correlation becomes the correlation between the two items, which is 0.63. The Likert internal-consistency criterion is, thus, satisfied for all four scales.

The pattern of correlations for each item across the four scales supports item discriminant validity for three of the scales. All but the two role functioning items correlate more highly with their hypothesized scale than with the other three scales. The role functioning items correlate more highly with the physical than with the role functioning scale. While this might not be surprising, previous studies strongly suggest that these dimensions are conceptually distinct (Stewart, Ware, and Brook, 1978, 1981, 1982). For example, a sizeable number of people who report limitations on one scale do not report limitations on the other.

As a first step in testing whether to combine the physical and role measures or to score them separately, the two sets of items are merged into a single scale. Items in the combined physical/role functioning measure correlate substantially with the resulting 8-item total scale score (Table 16–1). Item-scale correlations range from 0.41 to 0.76. These items also discriminate well, correlating more highly with the combined physical/role functioning measure than with either mental or current health.

Scale Scoring

All scales are scored by computing the simple algebraic sum of item responses (after items are recoded to define a favorable health state). Scores for the physical functioning scale range from 0 to 6. Role functioning scores range from 0 to 2. Scores on the combined physical/

role functioning scale range from 0 to 8. Mental health scores range from 5 to 30, and current health perceptions scores range from 4 to 20. On all scales, higher scores indicate better health (e.g., no limitations, more favorable health perceptions).

Because the physical and role functioning items satisfy the criteria for both cumulative (Guttman, 1944) and Likert scales, either scoring method is appropriate. The Guttman scoring method is more difficult to implement because of the problem of scoring respondents who do not fall into a "perfect" scale type (Stewart, Ware, and Brook, 1982). The MOS therefore adopted the Likert method to gain one additional scale level (by scoring separately the two items combined for the Guttman scale) and to achieve a more simplified scale scoring procedure. In scoring all scales, the MOS replaces missing items with the average of completed items. Fewer than one percent of respondents are missing one or more items.

Table 16–2 presents raw scale means and standard deviations for the combined sample. Frequency distributions of scale scores appear in Tables 16–3 through 16–5. All possible scores are observed for each scale. As expected in a general population, score distributions are somewhat skewed, with most respondents scoring on the favorable side of the scale midpoint.

Reliability

Internal-consistency reliability estimates for the four scales appear in Table 16–2. Without exception, these reliability estimates exceed conventional standards for group comparisons. Despite the relatively small number of items in each scale, coefficients range from 0.76 to 0.88. These coefficients are higher than those observed when identical short-form scales are constructed from responses to the full-length versions of the original HIE survey (Davies and Ware, 1981; Davies, Sherbourne, Peterson, and Ware, 1988).

Validity

Table 16–2 presents product-moment correlations among the five scales and between the scales and two other health measures used to explore empirical validity. Without exception, the direction and the

Table 16–1 Descriptive Statistics and Item-Scale Correlations for Five Health Scales: Combined Samples (N = 2,008)

Abbreviated Item Content	Mean	SD	Physical Functioning
Vigorous activities	0.77	0.42	.63[a]
Bending, lifting, stooping	0.90	0.30	.71[a]
Moderate activities	0.92	0.27	.72[a]
Walking uphill	0.91	0.28	.74[a]
Walking 1 block	0.96	0.18	.55[a]
Eating, dressing	0.97	0.15	.41[a]
Nervous person	4.86	1.15	.18
Felt calm and peaceful	4.36	1.20	.15
Felt downhearted	5.03	1.03	.20
A happy person	4.64	1.03	.22
Felt down in the dumps	5.59	0.84	.20
Health kept from working	0.94	0.24	.65
Unable to do kinds of work	0.89	0.30	.71
Somewhat ill	4.45	1.08	.55
Healthy as anybody	4.17	1.13	.52
Feeling bad	4.31	1.16	.49
Health is excellent	4.14	1.14	.58

[a] Indicates hypothesized item groupings and correlations that were corrected for overlap.

Table 16–2 Summary of Reliability and Validity Results: Combined Samples

Scale/Item	k[a]	Mean	SD	Reliability[b]
Role functioning (R)	2	1.83	0.50	.76
Physical functioning (P)	6	5.45	1.24	.88
Physical/role functioning (PR)	8	7.28	1.65	.83
Current health (C)	4	17.09	3.67	.83
Mental health (M)	5	24.50	4.05	.82
General health (G)[c]	1	3.35	0.77	—
Bed days (B)	1	4.14	12.61	—

[a] Number of items in scale.
[b] Internal consistency reliability estimated using Cronbach's (1951) Alpha coefficient.

Mental Health	Role Functioning	Current Health Perceptions	Physical & Role Functioning
.19	.55	.55	.64[a]
.18	.62	.50	.72[a]
.20	.68	.52	.75[a]
.20	.66	.57	.76[a]
.19	.51	.41	.57[a]
.18	.35	.36	.41[a]
.60[a]	.15	.28	.18
.65[a]	.12	.27	.15
.65[a]	.19	.32	.21
.64[a]	.19	.33	.22
.54[a]	.17	.30	.20
.18	.63[a]	.52	.68[a]
.20	.63[a]	.60	.73[a]
.31	.54	.68[a]	.58
.27	.49	.64[a]	.54
.35	.45	.57[a]	.50
.33	.54	.72[a]	.60

INTERCORRELATIONS						
R	P	PR	C	M	G	B
—						
.76	—					
.87[d]	.98[d]	—				
.62	.66	.68	—			
.21	.24	.25	.39	—		
.52	.58	.59	.72	.33	—	
−.42	−.38	−.42	−.40	−.27	−.37	—

[c] Recoded so a high score indicates better health.
[d] Artificially inflated due to overlapping items.

Table 16–3 Frequency Distribution for Physical and Role Functioning Scales: Combined Sample

Scale	Score	N	%	Cumulative %
Role functioning	0	108	5	5
	1	124	6	12
	2	1,777	88	100
		2,009		
Physical functioning	0	15	1	1
	1	41	2	3
	2	58	3	6
	3	74	4	9
	4	88	4	14
	5	170	8	22
	6	1,562	78	100
		2,008		
Physical/role functioning	0	14	1	1
	1	28	1	2
	2	38	2	4
	3	41	2	6
	4	50	2	8
	5	57	3	11
	6	91	4	15
	7	140	7	22
	8	1,549	77	1,000
		2,008		

relative magnitude of these correlations correspond with hypotheses based on previous studies that used the longer versions of the scales. The physical and role functioning scales are highly correlated (0.76). The current health perceptions scale, hypothesized to reflect variation in both physical and mental health, correlates substantially with both scales and more strongly with the physical and role functioning scales than mental health. As hypothesized, the current health perceptions scale correlates most highly with the single-item rating of health in terms of excellent, good, fair, or poor (EGFP; 0.72), which represents an alternative method of measuring the same health concept (Davies and Ware, 1981). The mental health and the physical and role functioning scales also correlate significantly with EGFP. Both correlate less strongly with EGFP, however, than with the current health perceptions scale, perhaps because of the lower reliability of the single EGFP item. As hypothesized, all five health scales correlate significantly and negatively with the measure of days spent in bed due to illness during the past twelve months.

Correlations between the five health scales and sociodemographic variables appear in Table 16–6. Without exception, the pattern of results corresponds with the MOS hypotheses.

Discussion

The goal was to construct a short-form health survey that would represent four of the more frequently measured health dimensions (physical functioning, role limitations due to poor health, mental health, and current health perceptions), demonstrate satisfactory psychometric properties, and reduce respondent burden relative to longer versions of the same scales. Such a measure would be comprehensive and more precise than single-item measures, yet short enough to be used in studies requiring a survey of limited length.

Table 16–4 Frequency Distribution for Current Health Perceptions: Combined Sample

Score	N	%	Cumulative %
4	14	<1	<1
5	22	1	2
6	19	<1	3
7	20	<1	4
8	34	2	5
9	16	<1	6
10	35	2	8
11	21	1	9
12	55	3	12
13	57	3	14
14	79	4	18
15	74	4	22
16	152	8	30
17	186	9	39
18	241	12	51
19	311	15	66
20	672	33	100

Table 16–5 Frequency Distribution for Mental Health Scale:
Combined Sample

Score	N	%	Cumulative %
5	2	<1	<1
6	1	<1	<1
7	3	<1	<1
8	2	<1	<1
9	2	<1	<1
10	7	<1	1
11	5	<1	1
12	8	<1	1
13	15	1	2
14	17	1	3
15	18	1	4
16	34	2	6
17	30	1	7
18	41	2	9
19	52	2	11
20	69	3	15
21	71	3	19
22	104	5	24
23	111	5	29
24	143	7	36
25	249	12	49
26	336	17	66
27	270	13	79
28	216	10	90
29	98	5	95
30	103	5	100

The survey achieves both breadth and depth of measurement and keeps respondent burden well within the limits required by most investigations. The MOS experience with this survey suggests that self-administration requires approximately three minutes for most respondents. Self-administration is used successfully with longer versions of the HIE measures (Stewart, Ware, and Brook, 1982; Davies, Sherbourne, Peterson, and Ware, 1988). Telephone administration, which is used in the current study, requires about three or four minutes. These administration times represent a reduction in respondent burden of approximately ninety percent relative to the full-length versions the scales are derived from.

The selected questionnaire items represent four of the most frequently surveyed general health dimensions (physical functioning, role limitations due to poor health, general mental health, and current health perceptions) (Ware, 1987). These items also measure a wide range of favorable and unfavorable health levels for each concept. All possible scale scores are observed for all measures in the current study. As expected for a general population, the score distributions are skewed, with most respondents scoring at the healthy end of the scales. Consistent with previous studies (Stewart, Ware, and Brook, 1978), this finding is most notable for the physical and role functioning scales. This result was expected from the outset; the scales are intended for use in both general and patient populations. Results from the MOS indicate that distributions of scores are less skewed for patients with chronic conditions (Stewart, Hays, and Ware, 1988).

A fifth scale that combines physical and role functioning items was also constructed, because of the high correlation between these two concepts. The MOS recommends scoring these two measures both singly and in combination. Further research is necessary to clarify the value of scoring and interpreting these two concepts separately.

The high correlation observed between the current health scale and the single-item rating of health (excellent to poor) is consistent with previous results (Davies and Ware, 1981). They perform much like alternate form measures of the same concept. Thus, the MOS recommends combining them into a 5-item scale in future studies (Stewart, Hays, and Ware, 1988).

Noteworthy omissions from this short-form battery are measures of limitations in social functioning due to poor health as well as pain. The

Table 16–6 Correlations Between Health Scales and Sociodemographic Variables: Combined Samples

Scales	Age	Sex[a]	Education	Income
Role functioning	−.25	−.07	.18	.22
Physical functioning	−.27	−.10	.22	.23
Physical/role functioning	−.26	−.10	.22	.23
Current health perceptions	−.23	−.07	.24	.23
Mental health	.11	−.07	.11	.14

Note: All are significant at $p < .01$.
[a] Scored 1 = male, 2 = female.

MOS recommends the addition of two or more items representing each of these important concepts in future studies. Examples of items with good face validity for each concept are presented elsewhere (Ware, 1987).

The results exceed expectations for these measures. A test in the MOS patient population was also successful (Stewart, Hays, and Ware, 1988). We conclude that attempts to construct short-form, multi-item scales for use in comprehensive health surveys are likely to prove successful. Given that respondent burden and data collection costs are major rate-limiting factors in the assessment of health outcomes, we strongly recommend continued development and evaluation of short-form health surveys for use in both general and patient populations.

17. Preliminary Tests of a 6-Item General Health Survey: A Patient Application

John E. Ware, Jr., Eugene C. Nelson,
Cathy D. Sherbourne, and Anita L. Stewart

To experiment with the extremes of the tradeoffs involved in using short-form and full-length scales, the MOS staff developed a short-form survey designed to be administered in less than two minutes. The tradeoffs include the choice between breadth and depth of measurement. The former is an issue of comprehensiveness and content validity; the latter is an issue of precision in measuring each health concept. To achieve breadth, the MOS selected six health concepts: physical, social, and role functioning; bodily pain; mental health in terms of psychological distress; and general health perceptions. Depth of measurement was limited to the precision that could be achieved using a single questionnaire item defining five or six levels for each concept.

The idea of achieving brevity through the use of single-item scales is not new. In fact, the most widely used health status measure is a single question which asks respondents to rate their health in general on an excellent-to-poor continuum. This item has been used by the National Center for Health Statistics for decades (NCHS, 1981) and has been studied extensively (Davies and Ware, 1981). In the search for the extreme of brevity in health assessment, others have adopted the strategy of one questionnaire item per concept (Gurin, 1960; Cantrill, 1965; Andrews and Withey, 1976; Wan and Livieratos, 1978; Spitzer, Dobson, Hall, et al., 1981; Davies and Ware, 1981; Coates, Gebski, Stat, et al., 1987; Nelson et al., 1987, 1989, 1990a, 1990b).

This chapter presents a description of the survey instrument designed to measure the six health concepts using a single-item measure for each (Table 17–1) (see pages 373–375 in the Appendix). Four of the single-item measures studied are identical or nearly identical to the

Table 17–1 Definitions of M O S 6-Item General Health Survey
Measures

Label	Definition
Physical functioning	Extent to which health problems limit everyday physical activities
Role functioning	Difficulty doing daily work during past 4 weeks, inside or outside the house, due to physical health or emotional problems
Social functioning	Extent of limitations in normal social activities due to physical health or emotional problems during past 4 weeks
Psychological distress	Amount of time in past 4 weeks bothered by emotional problems (feeling anxious, depressed, or irritable)
Current health perceptions	Overall rating of health as excellent, very good, good, fair, or poor
Pain	Intensity of bodily pain during past 4 weeks

C O O P charts, that added illustrations to items measuring role functioning, social functioning, pain, and psychological distress in the M O S
(Nelson, Landgraf, Hays, et al., 1990a). A summary and discussion of
three issues is presented: the logic underlying the selection and origin of
each item; preliminary tests to learn if ordered levels of health are
defined by each item; and preliminary tests of the validity of each item in
discriminating the health concept it was selected to measure from other
health concepts. For the latter tests, six multi-item M O S scales were
used as criteria.

Physical Functioning

The single-item rating of physical functioning focuses on limitations
during the past 4 weeks on everyday physical activities (such as walking
and climbing stairs) due to health problems. Five levels of limitations
are defined: not at all, slightly, moderately, quite a bit, and extremely.
Strenuous physical activities relative to self-care activities of daily living
were assessed because limitations in these activities are much more
prevalent.

The frequency and percentage of respondents and the mean physical functioning scores at each of the five levels of physical functioning defined by the item are shown in Table 17–2. Nearly half of the respondents were not limited at all. The rest were well distributed across the other four categories. Among those reporting any limitation, the great majority reported slight or moderate limitations. Only 2.1% reported extreme limitations.

The ordinality of the five levels of physical functioning defined by the single-item scale is strongly supported by the last column of Table 17–2 showing mean physical functioning scores for those at each level defined by the item. These means range from a high of 89.3 for the "not at all limited" level to a low of 12.0 for those who chose the "extremely limited" level. Differences between levels varied considerably, ranging from 15 to 25 points. The fact that the mean physical functioning score for the "not at all" level is well below 100, a perfect physical functioning score, suggests that a noteworthy number of physical limitations may have been missed by the single-item measure.

Social Functioning

Social functioning was measured by an item that asks about the extent of interference in normal social activities (with friends, family, neighbors, or groups) due to physical health or emotional problems. The extent of interference was defined in terms of five levels: not at all, slightly, moderately, quite a bit, and extremely. Fifty-two percent of those eligible for the MOS panel reported no limitations in response to this item.

Table 17–2 Frequency and Percentage of Respondents and Mean Physical Functioning Scores at Each Scale Level of Physical Functioning ($N = 3,036$)

Item Levels	f	%	Mean Physical Functioning
1–Not at all	1,489	49.0	89.3
2–Slightly	704	23.2	71.5
3–Moderately	439	14.5	56.3
4–Quite a bit	339	11.2	37.4
5–Extremely	65	2.1	12.0

Note: Physical functioning scale is favorably scored.

Table 17–3 Frequency and Percentage of Respondents and Mean Social Activity Limitations Due to Health Scores at Each Level of Social Functioning ($N = 3,053$)

Item Levels	f	%	Mean Social Activity Limitations
Extremely	61	2.0	18.2
Quite a bit	214	6.9	33.8
Moderately	366	11.9	43.8
Slightly	824	27.0	58.6
Not at all	1,588	52.0	70.0

Note: Social activity limitations scale is favorably scored.

As hypothesized, social functioning as defined by the scale for social activity limitations due to health (chapter 9) was much lower for those reporting that their physical and emotional health interfered "extremely" with their social activities than for those reporting that they were limited "not at all" (70.0 versus 18.2). The intervals between the five levels defined by the single-item scale were fairly equal (15, 10, 15, 11). The groups defined by this single item seem to differ well, on average, in terms of social functioning as defined by the longer-form social activity measure.

Role Functioning

Role limitations were assessed using an item that asked about difficulty in performing daily activities as a result of physical health or emotional problems: none at all, a little bit, some, quite a bit, or could not do daily work. A second item was administered in the MOS to explore whether any difficulties reported were due mostly or entirely to physical or emotional causes.

The frequency and percentage of respondents choosing each of the five levels of difficulty are given in Table 17–4. A substantial percentage of respondents reported at least a little difficulty in performing their daily work (61%). As shown in Table 17–5, about 54% of those attributed their limitations entirely to physical health problems, while 21% attributed their limitations entirely to emotional problems, and another 25% attributed the limitations to both types of problems.

The validity of the single-item role functioning measure was evaluated in terms of the strength of its relationship with the two full-length MOS role functioning measures (chapter 12). Mean role scale scores for these two measures are shown for those at each level of the single-item scale (last two columns of Table 17–4). As hypothesized, the mean role-physical scale scores for those reporting that they could not do daily work was substantially lower (14.1) than the mean scale score for those reporting that they were not at all limited in doing their daily work (90.0). Mean role-emotional scale scores also decreased substantially for those reporting inability to do daily work (37.7) relative to those reporting no limitations (91.8). The range of role scale scores reflected across levels of the single-item scale is large, and the intervals between levels defined by the single-item scale are not equal as defined by the full-length scales.

To evaluate the usefulness of the second single-item measure in improving the discriminations between physical and emotional causes of role limitations, the MOS calculated mean scale scores for both role

Table 17–4 Frequency and Percentage of Respondents and Mean Role Functioning Scores at Each Level of Role Functioning (N = 2,940)

Item Level	f	%	MEAN ROLE FUNCTIONING Emotional	Physical
None at all	1,134	38.6	91.8	90.0
A little bit	790	26.9	71.1	66.4
Some	575	19.6	52.3	45.5
Quite a bit	365	12.4	40.0	28.1
Could not do	76	2.6	37.7	14.1

Note: Role scales are favorably scored.

Table 17–5 Frequency and Percentage of Respondents Reporting Physical and Emotional Causes for Role Limitations

Reported Causes	f	%
Mostly or entirely physical	186	54
Mostly or entirely emotional	723	21
Physical and emotional about equally	861	25

scales for those reporting mostly physical, mostly emotional, and equal physical and emotional causes for their role limitations (Table 17–6). As hypothesized, the pattern of scores based on the role-physical and role-emotional scales varied for groups of respondents who attributed their problems to physical causes, emotional causes, or the two combined. The mean score of the role-physical scale was substantially lower for persons reporting mostly physical causes for their limitations (48.1 and 43.0 versus 71.4). The mean role-emotional scale was substantially lower for persons reporting emotional causes (40.1 and 37.5 versus 76.2). The results in Table 17–6 suggest that the two single-item role functioning measures scored in tandem will achieve better validity in discriminating the effects of physical and emotional problems than the first single-item measure, which captures limitations due to either kind of health problem.

Bodily Pain

For the single-item pain measure the MOS chose a categorical rating of the severity of bodily pain during the past four weeks and offered six response choices ranging from "none" to "very severe" (Table 17–7). Frequency distributions for the pain item ("how much bodily pain have you generally had during the past 4 weeks?") are shown in Table 17–7. The single-item measure detected a substantial amount of pain experienced by these patients, as indicated by the item responses. Approximately 78% of the MOS sample reported that they had experienced some pain during the preceding four-week interval. Thirty-one percent reported moderate, severe, or very severe pain.

Table 17–6 Mean Role Scale Scores for Respondents Reporting Physical and Emotional Causes for Their Role Limitations

Difficulty Attributions	Mean Role—Physical	Mean Role—Emotional
Mostly physical causes	48.1	76.2
Physical and emotional about equal	43.0	40.1
Mostly emotional causes	71.4	37.5

Note: Role scales are favorably scored.

Table 17–7 Frequency and Percentage of Respondents and Mean Pain
Severity Scores for Each Level of Bodily Pain (N = 2,928)

Levels	f	%	Mean Pain Severity
None	655	22	3.30
Very mild	776	26	12.19
Mild	593	20	21.89
Moderate	689	24	38.76
Severe	179	6	59.43
Very severe	36	1	75.38

Note: Pain scale is negatively scored.

As hypothesized, the mean level of pain severity, as defined by a full-length MOS pain severity scale (chapter 13), was substantially lower for those reporting no or mild bodily pain than the mean levels of pain for those reporting very severe bodily pain (3.30 versus 75.38, Table 17–7). A fairly wide range of pain severity scores is represented across the categories defined by the single-item measure. Intervals between means for those at each level of the single-item measure are not equal. The largest difference between mean pain severity scores is between the moderate and severe pain categories defined by the single-item measure. These differences in the size of the intervals between item levels should be taken into account when scoring those levels.

Mental Health

A difficult step in choosing one item to represent general mental health was the choice among the three major components of mental health defined by MOS scales: psychological distress, psychological well-being, and cognitive functioning. All components are important; however, the most clinically and socially relevant is likely to be psychological distress.

The psychological distress item selected asked about the extent to which the respondent had been bothered by emotional problems (such as feeling anxious, depressed, or irritable) during the past four weeks. Five response choices were offered: not at all, slightly, moderately, quite a bit, and extremely. This description of emotional problems attempts to represent the content of widely used general mental health measures in terms of psychological distress (chapter 7).

The frequencies and percentages of respondents and mean MHI-32 scores for persons at each of the five levels defined by the single-item scale are shown in Table 17–8. Approximately 71% were bothered at least slightly by emotional problems during the past 4 weeks. Over half of the sample (54.3%) were bothered only slightly or moderately, and 16.4% were bothered either quite a bit or extremely.

The order of the five categories defined by the single-item scale, from "not at all" to "extremely," is strongly supported by the means observed for the favorably scored MHI-32, which is the most complete summary MOS mental health scale (chapter 7). These means ranged from a high of 82.8 for those in the "not at all" category to a low of 37.7 for those in the "extremely" category (Table 17–8). The levels in between are ordered as hypothesized, and the intervals are roughly equal between categories, from nine to thirteen points on the MHI. Differences in psychological well-being assessed by MHI-32 but not captured by the single-item measure may account for the mean of 82.8 observed for those who reported being not at all bothered in response to the item.

General Health Perceptions

The most widely used measure of health perceptions is a single item asking about current health in general ("In general, would you say your health is excellent, good, fair, or poor?"). Because of the widespread use of this item, it is important to understand how good it is. Some studies have already addressed this issue. Davies and Ware (1981) evaluated the interval properties of the four responses and the frequency distribution of this single item based on the HIE general population. Based on their findings, they recommended incorporating an additional response choice ("very good") at the positive end of the scale. The MOS adopted this recommendation and tested the resulting 5-level scale based on a single-item measure. The predictive validity of this item has also been tested (Manning, Newhouse, and Ware, 1982).

The frequency and percentage of respondents who chose each of the five item categories are shown in Table 17–9. Because the item was also administered to the MOS screening sample, mean scores are presented for both samples. This item achieved the closest approximation to a

Table 17–8 Frequency and Percentage of Respondents and Mean
MHI-32 Scores for Each Level of Psychological Distress (*N* = 2,935)

Level	*f*	%	Mean MHI-32
1–Not at all	859	29.3	82.8
2–Slightly	1,070	36.4	73.5
3–Moderately	526	17.9	62.6
4–Quite a bit	399	13.6	51.6
5–Extremely	81	2.8	37.7

Table 17–9 Frequency and Percentage of Respondents and Mean
Current Health Scores for Each Level of Self-Rated Health

Level	*f*	%	MEAN CURRENT HEALTH		RECOMMENDED SCORING	
			Screening Sample	Baseline Sample	1–5 Scale	0–100 Scale
Excellent	186	6.1	87.9	86.9	5.00	100
Very good	852	27.9	75.5	75.4	4.36	84
Good	1,304	42.7	57.6	55.9	3.43	61
Fair	620	20.3	30.0	30.6	1.99	25
Poor	92	3.0	10.8	10.8	1.00	0

normal distribution of responses observed for any of the single-item
scales. The distribution is quite symmetrical, with only 6.1% and 3.0%
scoring in the highest and lowest categories. The mean 7-item current
health scale score for respondents at each of the five item levels is also
shown in Table 17–9 for both screening and baseline samples. The
means are remarkably similar, despite differences in the two samples.
The intervals between means for each pair of categories are fairly
unequal—12, 18, 28, and 19 in the screening sample and 12, 19, 25,
and 21 in the baseline sample. Similar results were observed in the HIE
(Davies and Ware, 1981).

Because of the widespread use and importance of this item, the MOS
gave considerable attention to how better to approximate an interval
scale using this item. To do so, the mean score on the current health
scale was assigned to the item responses and scores were then trans-

formed back to a 1–5 scale and to a 0–100 scale. Table 17–9 shows the recommended scoring. Because the intervals were so similar for the two samples, the MOS used the screening sample as the basis. The single-item measure correlated 0.70 with the full-length current health scale.

Discriminant Validity

As discussed above, substantial correspondence was observed between each of the six single-item scales and the full-length MOS scales they were selected to represent. The MOS also conducted preliminary tests of the validity of each single-item measure in discriminating among health concepts.

Results of correlational tests are presented in Table 17–10 using data for the baseline sample. The correlation in each column that should be highest is underlined. These are the correlations between each single-item measure and the multi-item MOS scale measuring the same concept. These correlations were without exception substantial, ranging from 0.71 to 0.83 with a median of 0.75. Each single-item scale correlated significantly higher with its corresponding MOS scale than with measures of other MOS health concepts. The median of the thirty off-diagonal correlations, which should be lower than the diagonal (underlined) correlations in Table 17–10, is 0.58.

These results support the discriminant validity of the single-item scales. In support of their construct validity, the pattern of correlations among the single-item scales is similar to the pattern observed among their full-length counterparts. The lowest correlations for both are between physical functioning and mental health; among the highest for both are correlations between physical, social, and role functioning.

Discussion

These preliminary tests of single-item measures of six general health concepts have yielded favorable results. The resulting 6-item survey should be evaluated further. Future studies should take into account the unequal intervals between levels when the items are scored and should focus on precision issues.

With response to precision, it is likely that the coarseness of single-item measures will limit their usefulness for purposes of detecting small to moderate differences between groups (McHorney, Ware, Rogers, et al., 1992). Coarseness and limits on reliability and the resulting large confidence intervals around scores based on single-item measures raise questions about their use in monitoring changes in health for individual patients over time. These issues should be addressed in longitudinal studies.

According to psychometric theory, the score based on a multi-item scale, even a short-form one, is more reliable than a score for a single-item scale (Cronbach, 1951). Consistent with this theory, five single-item measures of general mental health (MHI-5), each with a reliability of 0.64, achieve a scale score reliability of 0.90 when aggregated using the method of summated ratings. This example uses data from the MOS as follows: $N = 3,445$ and scale range $= 0$–100 for both measures: SD $= 27.9$ for single-item measures; SD $= 21.1$ for MHI-5. The 5-item scale also measures twenty-six levels of mental health, as opposed to only five levels for the single–item scale.

This gain in precision, with the multi-item scales, is important because it is a key factor in determining the confidence with which one can interpret scores for individual patients. The 95% confidence interval around a patient's score, based on a single MHI item with a reliability of 0.64, is about ± 32.8 points as opposed to ± 13.1 points for a 5-item scale measuring the same concept. Because the 95% confidence interval around an individual score is more than halved by MHI-5, relative to the single-item scale, the multi-item scale will detect a much smaller difference or change.

Further research is necessary to understand better other tradeoffs involved in using short- versus long-form versions of health scales. Most reports of empirical tests to date have compared instruments that vary in a number of different ways, including the length of the measures, the concepts represented, and the methods of scale construction and enumeration (Read, Quinn, and Hoefer, 1987; Liang, Fossel, and Larson, 1990). The results are difficult to interpret because there are many reasons that might explain the differences (Liang, Fossel, and Larson, 1990).

The HIE comparisons between short- and long-form measures in terms of predictive validity (Manning, Newhouse, and Ware, 1982) clearly indicate that multi-item scales, even short ones, are more valid than single-item measures, and that longer and more comprehensive questionnaires are the most valid. However, these analyses leave unanswered the very important issue of whether or not a short-form

Table 17–10 Correlations among Single-Item Measures and with Full-Length MOS Scales (*N* = 3,445)

Full-Length Scales	Physical Functioning	Social Functioning
Physical functioning (*k* = 10)	<u>.74</u>	.44
Social activity limitations due to health (*k* = 4)	.50	<u>.83</u>
Role functioning (*k* = 10)	.62	.58
Effects of pain (*k* = 6)	.54	.52
MHI (*k* = 18)	.24	.59
Health scale (*k* = 7)	.59	.54

measure is good enough and, if so, for what kinds of studies. Recent comparisons between 18-item, 5-item, and single-item scales from the Mental Health Inventory are examples of the kinds of studies useful for addressing this issue (Weinstein, Berwick, Goldman, et al., 1989; Berwick, Murphy, Goldman, et al., 1991). The latter study focuses on the MHI-5. A recent publication compares the single-item and multi-item measures from the MOS in terms of their discriminant validity in relation to clinical criteria (McHorney, Ware, Rogers, et al., 1992).

Any health survey designed for use among the young and the old as well as across sick and well populations represents a substantial compromise. If six health concepts are to be measured in less than two minutes, on average, it is impossible to attain a great level of detail using single-item measures. Single-item measures are likely to have at least two kinds of problems: ceiling and floor effects which are, respectively, problems of substantial numbers of people getting the highest or lowest possible scores in one population or another. Problems with floor effects were found for single-item measures from the 20-item MOS Short-Form General Health Survey in persons previously admitted to a public hospital (Bindman, Keane, and Lurie, 1990).

Like other MOS questionnaires, the 6-item form was designed for self-administration, telephone administration, or administration during a face-to-face interview. All three administration methods have been used successfully; however, different forms and instructions are required.

The most popular health surveys are likely to be those that achieve

| SINGLE-ITEM MEASURES | | | |
Role Functioning	Bodily Pain	Psychological Distress	General Health Perceptions
.61	.54	.16	.59
.69	.42	.55	.44
.71	.53	.39	.52
.59	.71	.35	.45
.51	.29	.77	.29
.63	.51	.41	.76

brevity and comprehensiveness. These two competing measurement goals were achieved here by constructing single-item scales for six health concepts. The preliminary results reported here for these scales support their use in studies based on *group*-level analyses. Further tests are required before conclusions can be drawn. Longitudinal tests are needed to address the appropriateness of using single-item measures in monitoring outcomes for individual patients. It is hoped that publication of this 6-item survey will facilitate such studies.

V

The Validity of
MOS Measures

Validity is perhaps the most important attribute of health measures because it pertains to the extent to which measures contain the information intended and to the meaning of scores. Part V discusses the validity of health measures.

Chapter 18 provides an overview of the essential steps in validating health measures, describes the present MOS approaches to validity, and suggests approaches that can be undertaken in the future. It is useful as a methodological guide to others attempting to validate health measures.

Chapter 19 presents analyses pertaining to construct validity that are designed to answer five questions: (1) could the two MOS theoretical dimensions of health, physical and mental, be confirmed empirically? (2) would each measure relate to these two dimensions in hypothesized ways? (3) what is the relationship between physical and mental health? (4) are the health measures biased by socially desirable responding? and (5) do the health measures predict subsequent utilization of services in hypothesized ways? Some of the construct validity analyses are reported in an article published in *Psychological Assessment: A Journal of Consulting and Clinical Psychology* entitled "The Structure of Self-Reported Health in Chronic Disease Patients" (Hays and Stewart, 1990).

Several articles that address validity are summarized in this introduction because they contribute important information regarding the validity of the MOS measures. Preliminary evidence of the construct validity of the 20-item MOS Short-Form General Health Survey is published in *Medical Care* in an article entitled "The MOS Short-Form General Health Survey: Reliability and Validity in a Patient Population" (Stewart, Hays, and Ware, 1988). In this article, the construct validity of the measures was supported in terms of correlations among the measures, their usefulness in comparing patient and general population samples, and correlations between health measures and socio-demographics which all corresponded to hypotheses.

Additional evidence of the validity of the 20-item MOS Short-Form General Health Survey is provided in two studies published in the *Journal of the American Medical Association,* "Functional Status and Well-Being of Patients with Chronic Conditions" (Stewart, Greenfield, Hays, et al., 1989) and "The Functioning and Well-Being of Depressed Patients" (Wells, Stewart, Hays, et al., 1989). These two studies illustrate one type of application of MOS measures: the description of the functioning and well-being associated with various chronic conditions. One article describes differences in these outcomes associated with several chronic medical conditions (Stewart, Greenfield, Hays, et al., 1989), and the other describes differences in these outcomes associated with depression relative to several chronic medical conditions (Wells, Stewart, Hays, et al., 1989). The latter article also contrasts the functioning and well-being of patients seen by general medical providers and mental health providers and contrasts these outcomes in patients with depressive disorder and patients with depressive symptoms and no disorder. In addition to the substantive findings of both studies, the results support the validity of the MOS measures.

The first clinical application (Stewart, Greenfield, Hays, et al., 1989) evaluated the relative decrements in functioning and well-being associated with hypertension, diabetes, myocardial infarction, congestive heart failure, arthritis, chronic lung problems, back problems, gastrointestinal disorders, and angina in 9,385 patients of medical providers. Scores were compared to two groups: patients with no chronic conditions and a general population sample. The methods used allowed estimation of the unique impact of each chronic condition on functioning and well-being, controlling for comorbidities and patient characteristics (age, education, income, and sex). The validity of the measures is supported in the sense that the measures discriminated between the comparison groups and the various chronic condition groups, and the profile of functioning and well-being among the different conditions corresponded to clinical expectations. For example, limitations tended to be greater for the more serious conditions. The magnitude of the differences associated with various chronic conditions also provides information regarding the meaning of score differences. For example, a 9-point difference in physical functioning (on a 0–100 scale) is equivalent to the effect of having arthritis or back problems.

The second study (Wells, Stewart, Hays, et al., 1989) included all 11,242 patients from the screening sample who completed the short-form survey, including patients of mental health providers. In addition to the nine chronic medical conditions defined in the first study, the second study identified patients with current depressive disorder as well as patients with depressive symptoms. Several approaches were taken in this study to identify limitations in functioning and well-being associated with depression. Again, the pattern of limitations associated with depression compared to limitations associated with the chronic medical conditions corresponded to clinical expectations, although less is known about the functioning and well-being of depressed patients. Further, an analysis to address the concern that depressed patients may overreport negative health states revealed that their reports were as highly predictive of bed-days and utilization as reports of nondepressed patients, suggesting that these self-reports are of considerable clinical and social consequence.

The findings reported in these articles are significant to complete an understanding not only of the validity but also of applications of the MOS measures.

18. Methods of Validating
MOS Health Measures

Anita L. Stewart, Ron D. Hays,
and John E. Ware, Jr.

Definition and Kinds of Validity

Validity refers to the extent to which a score measures what it is intended to measure and does not measure what it is not intended to measure (Anastasi, 1976) and to the extent to which a measure is useful scientifically (Nunnally, 1978). Validity studies increase understanding of the meaning of a score and the meaning of differences or changes in that score (Ware, 1984). Validating a health measure or a set of health measures is the process of accumulating many different kinds of evidence to determine the most appropriate interpretations(s) of a health score.

Since each piece of evidence only adds or takes away support for a particular interpretation, there is no clear point at which measures are considered valid. Therefore, the validation of health measures cannot be thoroughly assessed in a single study. Because health measures can be used for different purposes, their validity needs to be evaluated separately for each purpose. Health measures that are valid for one purpose (e.g., measuring outcomes) will not necessarily be valid for another (e.g., predicting demand for services) (Ware, Brook, Davies, et al., 1981).

A variety of different approaches help give understanding to the meaning of health measures. No standard guidelines are available for validating health measures. Thus, standards have been derived from those used to validate psychological and educational measures. Three categories of validity evidence are identified by the American Psychological Association, the American Educational Research Association, and the National Council on Measurement in Education (American Psychological Association [APA], 1985): content related, criterion related, and construct related. Content-related validity is a more qualitative approach than the other two, which are based on studies of empirical relationships. Nunnally (1978) refers to the same three types, labeling the second one predictive validity. These categories are intended as conveniences rather than to suggest that there is a rigid distinction among them (APA, 1985). Evidence of one type of validity is often evidence of another. Empirical approaches to validity include known groups, predictive, convergent/discriminant, multitrait-multimethod, and factorial. Depending on the purpose of the measure, some of these are criterion-related approaches under some circumstances and construct-related approaches under other circumstances. Four additional approaches provide useful validity information: evaluation of the interpretability of scores, the need for additional measurement using incremental validity analysis (Sechrest, 1967), examination of whether measures contain response bias, and validity generalization. The MOS has adopted a definitional structure (see Table 18–1) that best serves the validation of health measures based on an evaluation of the many different ways of defining validity.

This chapter presents an overview of the essential steps necessary to validate health measures and indicates the types of validation studies that have been performed on the MOS measures.

Content validity pertains to how well items in a measure, or concepts in a set of measures, sample a specified universe or domain of content (APA, 1985; Nunnally, 1978; Ware, 1984, 1987). Evaluation of how well the important aspects of a concept are being measured can be assessed at the level of an entire battery of health measures, within the components of a particular health concept, or within a single scale.

To perform content validation requires a definitional standard against which the concepts or items are compared. Standards can be based on well-accepted theoretical definitions, on existing accepted standards, or on interviews with those experiencing the types of problems studied. In developing the Sickness Impact Profile, for example, patients were interviewed to determine the full range of impact of disease on behavior (Gilson, Gilson, Bergner, et al., 1975). Ware (1987) has provided a set of minimum standards by which to evaluate the content validity of a battery of health measures based on an extensive review of existing measures.

Content validity is important during the construction and develop-

Table 18–1 Overview of Approaches to Testing Validity

Type of Validity	Definition and Examples
Content validity	**Are all relevant concepts represented in the measure or set of measures?**
Content validity of a battery	Are all aspects of functioning and well-being represented in the set of health measures?
Content validity of a scale	Are all aspects of a definition of a concept represented in a scale?
Criterion validity	**Does the measure correlate highly with the "gold standard" measure of that concept?**
Criterion validity	Does a new measure of depression correlate with the "gold standard" measure (e.g., Diagnostic Interview Schedule of the DSM-III)?
Criterion-related validity	Does a short-form measure of physical functioning correlate highly with a validated long-form measure of physical functioning?
Predictive validity	Do scores on a measure of health perceptions predict whether or not people use any health services in the following year?
Construct validity	**Do the measures correlate with measures of other variables in hypothesized ways?**
Convergent validity	Does a measure of pain intensity correlate with a measure of the effects of pain?
Discriminant validity	Does a measure of physical functioning correlate lower with a measure of mental health than with a measure of mobility?
Multitrait-multimethod approach	Does a self-reported measure of depression correlate higher with an observer rating of depression than it does with a self-reported measure of anxiety?
Known groups validity	Is the mean health perceptions score significantly lower for a group of patients than for a general population sample, as hypothesized?
Factorial validity	Are two underlying constructs (factors) of physical and mental health defined by the MOS health measures, as hypothesized?
Interpretability of scale scores	**What is the meaning of a score or a change (or difference) in a score?**
	What is the difference in mean health perceptions scores as a function of having arthritis?
	What is the amount of change in a physical functioning score achieved by providing an effective pain relief medication for angina?

Table 18–1 (*Cont.*)

Type of Validity	Definition and Examples
Incremental validity	Is a substantial gain in information achieved by adding items to a scale or scales to a battery of health measures?
	Does a mobility measure add a substantial amount of information over and above a physical functioning measure?
Response bias	Are scores systematically lower or higher due to response bias?
	Are scores of social functioning significantly correlated with a measure of socially desirable responding?
Validity generalization	Are the measures valid in different populations?
	Are the correlations among the measures similar in a patient population and a general population?

ment of measures (APA, 1985; Nunnally, 1978) and is a prerequisite to empirical validity. If the content of a concept is not adequately reflected, it is difficult to establish the more empirical types of validity.

The content validity of the MOS health measures was evaluated in terms of individual measures, the more common approach, and in terms of the entire set of measures to determine how well the set represents a comprehensive definition of health and to assure that the measures are not confounded with each other (Ware, Brook, Davies, et al., 1981).

For the entire MOS battery, the literature was relied on for the definitional standard of content validity because most relevant health concepts have been identified. For particular concepts, such as psychological distress/well-being, content validity studies ascertained whether all components were represented (e.g., whether they included depression, anxiety, positive affect). Within each scale, content validity determined whether the items were comprehensive in terms of the definition of that scale (e.g., whether all aspects of physical functioning were represented). For new measures, a large item pool was first created from several existing key instruments from which pilot study items were selected. Pilot studies typically were of measures with a large number of items. In evaluating pilot study results, one of the MOS criteria for retaining items was comprehensiveness (i.e., to represent the fullest range of components of each measure). Comprehensiveness at the item level also included attention to the range of levels tapped by items in the scale. For example, the MOS assured that the physical functioning scale reflected the performance of a full range of activities, from simple self-care to more difficult or vigorous ones.

Criterion and Construct Validity

Criterion validity demonstrates that test scores are systematically related to one or more outcome criteria (APA, 1985). One type of criterion validity involves the testing of a new measure in terms of how well it predicts an accepted "gold standard" measure. In the MOS, for example, a short screening measure of depression was developed by selecting items that best correlated with the gold standard measure of depression (Burnam, Wells, Leake, et al., 1988). Another type of criterion is some future event (e.g., poor health, death) that is predicted with the health measures.

Criterion validity is assessed by using scores on one measure to predict scores on the criterion (Anastasi, 1976; Cronbach, 1970). The higher the correlation between the measures, the stronger the evidence favoring criterion validity (Nunnally, 1978). MOS single-item measures were correlated with their respective long-form measure, which is considered a form of criterion-related validity.

When a measure is used to estimate some behavior external to the measure itself, the behavior is referred to as the "criterion," and the analysis is termed predictive validity (Nunnally, 1978). The predicted behavior can be concurrent in time or a future prediction. The latter is more common in health studies. If measures are to be used to identify patients likely to use a lot of health care services or patients at risk of poor health in the future (who thus may be in greater need of care), then the validity of the measures must be tested in terms of their ability to predict subsequent utilization and subsequent health. The prediction can be made in terms of group membership (e.g., those who have had any hospitalizations) or in terms of a continuous measure (amount of expenditures for health care). In general, the higher the correlation, the better. For the MOS measures, predictive validity tests involved examining the correlations between the measures and subsequent utilization (chapter 19).

The use of scores to predict some future event, such as utilization, can be considered criterion-related validity if the purpose of the score is to identify people who will be high utilizers. The same analysis can be considered evidence of construct validity if the purpose of the analysis is to confirm a hypothesis that a health measure is associated with subsequent utilization.

Construct Validity The basic issue in studies of construct validity is whether the health measure relates to other measures in ways consistent with plausible hypotheses. Patterns of relationships are hypothesized between the measure being validated and measures of other variables, and data are analyzed to see if the hypothesized patterns are confirmed empirically (Cronbach and Meehl, 1955; Nunnally, 1978). Hypotheses are usually stated regarding the direction and sometimes the strength of relationships that might be expected based on theory and literature. Validity is supported when the associations conform to the hypotheses. It is important that hypotheses be firmly grounded in theory. If the logic of the hypotheses is poorly thought through, a null finding might be taken as an indication of poor validity when in fact it reflects a true situation (McDowell and Newell, 1987).

Variables most often used to test patterns of relationships for health measures are utilization of health services, other general health measures, clinical measures, and mortality. Early studies of the validity of health measures included age as a validity variable, but because age does not consistently correlate with many health variables, we no longer consider it a good validity indicator.

The correlation of health measures with clinical status measures is a type of construct validity because certain measures of functioning or well-being can be hypothesized to be correlated with certain clinical measures. In this case, the clinical measures are not regarded as criteria but rather as constructs that should be related to the health measures. The best clinical measures for this purpose are those for which a strong hypothesis can be stated. The MOS examined the decrement in functioning and well-being associated with the presence of a variety of chronic medical conditions and depression to determine whether the decrement corresponded to the hypotheses about relative effects of those conditions (Stewart, Greenfield, Hays, et al., 1989; Wells, Stewart, Hays, et al., 1989). This process can also be considered a type of known-group validity.

For new measures, the evaluation of correlations of that measure with other measures provides the first step in beginning to understand the meaning of measures. In such cases, relationships between the new measures and other health concepts were evaluated. In these cases, the MOS was less interested in testing hypotheses about the nature of the relationships than in building a knowledge base about the meaning of the measures. For example, because the sleep measures are new, the purpose of the MOS studies of the relationships between the sleep measures and a variety of other health measures was to understand better the meaning of the sleep measures.

Convergent Validity The most commonly used type of construct validation is convergent validity, which focuses on the extent to which several measures of the same concept correlate with each other. Convergent validity at the item level was an essential part of the MOS method of scale construction (chapter 5).

Most of the MOS measures of functioning and well-being were based on the same method (self-report), but because the MOS often developed several subscales pertaining to the same construct, the convergent validity of those subscales was evaluated. For example, measures of physical functioning, mobility, and satisfaction with physical abilities were expected to correlate at least moderately with one another because they all assess physical functioning. Product-moment correlation coefficients and factor analysis were used to test these relationships. In factor analysis, measures that in fact are assessing the same underlying construct should correlate with, or load on, the same factor.

Discriminant Validity It is also important to demonstrate that a measure does not correlate with other measures that are intended to be different. For example, a measure of physical functioning would not be expected to be highly related to a measure of depression or of loneliness. Because all health measures are somewhat related, significant correlations are often observed among nearly all measures, especially in large samples like the MOS. Thus, discriminant validity is usually tested in relation to the correlations observed in the convergent validity studies. That is, the appropriate test is whether measures correlate lower with measures to which they are not expected to be related than they do with measures to which they are expected to be related.

Because item convergence and discrimination were an essential part of scale construction in the MOS, the discriminant validity of many of the measures was enhanced as a result of this process. Additional discriminant validity studies were then conducted using the final measures.

Multitrait-Multimethod Approach When more than one method of data collection or scale construction has been used, a variant of discriminant validity is possible. This elegant approach—the multitrait-multimethod (MTMM) procedure developed by Campbell and Fiske (1959)—blends convergent and discriminant validity. An MTMM matrix comprises intercorrelations of two or more health concepts (traits) measured by two or more methods. In the MTMM approach, a measure is expected to correlate significantly higher with other measures to which it should be (i.e., theoretically) related than with other measures to which it should not be related. Because all measures reported here are based on self-report, MTMM studies were not performed.

Known-Groups Validity Because one of the purposes of generic health measures is to detect the impact of disease and treatment on patient functioning and well-being, one test is how well the measures discriminate between groups known to differ in that health concept because of a particular disease. Known-groups validity involves comparisons of mean scores on a health measure across groups known to differ in the concept being validated (Kerlinger, 1973). For example, it was hypothesized that mean physical functioning would be lower in a group of patients than in a general population. Similarly, mean perceived health might be expected to be poorer in groups with a more severe disease (e.g., heart disease, cancer) than in those with a less severe disease (e.g., back problems, hypertension). Again, the evaluation of the generic measures in relation to clinical measures, such as the presence of various diseases, is especially useful in bridging the gap between these measures and those more familiar to clinicians. To represent a test of validity, it is important that the defined groups be clearly known to differ in the concept or construct being tested.

The MOS tested mean scores for the same measures administered to a patient sample and a general population sample for six short-form measures (Stewart, Hays, and Ware, 1988). Mean role limitations due to emotional problems scores were compared across groups of patients with and without depression. The MOS also determined the extent to which measures discriminated among nine chronic medical conditions defined in terms of physician report and patient report (Stewart, Greenfield, Hays, et al., 1989) as well as depression (Wells, Stewart, Hays, et al., 1989).

Factorial Validity When factor analysis is used to evaluate the structure of a set of scales, tests of the validity of the measures in relation to the underlying constructs can be performed. The same logic that leads to predictions about relationships among a set of variables can be applied to a particular concept. For example, if one underlying concept is expected to be represented by a set of measures (e.g., health perceptions), then one dimension or factor should be observed empirically using that set of measures.

The validity of a large set of measures was tested by evaluating their interrelationships in terms of their underlying structure, empirically testing the conceptual framework of health (chapter 2). Essentially, the MOS tested the presence of two underlying health dimensions: physical and mental health. Three patterns of correlations between measures and factors were hypothesized, namely, that some measured primarily physical health, others measured primarily mental health, and some measured both. Hypotheses were tested using confirmatory factor analysis, an analytic extension of exploratory factor analysis that allows for evaluation of a specific structure as defined by a pattern of factor loadings and factor intercorrelations (Long, 1983).

The Interpretability of Scale Scores

One aspect of validity pertains to how to interpret the score. Understanding what scale scores mean is confounded by two questions: the meaning of different scale levels (e.g., what does a score of 2 or of 71 mean?) and the meaning of differences or changes in scale units (e.g., is a 5-point difference meaningful?).

Meaning of Score Values For single-item measures with verbal response categories, the meaning of each score is quite clear. For example, the rating of health as excellent, very good, good, fair, or poor usually has scores ranging from 1 to 5; thus, each numeric score has a verbal interpretation. However, when multiple items are combined into a score, scores are possible over a broad range of numbers, and the score has no inherent meaning. The MOS provided several aids to understanding the meaning of scores. First, because the first clue to the meaning of the scale score itself (e.g., a group mean) comes from its relation to the endpoints, most measures were transformed to 0–100 scales, where the minimum possible score is 0 and the maximum 100. This process eliminates the problem of trying to interpret scores reported in many journal articles that all have different units.

Second, all measures were labeled to reflect the direction of scoring of the measure, and information on the direction of scoring is provided in all variable labels and tables so that it is immediately apparent whether a high score means better health or poorer health. This facilitates interpretation of correlations and of differences in mean scores. For example, if a variable is labeled "pain severity," then a high score indicates more pain, and a high score on "physical functioning" indicates better functioning.

Third, the MOS used a normative approach. When scales are normed in a general population or in some representative sample, the mean and the standard deviation become the "norm" against which scores of various subgroups can be compared. For the MOS Short-Form 20-item General Health Survey, two such normative samples are provided: a general population (chapter 16), and a representative sample of patients visiting a variety of providers (Stewart, Hays, and Ware, 1988). These can thus be used as comparison groups against which to compare scores obtained in other populations and samples. The MOS sample on which the other measures were developed consists of patients selected because they have one or more of the MOS chronic conditions. This sample is thus less "normative" than those available for the short form. Nevertheless, some understanding of the meaning of scores in other samples can be obtained by comparing them to the overall MOS sample mean and standard deviation.

Finally, some single-item measures have verbal descriptive categories for the different response choices. By calculating mean multi-item scale scores for the various descriptive categories, the meaning of the multi-item scale scores is better understood (Deyo and Patrick, 1988). To be useful, the verbal descriptor scale must be one that is itself reliable and valid. For selected concepts, mean multi-item scale scores were calculated for each level of the parallel single-item measures (e.g., mean physical functioning scores for the five levels of the single-item physical functioning measure). Although this calculation was done to understand the properties of the single item, the same results can also facilitate interpretation of the meaning of the various multi-item scale scores.

Meaning of Score Differences Because the main purpose of using health measures is usually to determine whether various treatments or types of health care are effective, it is of great interest to understand the meaning of a difference in scores or a change over time. For example, what is the meaning of a 5-point or a 10-point change in that score? Or perhaps better, what is the meaning of a difference in the amount of 0.1 standard deviation units, or of 0.5 standard deviation units? Such knowledge provides very important information that can be used in designing subsequent studies with enough precision to test hypotheses. However, a 5-point difference at one end of the scale may not mean the same thing as a similar difference at the other end of the scale. That is, a 5-point improvement at the severe end of the scale may mean far more to patients than a 5-point improvement at the healthy end of the scale.

This evaluation can be referred to as the calibration of measures or effect size analysis (Ware, 1984). Calibration involves documenting the meaning of differences in health scores by expressing them in terms that are relevant to patients, clinicians, or society. An example of such an analysis is to determine the percentage of those who received mental health care whose scores on psychological distress improved, or to examine the change in a score resulting from the onset of an acute chronic condition.

Deyo and Patrick (1988) discuss several issues regarding the responsiveness of scales to clinically meaningful changes, which can be regarded as evidence of the meaning of score differences. Deyo and Inui (1984) and Deyo and Centor (1986) present some very useful methods for testing the sensitivity of scale scores to clinical changes. For example, Deyo and Inui (1984) compared scores on various dimensions of the Sickness Impact Profile to clinical judgments of improvement or deterioration.

The MOS has contributed some information on the meaning of some of the health scores by documenting the unique decrements in health due to each of nine chronic medical conditions (Stewart, Greenfield, Hays, et al., 1989). For example, the presence of hypertension was reflected in a 3-point decrement in the current health perceptions measure.

Incremental Validity

In selecting a battery of measures, the uniqueness of each measure is an important consideration. This is an issue of incremental validity. Empirical studies of incremental validity address two basic issues: whether a long-form measure contributes sufficiently more information over and above a short-form measure and whether the addition of another health concept to a comprehensive battery contributes sufficiently more information over and above the initial set of concepts to justify the additional respondent burden and data-collection costs.

Short-form measures of health are less expensive to administer and are more popular with respondents; however, it is important to know that the use of short-form measures does not result in a serious loss of information compared to long-form measures. Thus, it is helpful to test the incremental validity of the long-form measures in relation to the short-form measures (Sechrest, 1967). In such tests, the increment in predictive power associated with the long-form measure is compared with the short-form one. For example, perceived current health could be predicted with a short-form physical functioning measure and then a long-form physical functioning measure added to the model to determine whether it significantly increases the variance explained. If it does, the long-form measure contributes a significant amount of additional information. The gain in predictive ability of the long-form measure must be weighed against its added cost or burden. In doing such tests, it is important to assure that any gains in prediction are not due simply to improved reliability (with additional items) rather than to the improved validity achieved by adding concepts or enriching a concept.

When the initial measures were being developed, the incremental validity of the MOS long-form measures was tested in several pilot studies using this method. The reasoning was that if an acceptable short-form measure contained as much information as the long form, then resources need not be expended on the long-form measure.

Response Bias

Two possible sources of bias that sometimes threaten the validity of health surveys and that often go along with self-reported methods (Bentler and Eichberg, 1975) are socially desirable response set (SDRS) and acquiescent response set.

Socially Desirable Response Set (SDRS) Socially desirable responding, a tendency to describe oneself in socially desirable or favorable terms, is among the most important sources of response bias in self-report research. Socially desirable responding affects the validity of self-reports because it results in underreporting of socially undesirable characteristics or overreporting of socially desirable behavior (Nunnally, 1978). There are two basic approaches to handling SDRS: minimizing its occurrence in the design of the question asked and measuring it so its effects can be evaluated and controlled for.

A number of instruments have been developed to measure the tendency to give socially desirable responses (Crowne and Marlowe,

1960; Jacobsen, Brown, and Ariza, 1983). These SDRS measures are typically included in the same questionnaires as the health measures. The correlations between the health measures and the SDRS measures are evaluated to determine the extent to which SDRS is present in other self-report measures (Crowne and Marlowe, 1960; Edwards, 1970). If SDRS is significantly correlated with a self-report measure, SDRS can be statistically controlled for in analyses involving that measure. Using such measures, SDRS has been found to be significantly correlated with depression, symptoms, life satisfaction, health-related behavior, problem drinking, and life events (Klassen, Hornstra, and Anderson, 1975; Kristiansen and Harding, 1984).

In the MOS, a brief SDRS measure was developed (Hays, Hayashi, and Stewart, 1989) and included in the validity studies combined with an evaluation of the relationship between SDRS and each of several health measures (chapter 19). Statistically significant correlations of SDRS with health measures are regarded as indicative of a problematic degree of SDRS in the measure.

By selecting appropriate methods for measuring those characteristics most likely to be susceptible to socially desirable responding, its occurrence in these measures can be minimized. For example, SDRS tends to be less problematic in mail surveys than it is in telephone and face-to-face interviews (Dillman, 1978). Because items differ in their susceptibility to social desirability responding (Edwards, 1970), its effects can be minimized when items are written. Thus, in developing item stems and response choices, the potential influence of SDRS was minimized wherever possible, following the recommendation of Smith (1967). Value-laden words were avoided and instructions were written to facilitate accurate, socially undesirable responses. Johnson's (1981) suggestion that "the best strategy for designing a valid scale is not to make lying or misrepresentation difficult, but to make self presentation as easy as possible" was adopted. Sometimes item response choices were reversed to put the one that was least "desirable" first. A response option that appears to the extreme left in a row of options tends to be selected more often than when it appears on the extreme right (Mathews, 1929).

Acquiescent Response Set Two types of acquiescent responding have been noted: agreement acquiescence and acceptance acquiescence (Bentler, Jackson, and Messick, 1971). Agreement acquiescence is a tendency of respondents to agree with statements regardless of content. Acceptance acquiescence refers to a tendency to accept characteristics as descriptive of oneself. Thus, acceptance acquiescence is denoted by agreement with items that describe characteristics and disagreement with items that deny characteristics. Acquiescence tends to occur more often when questions are ambiguous, lengthy, complicated, or otherwise difficult to understand. It also occurs more frequently in people with less education (Converse and Presser, 1986).

Both forms of acquiescence can be minimized by keeping questions simple, clear, and short, which the MOS attempted to do wherever possible. Agreement acquiescence can also be minimized by using several items to measure each concept, some with favorable wording and some with unfavorable wording (e.g., "do you have energy?" "do you feel tired?"). When these items are summed into a multi-item scale, agreement acquiescence tends to cancel out. The latter has been demonstrated for measures of health care attitudes (Ware, 1978). In selecting a final set of items for each measure, the MOS attempted wherever possible to achieve a balance between positively and negatively worded items. In some cases, however, this was impossible because some concepts are by definition negative (e.g., psychological distress is measured using only negatively worded items).

Validity Generalization

Given that the MOS wanted these generic measures to be appropriate for both patient and general populations and for severely ill as well as mildly ill groups, an important question is whether the validity of the measure is the same across these different groups. That is, can the validity evidence obtained with one type of sample be generalized to other samples, or must additional evidence be obtained in the new sample (APA, 1985)? Average scores were expected to differ in different groups, but the meaning of the scores should be stable across the groups (as reflected in the patterns of correlations and other empirical validity evidence). As evidence accumulates of similar validities in samples other than the MOS, validity generalization is increasingly assured. To the extent that the measures have different meanings in different groups, validity studies in different samples need to be performed until the generalizability is assured.

For many of the measures, the MOS had considerable prior experience in a general population (in the Health Insurance Experiment). Wherever this was the case, correlations among measures were compared with those obtained in the HIE to assure generalizability. The MOS evaluations of the structure of the short-form health measures were compared between two populations (Stewart, Hays, and Ware, 1988).

Discussion

This chapter provides both a methodological guide to the assessment of the validity of health measures and a summary of the approaches to validation that were taken in the MOS. Because many of the standards for validating health measures have been derived from those for validating measures in education and psychology, specific standards for validating health measures need to be developed. The issues in health assessment are more specific, and the validation process depends more on the purpose of the measure. Such new guidelines could provide needed clarity and increase the quality of available health measures. Such standards could be published, as are those in psychology and education (APA, 1985). The methods outlined in this chapter are intended to provide a first step toward such guidelines. We agree with McDowell and Newell (1987) that the validation of health measures is to a large extent an art form. If specific standards were outlined for health measures in particular and contributions obtained from a variety of investigators in health measurement, the "art" could be reflected in those standards.

The approach to validity outlined in this chapter is comprehensive and represents an ideal toward which to strive. When a reliable and variable measure has been subjected to preliminary validity studies, it can be used in analytic studies. Such studies can become sources of new validity information at the same time as they answer important clinical and policy questions. Because of the importance of validity, and because relatively little attention is generally given to validating health measures, future studies should incorporate some validation strategies.

The validity studies presented in this book are based on self-report data, and most are based on cross-sectional analysis. Because of the importance of using multiple perspectives, additional validity studies currently underway include tests of associations of these health measures with other measures based on clinical assessment as well as on measures occurring at a later point in time. For example, the relationship of these measures to measures of disease severity defined in terms of both physician-reported information and an independent clinical assessment will be tested. The MOS will evaluate the measures in relation to subsequent mortality and to changes in disease severity over time using prospective data.

Many of the health measures presented here are derived from measures that have been widely used and validated. The validity history of a measure is thus an important component. The prior validation evidence for those measures with a prior history (e.g., health perceptions and psychological distress/well-being) was reviewed.

The methods of validity presented in this chapter and applied in the MOS pertain primarily to tests of validity for measures to be used for research purposes. If measures are to be used for purposes of assessing individual patients in the offices of clinicians, additional standards are needed. For example, if a measure is to be used to identify patients in need of particular clinical interventions, then validation studies must be designed to assure that the measure is capable of doing so accurately. These types of studies are one of the next steps needed as the demand for measures that can be used by clinicians in everyday practice increases.

19. Construct Validity of MOS Health Measures

Ron D. Hays and Anita L. Stewart

The construct validity of a set of nineteen of the most direct measures of health was examined in terms of the interrelationships among the health measures and their relationships to selected validity measures. These analyses are based on self-reported measures. The approach to validation reported in this chapter was designed to answer five questions: (1) could two theoretical dimensions of health, physical and mental, be confirmed empirically? (2) would each measure relate to these two dimensions in hypothesized ways, assuming that physical and mental health are correlated? (3) what is the relationship between physical and mental health? (4) are the health measures biased by socially desirable responding? and (5) do the health measures predict subsequent utilization of services in hypothesized ways?

The first two questions require a hypothesis for the two theoretical constructs of physical and mental health, which are not directly measurable but can be defined by two or more measures. The constructs of physical and mental health were measured in terms of a subset of eight of the nineteen health measures considered to be the purest measures of health status. In selecting this set, we depended on the face validity of the measures as well as on prior experience with similar measures. This chapter is intended to be supplemented by a published article, "The Structure of Self-Reported Health in Chronic Disease Patients," by Ron D. Hays and Anita L. Stewart, which appeared in *Psychological Assessment: A Journal of Consulting and Clinical Psychology* (1990) 2:22–30.

Testing for the Number of Dimensions of Health Exploratory factor analysis was used to provide a preliminary examination of whether two factors explain adequately the relationships among the measures. Multiple criteria, described in chapter 5, were examined (Guttman's weakest lower bound, the scree test, the Tucker-Lewis reliability coefficient). Confirmatory methods provided additional confirmation regarding the number of dimensions.

Relationship of Each Measure to Physical and Mental Health and Intercorrelation Between Physical and Mental Health Confirmatory analytic procedures were employed to address the second and third questions. Confirmatory methods involve testing a priori hypotheses about the relationships among the measures. Three types of confirmatory analyses were employed: bivariate correlations, multitrait scaling analysis, and structural equation modeling. Two types of hypotheses were specified: the measurement model, specifying how each measure relates to the physical and mental health constructs, and the structural model, specifying how the underlying constructs of physical and mental health relate to one another.

A summary of the nineteen most direct measures, including the direction of scoring, the number of items in each measure, the mean and standard deviation, the internal-consistency reliability (for multi-item measures) is presented in Table 19–1. The MOS hypothesized for each measure whether it would represent primarily physical health (P), mental health (M), or both (PM). Hypotheses for the measurement model were based on previous research (R. D. Hays, unpublished manuscript; Ware and Allen, 1986; Ware, Davies-Avery, and Brook, 1980) for most of the measures. For example, we hypothesized that physical functioning primarily measured physical health (Ware, Davies-Avery, and Brook, 1980). For measures with which we had no prior experience on which to base a hypothesis (e.g., sleep), hypotheses were based on content.

Hypotheses for the structural model were also based on previous research (Ware, Davies-Avery, and Brook, 1980), which specified a positive correlation between physical and mental health (i.e., an oblique as opposed to an orthogonal model). The MOS also examined two important plausible alternative models: a model hypothesizing that physical and mental health are orthogonal (uncorrelated) and one hypothesizing a single dimension of health (i.e., that physical and mental health are perfectly correlated).

Four of the purest measures of physical health (physical functioning, satisfaction with physical ability, mobility, and role limitations due to physical health) and four of the purest measures of mental health

Table 19–1 Summary of Most Direct Health Measures Included in Construct Validity Studies (N = 3,211)

Health Measures	Scoring[a]	Hypothesized Construct	k[b]	Mean	SD	R_{tt}[c]
Role limitations due to physical health	(−)	P	7	35.8	34.4	.86
Physical functioning	(+)	P	10	73.2	26.4	.92
Satisfaction with physical ability	(+)	P	1	61.0	25.8	n/a
Mobility	(+)	P	2	93.3	16.1	n/a
Unable to work due to health	(−)	P	1	0.2	0.4	n/a
Effects of pain	(−)	P	6	22.0	24.1	.91
Pain severity	(−)	P	5	0.0	0.9	.86
Depression/behavioral-emotional control	(−)	M	13	19.3	18.3	.95
Positive affect	(+)	M	7	61.2	22.8	.94
Anxiety	(−)	M	6	24.5	19.3	.92
Feelings of belonging	(+)	M	3	70.6	26.3	.87
Role limitations due to emotional problems	(−)	M	3	30.0	39.2	.83
Cognitive functioning	(+)	M	6	82.4	16.5	.87
Physical/psychophysiologic symptoms	(−)	PM	8	24.9	17.4	.75
Energy/fatigue	(+)	PM	5	55.4	22.0	.88
Social activity limitations due to health	(−)	PM	4	34.8	19.2	.77
Sleep problems index II	(−)	PM	9	0.0	0.7	.86
Current health perceptions	(+)	PM	7	56.9	24.6	.88
Health distress	(−)	PM	6	20.0	22.6	.94

[a] P = hypothesized to measure primarily physical health; M = hypothesized to measure primarily mental health; PM = hypothesized to measure physical and mental health about equally. A (+) high score indicates better health; a (−) high score indicates poorer health. N/a = not applicable.
[b] k = number of items.
[c] R_{tt} = internal-consistency reliability.

(depression/behavioral-emotional control, anxiety, feelings of belonging, and positive affect) were selected as criteria. Bivariate (Pearson product-moment) correlations between each health measure and these criteria were examined. The MOS hypothesized that the pattern of correlations would correspond to the hypotheses about each measure. Measures hypothesized to measure only physical health were expected to be more strongly correlated with the pure physical health measures than with the pure mental health measures. Measures hypothesized to measure only mental health were expected to be more strongly correlated with the pure mental health measures than with the pure physical health measures. Measures hypothesized to measure both physical and mental health were expected to correlate about equally with the pure physical and the pure mental health measures.

For the multitrait scaling analyses, the physical and mental health dimensions were operationalized as aggregate indexes formed by summing across all measures of the dimension after standardizing the indicators and scoring each of them in a consistent direction. Measures hypothesized to represent both physical and mental health were included in both indexes. Correlations between each of the health measures and the aggregated indexes were computed. All correlations between measures and indexes were corrected for indicator overlap (Howard and Forehand, 1962). We expected that hypothesized measures of physical health would correlate higher with the physical health index than with the mental health index and that hypothesized measures of mental health would correlate higher with the mental health index than with the physical health index. Measures defining both physical and mental health were expected to correlate similarly with the two health indexes. Visual inspection of the pattern of correlations was deemed sufficient for this preliminary evaluation of the relationships between each measure and the physical and mental health constructs. The basic limitation of multitrait scaling analysis is that constructs are formed by adding together observed variables that are measured with error. A method that allows explicit control of error in variables is preferable.

Confirmatory factor analysis can be used to estimate "error-free" constructs, which are composed of the portion of observed variables that is common or correlated with other variables. These constructs are called latent or unobserved variables because they are indirectly measured. Confirmatory factory analysis is a subtype of the more general structural equation modeling (SEM) analytic procedure. To use the SEM methodology, a model must be hypothesized to explain the observed interrelationships among measured variables of interest. The methods of the SEM approach are described in Hays and Stewart, 1990.

Using multitrait scaling and SEM methods, four basic questions were asked in testing the hypotheses:

(1) Do measures relate to physical and mental health in the hypothesized direction?

Multitrait scaling: Is the correlation between the measure and the index (corrected for overlap) greater than 0.40 and in the hypothesized direction?

SEM: Is the parameter estimate for each measure that is hypothesized to have a nonzero relationship with the construct statistically significant and in the hypothesized direction?

(2) To what extent does each measure assess physical or mental health?

Multitrait scaling: The larger the correlation (in the hypothesized direction) for each measure, the more indicative it is of the dimension.

SEM: The larger the parameter estimate (in the hypothesized direction) for each measure, the more indicative it is of the dimension.

(3) Do the theoretical constructs of physical and mental health relate to one another?

Multitrait scaling: Not applicable. Because the physical and mental health indexes are defined by several of the same measures, the degree of overlap does not allow for an independent evaluation of their interrelationship.

SEM: Tests the significance of the estimated correlation between the constructs.

(4) How well does the hypothesized model (measurement and structural models collectively) fit the data?

Multitrait scaling: Not applicable.

SEM: Goodness-of-fit measures are evaluated. Chi square is used to evaluate statistical significance—the lower the better. The goal is to achieve a nonsignificant chi square, indicating a nonsignificant difference between the hypothesized model and the data. Delta, rho, and comparative fit indices, which represent the proportion of possible covariation in the data explained by the model, should be greater than 0.90.

Testing for Socially Desirable Responding To evaluate whether the health measures are biased by socially desirable responding, the MOS tested whether each health measure was associated with a measure of a socially desirable response set (SDRS). SDRS was assessed by a 5-item measure, the SDRS-5, derived from the Crowne and Marlowe (1960) scale. Reliability for the measure was 0.68 in the MOS (Hays, Hayashi, and Stewart, 1989). The SDRS-5 is designed to appear as if it is assessing the respondent's relationship with others and is not easily detected by respondents as an SDRS measure. To determine the associations between SDRS and the observed measures of physical and mental health,

Pearson product-moment correlations were computed between the SDRS-5 scale and the health measures. Nonsignificant associations of each measure with SDRS suggested valid, nonbiased measures. The correlation of SDRS with each of the measures was examined, adjusting for lack of perfect reliability (Guilford, 1954). The adjusted correlations are calculated by dividing the raw correlations by the square root of the product of 0.68—reliability of the SDRS-5 scale—and the reliability of the health measure. SDRS was also included in the SEM analyses so that its relationship with the latent measures of health could be examined.

Predicting Utilization of Services Evaluation of whether measures predict use of health services is a common approach for evaluating their validity. Newcomb and Bentler (1987) examined the associations between health perceptions (physical hardiness), subjective health problems (happiness with health, perceived major health problems, difficulty with health), symptoms, and health service utilization (nights in hospital, number of hospitalizations, times seen by a physician for an emergency, times seen by a physician for illness) using confirmatory factor analysis. Subjective health problems and symptoms correlated $r = 0.28$ with utilization; worse health perceptions correlated $r = 0.12$ with utilization. However, in their study utilization was postdicted by the health status variables in a cross-sectional analysis. Manning, Newhouse, and Ware (1982) demonstrated that cross-sectional analysis can lead to bias (and the direction of the bias cannot generally be known a priori) in estimation of parameters in utilization studies.

Mental health has been shown to be predictive of use of mental health services and the level of care received from mental health specialists (Ware, Manning, Duan, et al., 1984). Physical and role functioning have been found to have effects on use of mental health services that are distinct from the effects of mental health (Ware, Manning, Duan, et al., 1984). Individuals with physical or role limitations tend to be heavier utilizers of general medical services (Manning, Newhouse, and Ware, 1982) and more likely to be hospitalized (Cafferata, 1987; Weinberger, Darnell, Tierney, et al., 1986) than those without these limitations. Depressive symptoms have also been linked to increased likelihood of hospital admission during the following year (Weinberger, Darnell, Tierney, et al., 1986).

Four measures of utilization of services were selected as validity variables in studies of the predictive validity of the measures. These utilization measures, assessed one year after the health measures, were based on self-reports and included: (1) overnight stays in a hospital, nursing home, or convalescent home during the last twelve months, (2) visits to a doctor or other health professional in the last six months, (3) visits to a mental health specialist in the last six months, and (4) visits to a medical doctor other than a psychiatrist to discuss personal or emotional problems in the last six months. For each validity variable, both a dichotomous (o = none, 1 = 1 or more) and a continuous indicator (number of overnight stays, visits) were derived. The dichotomized measure of any visits to a doctor was very skewed, with 91% of respondents reporting at least one visit. Thus, this measure may be problematic in these tests.

If the health measures are valid, they should be significantly correlated with all measures of utilization. Measures of physical health were hypothesized to be more highly correlated than measures of mental health with overnight stays and doctor or health professional visits, and measures of mental health were hypothesized to be more highly correlated than measures of physical health with visits to mental health specialists and with doctor visits to discuss personal or emotional problems.

Results of Construct Validity Analyses

Evaluating the Number of Dimensions of Health Guttman's weakest lower bound, the Tucker-Lewis reliability coefficient (0.95) and Cattell's scree test supported a two-factor solution. Two factors were rotated that corresponded to physical and mental health.

Evaluating the Physical and Mental Health Constructs Bivariate correlations between each of the health measures and the purest health measures revealed a pattern consistent with hypotheses: measures of physical health correlated higher with the pure physical health measures than they did with the pure mental health measures and vice versa (see Table 19–2). Measures hypothesized to measure both physical and mental health correlated about equally with the physical and mental health criterion measures. One exception to our hypotheses was that effects of pain, hypothesized to measure primarily physical health, correlated substantially with mental health indicators.

Results of the multitrait scaling analysis are shown for the physical and mental health indexes in Table 19–3. Correlations between scales and the indexes they are hypothesized to represent are indicated by

Table 19–2 Correlations between Each Health Measure and Purest Measure of Physical and Mental Health (N = 1,980)

	PHYSICAL		
Health Measures[a]	ROLEPH (−)	PFI (+)	PFSAT (+)
Role limitations due to physical health (P)(−)	—	−.65	−.59
Physical functioning (P)(+)	−.65	—	.64
Satisfaction with physical ability (P)(+)	−.59	.64	—
Mobility (P)(+)	−.48	.58	.41
Unable to work due to health (P)(−)	.45	−.49	−.37
Effects of pain (P)(−)	.67	−.54	−.55
Pain severity (P)(−)	.57	−.49	−.50
Depression/behavioral-emotional control (M)(−)	.33	−.14	−.33
Positive affect (M)(+)	−.34	.16	.41
Anxiety (M)(−)	.32	−.17	−.34
Feelings of belonging (M)(+)	−.20	.05	.23
Role limitations due to emotional problems (M)(−)	.45	−.22	−.33
Cognitive functioning (M)(+)	−.39	.24	.32
Physical/psychophysiologic symptoms (PM)(−)	.56	−.48	−.53
Energy/fatigue (PM)(+)	−.63	.53	.62
Social activity limitations due to health (PM)(−)	.55	−.43	−.50
Sleep problems index II (PM)(−)	.47	−.33	−.41
Current health perceptions (PM)(+)	−.60	.59	.65
Health distress (PM)(−)	.54	−.44	−.54

[a] P = hypothesized to measure primarily physical health; M = hypothesized to measure primarily mental health; PM = hypothesized to measure physical and mental health about equally. A (+) high score indicates better health; a (−) high score indicates poorer health.

footnote "c" and are corrected for overlap. The matrix of correlations provides support for the hypothesized dimensions of health. The final column in Table 19–3 provides the difference, in absolute magnitude, between the correlations of each measure with the indexes. This column shows that the indicators that were hypothesized to represent physical health but not mental health correlated substantially higher with the physical health index than they did with the mental health index (i.e., there was a positive difference between correlations). Similarly, the measures hypothesized to represent mental but not physical health

	MENTAL			
MOB (+)	DEPBC (−)	POS (+)	ANX (−)	BEL (+)
−.48	.33	−.34	.32	−.20
.58	−.14	.16	−.17	.05
.41	−.33	.41	−.34	.23
—	−.25	.22	−.26	.08
−.44	.20	−.18	.18	−.09
−.46	.43	−.41	.43	−.24
−.37	.29	−.30	.32	−.16
−.25	—	−.84	.80	−.66
.22	−.84	—	−.72	.73
−.26	.80	−.72	—	−.51
.08	−.66	.73	−.51	—
−.24	.65	−.57	.56	−.44
.28	−.74	.62	−.72	.49
−.36	.44	−.41	.48	−.29
.41	−.53	.58	−.50	.38
−.47	.65	.61	.55	.43
−.34	.57	−.54	.57	−.40
.43	−.43	.48	−.42	.30
−.44	.59	−.52	.54	−.35

correlated noticeably higher with the mental health index than with the physical health index (i.e., there were negative differences between correlations).

Measures defining both physical and mental health correlated about equally with physical and mental health. The current health measure, although correlating fairly evenly with physical and mental health, yielded the largest difference in correlations favoring physical health of the measures hypothesized to measure both physical and mental health. Role limitations due to emotional problems had a slightly smaller difference than did the other mental health indicators, suggesting that such role limitations reflect physical health to a greater extent than the other mental health measures do.

Table 19–3 Scale-Index Correlations for Health Measures
(N = 1,980)

| Health Measures[a] | INDEXES | | |
	Physical	Mental	Diff.[b]
Role limitations due to physical health (P)(−)	−.766[c]	−.590	.176
Physical functioning (P)(+)	.696[c]	.414	.282
Satisfaction with physical ability (P)(+)	.712[c]	.573	.139
Mobility (P)(+)	.580[c]	.416	.164
Unable to work due to health (P)(−)	−.500[c]	−.352	.148
Effects of pain (P)(−)	−.773[c]	−.629	.144
Pain severity (P)(−)	−.667[c]	−.500	.167
Depression/behavioral-emotional control (M)(−)	−.540	−.837[c]	−.297
Positive affect (M)(+)	.538	.802[c]	−.264
Anxiety (M)(−)	−.527	−.764[c]	−.237
Feelings of belonging (M)(+)	.335	.588[c]	−.253
Role limitations due to emotional problems (M)(−)	−.494	−.651[c]	−.157
Cognitive functioning (M)(+)	.532	.732[c]	−.200
Physical/psychophysiologic symptoms (PM)(−)	−.706[c]	−.615[c]	.091
Energy/fatigue (PM)(+)	−.742[c]	.716[c]	.026
Social activities limitations due to health (PM)(−)	−.695[c]	−.735[c]	−.040
Sleep problems index (PM)(−)	−.612[c]	−.686[c]	−.074
Current health perceptions (PM)(+)	.773[c]	.645[c]	.128
Health distress (PM)(−)	−.704	−.705[c]	−.001

Note: Standard error of correlation = 0.02.
[a] P = hypothesized to measure primarily physical health; M = hypothesized to measure primarily mental health; PM = hypothesized to measure physical and mental health about equally. A (+) high score indicates better health; a (−) high score indicates poorer health.
[b] Diff. = difference (in absolute magnitude) between the two correlations in each row; a positive difference indicates that the correlation with physical health was larger; a negative difference indicates that the correlation with mental health was larger.
[c] Indicates hypothesized to relate to construct and, thus, corrected for overlap.

Results of the confirmatory factor analysis are summarized in Table 19–4. The hypothesized model fit the data well on practical grounds (delta = 0.95, rho = 0.94, comparative fit index = 0.93), but it was rejectable statistically because of the large sample size. All of the parameter estimates for the hypothesized model, except the correlation

Table 19–4 Standardized Parameter Estimates for Hypothesized Confirmatory Factor Analysis Model (*N* = 1,980)

Health Measures[a]	Physical		Mental	
Factor loadings				
Role lim. due phys. health (P)(−)	−.81	(−.84)	—[b]	—[b]
Physical functioning (P)(+)	.72	(.76)	—[b]	—[b]
Satisf. with phys. ability (P)(−)	.72	(.77)	—[b]	—[b]
Mobility (P)(−)	.58	(.61)	—[b]	—[b]
Depress./behav.-emot. control (M)(−)	—[b]	—[b]	−.92	(−.92)
Positive affect (M)(+)	—[b]	—[b]	.82	(.84)
Anxiety (M)(−)	—[b]	—[b]	−.85	(−.86)
Feelings of belong. (M)(+)	—[b]	—[b]	.60	(.61)
Correlations				
Unable to work due health (P)(−)	−.57	(−.53)	−.23	(−.26)
Effects of pain (P)(−)	−.79	(−.72)	−.48	(−.46)
Pain severity (P)(−)	−.68	(−.65)	−.34	(−.33)
Role limit. due emot. prob. (M)(−)	−.48	(−.50)	−.67	(−.65)
Cognitive funct. (M)(+)	.46	(.46)	.79	(.78)
Phys./psych. symptoms (PM)(−)	−.68	(−.68)	−.50	(−.49)
Energy/fatigue (PM)(+)	.77	(.76)	.59	(.60)
Soc. activ. limit. due health (PM)(−)	−.69	(−.65)	−.68	(−.66)
Sleep prob. index (PM)(−)	−.55	(−.52)	−.63	(−.59)
Current health percep. (PM)(+)	.77	(.79)	.49	(.51)
Health distress (PM)(−)	−.69	(−.70)	−.63	(−.58)
SDRS	−.05	(−.04)	.08	(.07)
Age	.00	(.00)	—	—
Income	−.02	(−.04)	—	—
Education	—	—	—	—
Gender	—	—	—	—

Note: Only the first 8 measures in the table were allowed to load on the physical and mental health latent variables. Maximum likelihood and arbitrary distribution theory (in parenthesis) estimates are provided. Dashes indicate that parameters were nonsignificant and therefore fixed at zero. Physical and mental health intercorrelated *r* = 0.46 (0.44). The correlation between age and physical health was not statistically significant. Standard errors for parameter estimates shown above ranged from 0.01 to 0.04. Nine correlated uniqueness terms and 60 correlations among measured variables were estimated, but they are not shown.
[a] P = hypothesized to measure primarily physical health; M = hypothesized to measure primarily mental health; PM = hypothesized to measure physical and mental health about equally. A (+) high score indicates better health; a (−) high score indicates poorer health.
[b] Fixed at zero a priori.

between age and physical health, were statistically significant and in the hypothesized direction. The correlation between age and physical health was included because it was significant in one of the subsample analyses (Hays and Stewart, 1990). The correlation between the physical and mental health latent variables was estimated to be 0.460. This moderate positive correlation indicates that physical and mental health are related but distinct constructs. More detail is presented in Hays and Stewart, 1990.

The correlations between the eleven health measures not included in the pure set and the physical and mental health constructs defined by the eight purest measures were consistent with the hypotheses. The measures hypothesized to define physical but not mental health correlated more strongly with physical health than with mental health. Similarly, the measures hypothesized to define mental health but not physical health correlated more strongly with mental than with physical health. The measures hypothesized to define both physical and mental health correlated about equally with the two constructs, except for current health, which correlated notably more with physical than with mental health.

The two alternative models were less satisfactory. The uncorrelated (orthogonal) model of health fit the data significantly less well than the hypothesized model. Thus, a correlated (oblique) model more closely fits the observed data than an orthogonal model. The one-factor model in which the correlation between physical and mental health was constrained at 1.0 was rejectable statistically and on practical grounds. Thus, a two-factor model more adequately represents the data than a one-factor model.

Association of Measures with SDRS   The raw zero-order correlations between SDRS and the health measures as well as correlations adjusted for unreliability are presented in Table 19–5. All raw correlations were statistically significant because of the large sample size, although all but three were less than 0.23 in absolute magnitude (a widely used criterion of meaningfulness—5% of the common variance). The strongest bivariate associations with SDRS (absolute magnitude ranged from 0.17 to 0.26) were observed for the mental health measures (e.g., anxiety, positive affect).

The confirmatory factor analysis model contains correlations between SDRS and physical health and mental health of −0.054 and 0.085, respectively. The relatively small correlation between SDRS and

Table 19–5 Correlations of Health Measures with Socially Desirable Response Set

Health Measure[a]	Raw Correlation	Correlation Adjusted for Unreliability
Role limitations due to physical health (P)(−)	−.04	−.06
Physical functioning (P)(+)	−.11[b]	−.14
Satisfaction with physical ability (P)(+)	.07	.11
Mobility (P)(+)	−.04[b]	−.06
Unable to work due to health (P)(−)	.05[b]	.08
Effects of pain (P)(−)	−.09	−.11
Pain severity (P)(−)	−.05	−.07
Depression/behavioral-emotional control (M)(−)	−.24	−.30
Positive affect (M)(+)	.26	.33
Anxiety (M)(−)	−.26	−.33
Feelings of belonging (M)(+)	.19	.25
Role limitations due to emotional problems (M)(−)	−.17	−.22
Cognitive functioning (M)(+)	.21	.27
Physical/psychophysiologic symptoms (PM)(−)	−.08	−.11
Energy/fatigue (PM)(+)	.09	.11
Social activity limitations due to health (PM)(−)	−.13	−.18
Sleep problems index II (PM)(−)	−.14	−.18
Current health perceptions (PM)(+)	.08	.10
Health distress (PM)(−)	−.11	−.14

Note: All correlations are statistically significant ($p < .05$).
[a] P = hypothesized to measure primarily physical health; M = hypothesized primarily to measure mental health; PM = hypothesized to measure physical and mental health about equally. A (+) high score indicates better health; a (−) high score indicates poorer health.
[b] These raw correlations are in the unhypothesized direction.

the mental health latent variable relative to the zero-order correlations reflects a difficulty in the model in reproducing these sample correlations (i.e., there are relatively large standardized residuals).

Predictive Validity Correlations between the eight validity variables measured one year following baseline and the nineteen health measures measured at baseline are presented in Table 19–6. These results provide

Table 19–6 Correlations between Health Measures and 12-Month Utilization Variables

Measure	PH[a]		
	ANYHOSP	NUMHOSP	ANYMED
Role limitations due to physical health (P)(−)	.159c	.060d	.015
Physical functioning (P)(+)	−.193c	−.096c	.000
Satisfaction with physical ability (P)(+)	−.152c	−.054d	−.028
Mobility (P)(+)	−.178c	−.072c	−.014
Unable to work due to health (P)(−)	.108c	.086c	.043
Effects of pain (P)(−)	.132c	.051d	.018
Pain severity (P)(−)	.107c	.040	.018
Depression/behavioral-emotional control (M)(−)	.028	.011	.001
Positive affect (M)(+)	−.026	−.020	−.007
Anxiety (M)(−)	.030	.017	.009
Feelings of belonging (M)(+)	.008	−.047	.015
Role limitations due to emotional problems (M)(−)	.023	−.008	−.015
Cognitive functioning (M)(+)	−.033	−.038	.045
Physical/psychophysiologic symptoms (PM)(−)	.129c	.064d	.038
Energy/fatigue (PM)(+)	−.147c	−.071c	−.044
Social activity limitations due to health (PM)(−)	.147c	.063d	−.005
Sleep problems index (PM)(−)	.087c	.067c	.020
Current health perceptions (PM)(+)	−.211c	−.089c	−.056d
Health distress (PM)(−)	.126c	.028	.046
X	.16	.30	.91
SD	.37	2.14	.29

[a]PH = Physical health-related utilization; ANYHOSP = Any overnight stays in hospital, nursing home, or convalescent home during last 12 months; NUMHOSP = Number of overnight stays in hospital, nursing home, or convalescent home during the last 12 months; ANYMED = Any visits to a doctor or other health professional in the last 6 months; NUMMED = Number of visits to a doctor or other health professional in the last 6 months.

[b]MH = Mental health-related utilization; ANYMHMH = Any visits to a mental health specialist

strong evidence in favor of the construct validity of health measures. Every measure of health was significantly correlated with half or more of the utilization variables.

The strongest relationships were observed between the measures of only mental health (depression/behavioral-emotional control, positive

PH[a]	MH[b]			
NUMMED	ANYMHMH	NUMMHMH	ANYMDMH	NUMMDMH
.103[c]	.043	−.012	.136[c]	.136[c]
−.053[d]	.116[c]	.107[c]	−.064[d]	−.118[c]
−.151[d]	−.085[c]	−.034	−.140[c]	−.116[c]
−.112[c]	−.023	.015	−.126[c]	−.160[c]
.039	−.017	−.002	.057[d]	.079[c]
.160[c]	.117[c]	.058[d]	.197[c]	.155[c]
.153[c]	.072[c]	.037	.162[c]	.140[c]
.312[c]	.454[c]	.387[c]	.239[c]	.181[c]
−.287[c]	−.405[c]	−.332[c]	−.207[c]	−.126[c]
.284[c]	.393[c]	.315[c]	.240[c]	.171[c]
−.237[c]	−.346[c]	−.306[c]	−.149[c]	−.115[c]
.213[c]	.297[c]	.244[c]	.179[c]	.154[c]
−.206[c]	−.296[c]	−.236[c]	−.184[c]	−.168[c]
.199[c]	.126[c]	.084[c]	.187[c]	.185[c]
−.221[c]	−.175[c]	−.140[c]	−.158[c]	−.133[c]
.257[c]	.285[c]	.239[c]	.216[c]	.176[c]
.192[c]	.190[c]	.135[c]	.194[c]	.193[c]
−.180[c]	−.103[c]	−.067[c]	−.160[c]	−.153[c]
.205[c]	.235[c]	.147[c]	.232[c]	.181[c]
7.17	.18	2.54	.17	.57
9.98	.38	8.15	.37	2.12

in the last 6 months; NUMMHMH = Number of visits to a mental health specialist in the last 6 months; ANYMDMH = Any visits to a medical doctor (other than a psychiatrist) to discuss personal/emotional problems in the last 6 months; NUMMDMH = Number of visits to a medical doctor (other than a psychiatrist) to discuss personal/emotional problems in the last 6 months.
[c]$p<.01$.
[d]$p<.05$.

affect, anxiety, cognitive functioning, feelings of belonging, and role limitations due to emotional problems) and visits to mental health specialists. The magnitude of the correlations between these measures and whether or not a visit for reasons of mental health occurred ranged from 0.30 to 0.45; the magnitude of the correlations between these measures and the number of visits to mental health specialists ranged from 0.24 to 0.39. Interestingly, the mental health measures were strongly related to the number of visits to doctors or other health professionals (absolute magnitude ranged from 0.21 to 0.31), but they were not associated with the dichotomized version of doctor visits (the range was 0.01 to 0.40). The lack of association between all the health measures and the dichotomized doctor visit measure may be due to the poor variability of this measure.

Discussion of Results

The consistency in results across the various methods provides strong verification of the MOS conceptualization of health. The examination and confirmation of two dimensions of health, physical and mental, by the health measures examined appears to diverge from the three dimensions of health (physical, mental, and social) defined by the World Health Organization and verified empirically (Ware, Davies-Avery, and Brook, 1980). In Ware et al.'s analysis, social health was operationalized in terms of the amount of social participation or level of social activity (e.g., number of visits to friends). The MOS social functioning measures are explicitly operationalized as indicators of physical and mental health rather than the extent of social activity (chapters 2, 9, and 12). If the analyses had included measures such as family and marital functioning, or number of visits to friends, a third dimension of social functioning or social activity might have been observed.

Aggregate indexes reflecting the two underlying physical and mental health dimensions may be appropriate for some analyses, although the unique information available in the separate measures may be obscured. Until the analyses necessary to determine the optimal scoring of such indexes have been completed, use of the separate measures is recommended.

Three of the six measures hypothesized to measure both physical and mental health tended to measure physical health slightly more than mental health: current health, physical/psychophysiologic symptoms, and energy/fatigue. Ware, Davies-Avery, and Brook (1980) found a more even pattern of loadings of current health on physical and mental dimensions. This in part can be due to discrepancies in defining the underlying constructs and methodological differences. In the MOS, physical health and mental health are defined in more complex terms than in the 1980 study by Ware, Davies-Avery, and Brook. In the MOS, physical health and mental health were allowed to correlate in the analysis, which was not true in the Ware et al. study. The use of orthogonal or oblique rotation affects conclusions drawn from data (Ford, MacCallum, and Tait, 1986). When constructs are known to be correlated, as are physical and mental health, an oblique (correlated) solution is more appropriate than an orthogonal (uncorrelated) solution. Ware and Allen (1986) found results consistent with those presented here when they allowed a correlation between physical and mental health.

Symptoms in the MOS were designed to be about equally representative of physical and mental health (i.e., it contains a mixture of physical and psychophysiologic symptoms—see chapter 15). This representation tended to be true in the bivariate and scale-index correlations, but it was less so in the SEM analysis. In the SEM analysis, physical/psychophysiologic symptoms correlated slightly higher with physical health than with mental health.

Energy/fatigue correlated more highly with physical health than it did with mental health in the SEM analysis, although its correlation with mental health was substantial. However, in the scale-index analysis and in the bivariate correlations, the scale tended to correlate about equally with physical and mental health. Ware, Davies-Avery, and Brook (1980) found that the Health Insurance Experiment vitality scale loaded more highly on mental health than it did on physical health. The MOS findings that the energy/fatigue concept represents both physical health and mental health may reflect successful efforts at unconfounding energy/fatigue from closely related mental health concepts such as depression. These findings could also be due to sample differences; the MOS sample includes more people with physical and mental health problems.

The zero-order correlations between each health measure and SDRS revealed that the mental health indicators are somewhat more highly correlated with SDRS than are the physical health indicators, consistent with Ware and Allen (1986), but the extent of SDRS bias was small.

The utilization variables were selected to provide a preliminary examination of validity and do not represent the universe of all possible validity variables. Nonetheless, the results corresponded with the hypothesized relationships in support of the predictive validity of the measures. The positive correlation between physical functioning and visits to mental health specialists was unexpected. However, patients of mental health specialists in the MOS are significantly younger, more likely to be white, and tend to be more educated than patients of general medical providers (Wells, Stewart, Hays, et al., 1989). Because of the MOS design and focus on chronic medical conditions and depression, the association of physical functioning with mental health visits may be due in part to the better physical functioning of mental health specialty patients in the sample.

The validity studies reported were limited to nineteen of the most direct health measures, and although the validity of the remaining measures is still unaddressed, these nineteen measures include all primary measures and those most likely to be used in the majority of analyses regarding functioning and well-being. Analyses of the validity of the remaining measures are planned for the future.

VI

Summary, Discussion, and

Future Directions

20. Summary and Discussion of MOS Measures

Anita L. Stewart, Cathy D. Sherbourne,
Ron D. Hays, Kenneth B. Wells,
Eugene C. Nelson, Caren J. Kamberg,
William H. Rogers, Sandra H. Berry,
and John E. Ware, Jr.

More than seventy survey measures of functioning and well-being developed for the MOS have been presented for use by other investigators. Twelve major concepts of functioning and well-being are represented (see Table 20–1). The goal was to develop a set of measures appropriate for diverse populations that could be used as a standard for comparisons of populations with different chronic health problems as well as for healthy populations. The MOS samples represent a wide range of ages, including many elderly. Some MOS patients were relatively well, having only mild hypertension, while others were quite ill, having severe and complicated heart disease and other comorbid problems. Many MOS patients had depression, either alone or in combination with a medical condition.

The MOS measures reflect the influence and contributions of many other investigators in the field of health assessment. The measures are based most directly on the health measures developed for the RAND Health Insurance Experiment (HIE), which in turn were based on the work of many others. Some MOS measures are similar and others identical to HIE measures, which, unlike the MOS, was limited to a nonaged general population. HIE measures were modified in the MOS to make them more appropriate for use in elderly and chronically ill populations. Although the total number of questionnaire items in the MOS is less than in the HIE battery, the MOS approach is comprehensive, and noteworthy improvements in specific measures have been achieved. In expanding and modifying the HIE measures, we drew upon the ideas and approaches of numerous others.

Table 20–1 Summary of Functioning and Well-Being Concepts

Concept	Chapter	Definition
Physical functioning	6	Performance of physical activities such as self-care, walking, climbing stairs, and vigorous activities
Mobility	6	Getting around in the community
Role functioning	12	Performance of usual role activities such as working at a job, housework, child care, community activities, and volunteer work
Social functioning	9–11	Functioning in normal social activities with family, friends, neighbors; marital functioning; sexual problems
Psychological distress/well-being	7	Positive and negative psychological states including anxiety, depression/behavioral-emotional control, feelings of belonging, positive affect
Cognitive functioning	7	Cognitive problems such as forgetfulness, difficulty concentrating
Health perceptions	8	Personal evaluations of health in general including current and prior health, health outlook, resistance to illness
Health distress	8	Psychological distress due to health problems
Energy/fatigue	8	Feelings of energy, pep, fatigue, tiredness
Sleep	14	Quantity, disturbance, adequacy of sleep
Pain	13	Subjective feelings of bodily distress or discomfort such as headaches or backaches
Physical/psychophysiologic symptoms	15	Subjective perceptions about the internal state of the body such as stiffness and coughing

Underlying Conceptual Framework

The MOS measures were based on a comprehensive conceptual model of health (chapter 2) which includes two overarching dimensions of health—physical and mental. These two dimensions are assessed from five perspectives: (1) clinical status, including diagnosed conditions and impairments; (2) physical functioning and well-being; (3) mental functioning and well-being; (4) social functioning and well-being; and (5) general health perceptions and satisfaction. Each of these five perspectives provides an essential and unique point of view regarding people's physical and mental health. The latter four perspectives, which were assessed using standardized patient questionnaires in the MOS, are covered in this book.

This two-dimensional conceptualization represents a noteworthy shift in direction from the prior work in the HIE, which defined three dimensions of health—physical, mental, and social (Ware, Brook, Williams, et al., 1980). Empirical results from the HIE indicated that several measures focusing primarily on social contacts had little to do with physical or mental health status or with perceptions of health in general (Ware, Brook, Williams, et al., 1980; Donald and Ware, 1982). The idea that physical and mental health "ends at the skin," whereas social activity measures extend the conceptual framework beyond the individual (Ware, Brook, Davies, et al., 1981), led us to change the three-dimensional conceptualization from the HIE framework to two dimensions. Within this framework, limitations in social and role activities due to health problems were assessed. Thus these measures are indicators of physical or mental health problems. This two-dimensional framework was supported empirically when the structure of the MOS measures was tested (chapter 19).

Some of the MOS measures assess physical health, some assess mental health, and others do not distinguish and are considered measures of both physical and mental health. As hypothesized, role and social limitations caused by health problems assessed one or both dimensions.

Methods of Constructing MOS Measures

The MOS multi-item measures were constructed using multitrait scaling, an analytic technique that assures the internal consistency of items in a particular scale and also assures that items do not overlap significantly with other conceptually similar scales. The satisfactory performance of questionnaire items in these tests of item convergence and item discrimination is an important and considerable strength of the MOS measures.

Because the MOS measures of functioning and well-being were constructed and evaluated in relation to each other as a complete set, each measure is as unique as possible. The measures are correlated because the health concepts they measure are correlated. Each MOS health scale, however, contains unique reliable variance, a property evaluated in relation to a comprehensive set of measures and health concepts. Therefore, in using the entire survey, investigators can be assured that redundancy is less likely than when scales are chosen from different instruments.

Progress has been made in the MOS in constructing more practical health measures. Scales of different lengths, including single-item scales, were constructed for key dimensions of health. These short-form measures are intended to provide choices to those facing tradeoffs between breadth and depth of measurement in selecting health measures for a particular study. In theory, the long-form measures yield scores with the greatest precision in terms of reliability and number of scale levels. Because they have fewer items, the short-form scales define fewer scale levels and may be less reliable. Their reliability and validity, however, appear to be adequate for some purposes. They have proven to be very useful so far. The six single-item general health measures are intended to provide a very short alternative to the multi-item scales when only a few minutes of questionnaire administration time is available.

Four Sets of MOS Measures

The largest set of MOS health measures included in a single questionnaire was administered in the baseline Patient Assessment Questionnaire. This 149-item questionnaire is called the MOS Functioning and Well-Being Profile (MOSFWBP). The MOSFWBP includes thirty-five scales and eight summary indexes that combine certain scales; it is recommended for use in studies desiring the "full set."

From this full set, a smaller subset, the MOSFWBP-C (Core Subset), contains twenty scales and four summary indexes constructed from 113 questions. The selection of the MOSFWBP-C is subjective, based on the content of the measures. The MOSFWBP-C includes measures that appear to define health most directly and, given our experience to date, are most likely to be affected by treatments for health problems or to detect changes in health. Measures that include information on personality factors or attitudes in addition to health were excluded from the MOSFWBP-C. For example, health concern (e.g., I often think about my health) and resistance to illness (e.g., I get sick easier than other people) were excluded. Similarly, health outlook may include information on pessimism or optimism in addition to health status. The MOSFWBP-C was included in tests of the construct validity of the measures (chapter 19). Subsequent empirical studies of validity, such as tests of their sensitivity to clinical changes in the severity of illness and of their ability to predict subsequent utilization and health, are needed to confirm these as the most direct and useful measures.

Two MOS options for those requiring extremely brief surveys are reported here. The 20-item MOS Short-Form General Health Survey, administered to the screening sample, measures six health concepts. The MOS 6-item General Health Survey consists of six self-administered, single-item measures which were administered to the baseline sample. A 36-item short form (SF-36) has also been constructed (Ware and Sherbourne, 1992) and has been evaluated favorably in preliminary studies (McHorney, Ware, Rogers, et al., 1992).

The content of the four sets and the number of items in each are compared in Table 20–2, organized according to concepts. The first rows of Table 20–2 summarize the total number of items in each set of measures and estimates the amount of time required to complete each set. The remaining rows in Table 20–2 refer to specific measures within each concept.

Definitions of the measures in the MOSFWBP are shown in Table 20–3, and those measures that are part of the MOSFWBP-C are indicated. Definitions of the measures included in the 20-item MOS Short-Form General Health Survey are shown in Table 20–4, and definitions of the 6-item General Health Survey are shown in Table 20–5.

Summary statistics on the MOSFWBP for the Patient Assessment Questionnaire (PAQ) baseline sample are shown in Table 20–6, including means, standard deviations, skewness, and reliability where applicable. Correlations among the measures are shown in Table 20–7; in this matrix only the largest version of each index was included. Summary statistics on the 6-item General Health Survey from the PAQ baseline sample are shown in Table 20–8. Because of the unusual nature of this sample, which consisted of patients with one or more chronic conditions, these statistics do not represent norms in the traditional sense. If the means were to be broken down by chronic conditions, poorer scores would be observed for those with more severe conditions and better scores for those with less severe conditions. The measures are highly reliable. Some measures are more skewed than others. Those

Table 20–2 Measures of Functioning and Well-Being Constructed for the MOS: Number of Items in Different Sets

Measure	SETS OF MEASURES			
	Full Set MOSFWBP	Core Subset MOSFWBP-C	20-Item Short Form	6-Item Survey
Total number of questions	149	113	20	6
Est. minutes to complete[a]	30–37	23–28	4–5	2–3
Physical functioning				
Physical functioning (+)	10	10	6	1
Satisfaction with physical ability (+)	1	1		
Mobility				
Mobility (+)	2	2		
Role functioning				
Role limitations due to physical health (−)	7	7		
Role limitations due to emotional problems (−)	3	3		
Unable to work due to health (−)	1	1		
Unable to do housework due to health (−)	1	1		
Role Functioning (+)			2	1
Social, family, sexual functioning				
Social activity limitations due to health (−)	4	4	1	1
Sexual problems (−)	5			
Satisfaction with family life (+)	3			
Overall happiness with family life (+)	1			
Marital functioning (+)	6			
Psychological distress/well-being				
Anxiety (−)[b]	6	6		
Depression/behavioral- emotional control (−)[b]	13	13		
Positive affect (+)	7	7		
Feeling of belonging (+)	3	3		
Psychological distress (−)[c]	22	22		1
Psychological well-being (+)[c]	10	10		
Mental health index (+)[c]	32	32	5	

Table 20–2 (*Cont.*)

Measure	Full Set MOSFWBP	Core Subset MOSFWBP-C	20-Item Short Form	6-Item Survey
	SETS OF MEASURES			
Cognitive functioning				
Cognitive functioning (+)	6	6		
Health perceptions				
Current health (+)	7	7	5	1
Prior health (+)	3			
Health outlook (+)	6			
Health concern	4			
Resistance to illness (+)	4			
Health perceptions index (+)c	23	13		
Health distress				
Health distress (−)	6	6		
Energy/fatigue				
Energy/fatigue (+)	5	5		
Sleep				
Sleep quantity	1			
Optimal sleep (+)	1			
Sleep disturbance (−)	4			
Sleep adequacy (+)	2			
Sleep somnolence (−)	3			
Sleep shortness of breath or headache (−)	1			
Snoring (−)	1			
Sleep problems index I (−)c	9	9		
Pain				
Effects of pain (−)	6	6		
Pain severity (−)	5	5	1	1
Days pain interfered (−)	1			
Overall pain index (−)d	12			
Physical/psychophysiologic symptoms				
Physical/psychophysiologic symptoms (−)	8	8		

a Pilot and main results and prior studies indicate additional time is needed to read the instructions and orient the individual to the questionnaire.

b Measure has alternate shorter version.

c Measure has alternate shorter version and is constructed from other measures.

d Measure is constructed from other measures.

Table 20–3 Definitions of 149-Item MOS Functioning and Well-Being Profile (MOSFWBP) Measures

Measure[a]	# of Items	Definition	Included in MOSFWBP-C
Physical functioning			
Physical functioning (+)	10	Extent to which health limits physical activities such as self-care, walking, climbing hills and stairs, bending, lifting, and moderate and vigorous activities	Yes
Satisfaction with physical ability (+)	1	Satisfaction with physical ability to do what wanted	Yes
Mobility			
Mobility (+)	2	Amount of time in bed or chair all or most of the day, and amount of time needs assistance getting around community	Yes
Role functioning			
Role limitations due to physical health (−)	7	Limitations in work or other regular daily activities due to physical health during past 4 weeks such as took frequent rests, limited in kind of work, had difficulty, or accomplished less than wanted	Yes
Role limitations due to emotional problems (−)	3	Limitations in work or other regular daily activities due to emotional problems during past 4 weeks including cut down amount of time spent, accomplished less than wanted, didn't do work as carefully as usual	Yes
Unable to work due to health (−)	1	Unable to work due to health (dichotomous measure)	Yes
Unable to do housework due to health (−)	1	Unable to do housework due to health (dichotomous measure)	Yes
Social, family, sexual functioning			
Social activity limitations due to health (−)	4	Limitations in normal social activities during past 4 weeks due to physical health or emotional problems, comparison of these limitations to those of others their age, and changes in social activities over last 6 months because of changes in physical or emotional condition	Yes

Table 20–3 (*Cont.*)

Measure[a]	# of Items	Definition	Included in MOSFWBP-C
Sexual problems (−)	5	Extent of problems during past 4 weeks including lack of interest, inability to enjoy sex, difficulty becoming aroused, difficulty having an orgasm (women), and difficulty getting or maintaining an erection (men)	No
Satisfaction with family life (+)	3	Satisfaction with family life in terms of cohesiveness, amount of support and understanding, amount talk things over	No
Overall happiness with family life (+)	1	Overall happiness with family life	No
Marital functioning (+)	6	Reports about relationship with spouse or partner (or person feel closest to) over past 4 weeks in terms of saying anything wanted, sharing personal feelings, feeling close, being supportive	No
Psychological distress/well-being			
Anxiety I (−)	6	Amount of time in past month very nervous person, bothered by nervousness, tense, high strung, difficulty calming down, rattled or upset, restless or fidgety	Yes
Anxiety II (−)[b]	3	Amount of time in past month very nervous person, tense, high strung, restless or fidgety	Yes
Depression/behavioral-emotional control I (−)	13	Amount of time in past month felt in low spirits, downhearted, depressed, moody, down in the dumps, nothing to look forward to, not in firm control of behavior, felt like crying, felt others better off if dead, not emotionally stable, thought about taking own life	Yes
Depression/behavioral-emotional control II (−)[b]	8	Amount of time in past month felt in low spirits, downhearted, depressed, moody, down in dumps, nothing to look forward to, not in firm control of behavior, not emotionally stable	Yes
Positive affect I (+)	7	Amount of time in past month been a happy person, generally enjoyed things, felt calm and peaceful, happy, satisfied, pleased, felt living was a wonderful adventure, cheerful and lighthearted, daily life interesting	Yes
Positive affect II (+)[b]	4	Amount of time in past month been a happy person, felt calm and peaceful, felt cheerful and lighthearted, daily life interesting	Yes

Table 20–3 (*Cont.*)

Measure[a]	# of Items	Definition	Included in MOSFWBP-C
Feelings of belonging (+)	3	Amount of time in past month felt relationships full, felt loved and wanted, felt close to people	Yes
Psychological distress I (−)	22	Amount of time during past month very nervous person, bothered by nervousness, tense, difficult calming down, anxious, rattled or upset, restless, fidgety, low spirits, downhearted, depressed, moody, depression interfered, down in dumps, nothing to look forward to, not in firm control, felt like crying, felt others better off if dead, not emotionally stable, thought about taking life	Yes
Psychological distress II (−)[b]	12	Amount of time during past month very nervous person, tense, anxious or worried, restless, fidgety, low spirits, downhearted, depressed, moody, down in dumps, nothing to look forward to, not in firm control, not emotionally stable	Yes
Psychological well-being I (+)	10	Amount of time during past month been a happy person, enjoyed things, calm and peaceful, satisfied, felt living was an adventure, cheerful, daily life interesting, love relationships full, felt loved, felt close to people	Yes
Psychological well-being II (+)[b]	5	Amount of time during past month been a happy person, calm and peaceful, cheerful, daily life interesting, felt loved	Yes
Mental health index I (MHI − 32) (+)	32	Includes depression/behavioral-emotional control, anxiety, feelings of belonging, positive affect	Yes
Mental health index II (MHI − 17) (+)[b]	17	Includes depression/behavioral-emotional control, anxiety, feelings of belonging, positive affect	Yes
Mental health index III (MHI − 5) (+)[c]	5	Amount of time during past month very nervous person, downhearted, down in dumps, happy person, calm and peaceful[b]	Yes
Cognitive functioning			
Cognitive functioning (+)	6	Amount of time in past month became confused, reacted slowly to things, had difficulty reasoning, forgetful, trouble keeping attention, and had difficulty concentrating	Yes

Table 20–3 *(Cont.)*

Measure[a]	# of Items	Definition	Included in MOSFWBP-C
Health perceptions			
Current health (+)	7	Ratings of overall current health (e.g., I have been feeling bad lately, my health is excellent)	Yes
Prior health (+)	3	Ratings of health in the past (e.g., never been seriously ill, so sick once thought I might die)	No
Health outlook (+)	6	Ratings of future health (e.g., good health is in my future, expect my health to get worse)	No
Health concern	4	Concern about health, often think about health	No
Resistance to illness (+)	4	Ratings of resistance to illness (e.g., my body resists illness, get sick easier than others)	No
Health perceptions index I (+)	23	Ratings of current health, health outlook, health distress, and resistance to illness	No
Health perceptions index II (+)	19	Ratings of current health, health outlook, and health distress	No
Health perceptions index III (+)	13	Ratings of current health and health distress	Yes
Health distress			
Health distress (−)	6	Amount of time in past month feeling distressed about health (e.g., discouraged by health, worry about health, afraid because of health)	Yes
Energy/fatigue			
Energy/fatigue (+)	5	Amount of time in past month felt full of pep, energetic, worn out, tired, and had enough energy to do things wanted to do	Yes
Sleep			
Sleep quantity	1	Average hours of sleep during past 4 weeks	No
Optimal sleep (+)	1	Dichotomous measure 1 = optimal (7 or 8 hours of sleep), 0 = all other amounts, on average, during past 4 weeks	No
Sleep disturbance (−)	4	Amount of time during past 4 weeks had trouble falling asleep, staying asleep	Yes
Sleep adequacy (+)	2	Amount of time during past 4 weeks got enough sleep to feel rested, got amount of sleep needed	Yes
Sleep somnolence (−)	3	Amount of time during past 4 weeks felt drowsy during day, had trouble staying awake, took daytime naps	No

Table 20–3 (*Cont.*)

Measure[a]	# of Items	Definition	Included in MOSFWBP-C
Sleep shortness of breath or headache (−)	1	Amount of time during past 4 weeks awakened short of breath or with a headache	Yes
Snoring (−)	1	Amount of time during past 4 weeks snored during sleep	No
Sleep problems index II (−)	9	Sleep disturbance, adequacy, somnolence, and awaken short of breath during past 4 weeks	Yes
Sleep problems index I (−)[d]	6	Sleep disturbance, adequacy, somnolence, and awaken short of breath during past 4 weeks	Yes
Pain			
Effects of pain (−)	6	Effects of pain on daily activities including ability to walk, sleep, work, recreation, and on mood and life enjoyment during the past 4 weeks	Yes
Pain severity (−)	5	Pain intensity (average and at its worst), frequency, duration during past 4 weeks	Yes
Days pain interfered (−)	1	Number of days during past 30 days pain interfered with things	No
Overall pain index (−)	12	Effects of pain on daily activities including ability to walk, sleep, work, recreation, and on mood and life enjoyment; pain intensity, frequency, duration; and number of days pain interfered, all during past 4 weeks	No
Physical/psycho-physiologic symptoms			
Physical/psycho-physiologic symptoms (−)	8	Frequency of occurrence of 8 general (nondisease-specific) symptoms including stiffness, pain, swelling, or soreness of muscles or joints; coughing that produced sputum; backaches; nausea, acid indigestion; heavy feelings in arms and legs; headaches; lump in throat, all during the past 4 weeks	Yes

[a] A (+) high score means better health; a (−) high score means poorer health.
[b] Shorter version of level I scale or index; part of 17-Item battery.
[c] Part of the MOS 20-Item Short-Form General Health Survey, a subset of the 17-item and the 32-item index.
[d] Shorter version of level II index.

Table 20–4 Definitions of 20-Item M O S Short-Form General Health Survey Measures

Measure	# of Items	Definition
Physical functioning	6	Extent to which health interferes with a variety of physical activities (e.g., sports, carrying groceries, climbing stairs, and walking)
Role functioning	2	Extent to which health interferes with usual daily activity such as work, housework, or school
Social functioning	1	Extent to which health interferes with normal social activities such as visiting with friends or group activities during past month
Mental health index[a]	5	General mood or affect, including anxiety, depression, and psychological well-being during the past month
Current health perceptions	5	Overall ratings of current health in general
Pain	1	Intensity of bodily pain in past 4 weeks

[a]Same as mental health index III (M H I − 5)

Table 20–5 Definitions of M O S 6-Item General Health Survey Measures

Measure	# of Items	Definition
Physical functioning	1	Extent to which health problems limit everyday physical activities
Role functioning	1	Difficulty doing daily work during past 4 weeks, inside or outside the house, due to physical health or emotional problems
Social functioning	1	Extent of limitations in normal social activities due to physical health or emotional problems during past 4 weeks
Psychological distress	1	Amount of time in past 4 weeks bothered by emotional problems (feeling anxious, depressed, or irritable)
Current health perceptions	1	Overall rating of health as excellent, very good, good, fair, or poor
Pain	1	Intensity of bodily pain in past 4 weeks

Table 20–6 Characteristics of MOSFWBP measures: PAQ Baseline Sample (N = 3,053)

Category/Scale[a]	# of Items	Mean	SD	Reliability	Skewness
Physical functioning					
Physical functioning (+)	10	73.2	26.4	.92	−0.1
Satisfaction with physical ability (+)	1	61.0	25.8	.63[c]	−0.4
Mobility					
Mobility (+)	2	93.3	16.1	.71	−3.3
Role functioning					
Role limitations due to physical health (−)	7	35.8	34.4	.86	0.5
Role limitations due to emotional problems (−)	3	30.0	39.2	.83	0.8
Unable to work due to health (−)	1	0.2[d]	0.4	n/a	1.8
Unable to do housework due to health (−)	1	0.2[d]	0.4	n/a	1.8
Social, family, sexual functioning					
Social activity limitations due to health (−)	4	34.8	19.2	.77	−1.0
Sexual problems (−)	5	27.2	32.0	.90	1.0
Satisfaction with family life (+)	3	62.2	28.7	.93	−0.5
Overall happiness with family life (+)	1	4.5[e]	1.2	.80[c]	−1.1
Marital functioning (+)	6	71.8	22.0	.82	−0.9
Psychological distress/ well-being					
Anxiety I (−)	6	24.5	19.3	.92	0.9
Anxiety II (−)	3	25.8	21.3	.86	0.9
Depression/behavioral-emotional control I (−)	13	19.3	18.3	.95	1.3
Depression/behavioral-emotional control II (−)	8	21.1	19.6	.94	1.2
Positive affect I (+)	7	61.2	22.8	.94	−0.5
Positive affect II (+)	4	60.7	23.3	.85	−0.5
Feelings of belonging (+)	3	70.6	26.3	.87	−0.7
Psychological distress I[b]	22	26.8	14.8	.97	1.1
Pscyhological distress II[b]	12	23.0	19.2	.95	1.1
Psychological well-being I (+)[b]	10	64.0	22.3	.94	−0.6
Psychological well-being II (+)[b]	5	63.0	22.9	.91	−0.6

Table 20–6 *(Cont.)*

Category/Scale[a]	# of Items	Mean	SD	Reliability	Skewness
Mental Health Index I (+)[b]	32	70.3	16.2	.98	−0.9
Mental Health Index II (+)[b]	17	72.8	19.5	.96	−0.9
Mental Health Index III (+)[b]	5	72.0	20.8	.90	−0.9
Cognitive functioning					
Cognitive functioning (+)	6	82.4	16.5	.87	−1.3
Health perceptions					
Current health (+)	7	56.9	24.6	.88	−0.3
Prior health (+)	3	56.2	33.3	.74	−0.3
Health outlook (+)	6	59.6	20.7	.87	−0.2
Health concern (−)	4	66.2	23.6	.73	−0.6
Resistance to illness (+)	4	68.0	22.2	.79	−0.8
Health perceptions index I (+)[b]	23	64.0	19.2	.93	−0.5
Health perceptions index II (+)[b]	19	64.7	19.2	.93	−0.6
Health perceptions index III (+)[b]	13	67.1	22.0	.94	−0.7
Health distress					
Health distress (−)	6	20.0	22.6	.94	1.3
Energy/fatigue					
Energy/fatigue (+)	5	55.4	22.0	.88	−0.3
Sleep					
Sleep quantity	1	6.9[f]	1.4	n/a	0.9
Optimal sleep (+)	1	0.6[g]	0.5	n/a	−0.2
Sleep disturbance (−)	4	0.0[h]	0.8	.84	0.9
Sleep adequacy (+)	2	60.8	25.3	.75	−0.6
Sleep somnolence (−)	3	26.5	19.8	.76	0.9
Sleep shortness of breath or headache (−)	1	13.3	21.8	n/a	1.8
Snoring (−)	1	31.4	30.2	n/a	0.8
Sleep problems index II (−)[b]	9	0.0[h]	0.7	.86	0.8
Sleep problems index I (−)[b]	6	28.3	18.2	.78	0.8
Pain					
Effects of pain (−)	6	22.0	24.3	.91	1.1
Pain severity (−)	5	0.0[h]	0.9	.86	0.3
Days pain interfered (−)	1	5.1[i]	8.2	.78[c]	1.8
Overall pain index (−)[b]	12	0.0[h]	0.8	.93	0.7

Table 20–6 *(Cont.)*

Category/Scale[a]	# of Items	Mean	SD	Reliability	Skewness
Physical/psychophysiologic symptoms					
Physical/psychophysiologic Symptoms (−)	8	24.9	17.4	.75	0.8

Note: All scores range from 0–100 except where otherwise indicated.
[a] A (+) high score indicates better health; a (−) high score indicates poorer health.
[b] Measure is constructed from other measures and should be used cautiously in analyses involving its components. See respective chapters for information on content.
[c] Alternate forms reliability (for single-item measures). Represents lower-bound estimates because of noncomparability of alternate forms.
[d] 0 = able, 1 = unable
[e] Scores range from 1–6
[f] Number of hours
[g] 0 = nonoptimal, 1 = optimal
[h] Standardized scores
[i] Number of days

most highly skewed should be used with caution, as ceiling (or floor) effects may be observed in which large numbers of people cannot get worse (or better) on the measure.

The summary statistics on the 20-item MOS Short-Form General Health Survey for the screening sample, shown in Table 20–9, can be considered more representative of patients in general and more normative than the PAQ baseline sample (Stewart, Hays, and Ware, 1988).

State-of-the-Art Advances of MOS Measures

The MOS health measures represent advances in the state of the art of measuring functioning and well-being. Improvements occur in two categories: an improved level of comprehensiveness across concepts, and specific improvements within various concepts, such as improved reliability, validity, and precision.

Comprehensiveness of the MOS Measures Because little is known about which concepts are most affected by disease and treatment and which are most important, the comprehensiveness of a health survey is crucial. An evaluation of the way in which the content of the MOS concepts compares with five other well-known health surveys is valuable. Table 20–10 lists the concepts measured in the MOS full set

(MOSFWBP), the 20-item Short-Form General Health Survey and the 6-item General Health Survey in comparison with the HIE and other well-known comprehensive health surveys, including the Sickness Impact Profile (SIP) (Bergner, Bobbitt, Carter, and Gilson, 1981), the Duke-UNC Health Profile (Parkerson, Gehlbach, Wagner, et al., 1981), the Nottingham Health Profile (Hunt and McEwen, 1980), and the Quality of Well-Being Scale (QWB) (Patrick, Bush, and Chen, 1973a). Table 20–10 shows that the MOS full set is more comprehensive than any other measure or set of measures.

Table 20–10 inadequately shows the variations in approach of different measures, but it does show the range of concepts covered. Some of the concepts tapped by these different surveys but not reflected in the table are covered more thoroughly by some surveys than others. For example, the SIP assesses physical functioning in terms of several subscales, whereas the QWB includes only one subscale. The SIP creates separate scores of body movement and ambulation, whereas the MOS approach combines these into a single physical functioning measure. The MOS has considerably expanded the HIE model of health to incorporate sleep, bodily pain, energy/fatigue, cognitive functioning, family functioning, and sexual functioning. Although the SIP is comprehensive with respect to various aspects of functioning (twelve subscales and two summary indexes are provided), it does not assess psychological distress/well-being, pain, symptoms, or health perceptions. The SIP includes two categories of functioning not included in the MOS measures: recreation/pastimes and communication. The SIP also includes eating problems, which are not assessed in the MOS.

The Duke-UNC Health Profile produces five scores pertaining to functioning, symptoms, and perceptions. The Nottingham Health Profile includes seven aspects of functioning, emotional well-being, symptoms, and perceptions. The QWB includes functioning and symptoms summarized into one score. Although separate QWB scores can be derived for the dimensions of functioning, this has not usually been done, and the reliability and validity of the separate QWB functioning scores has not been studied. Thus, health care interventions cannot easily be described in terms of their differential impact on different aspects of functioning and well-being using the QWB.

Specific Improvements Table 20–11 summarizes the more noteworthy improvements made in the MOS measures compared to the best existing prior measure of each concept. Six basic types of improvements were made: (1) the conceptualization of the measures (e.g., clarified the

Table 20–7 Correlations among Selected Measures (N = 3,445)

	1.	2.	3.	4.	5.	6.	7.	8.	9.	10.	11.	12.
1. Physical functioning	(.92)											
2. Satisfaction with physical ability	.63	(.63)										
3. Mobility	.58	.41	(.71)									
4. Role limitations due to physical health	.65	.59	.50	(.86)								
5. Role limitations due to emotional problems	.26	.35	.27	.49	(.83)							
6. Unable to work due to health	.50	.36	.48	.46	.24	(—)						
7. Social activity limitations due to health	.45	.52	.49	.55	.55	.38	(.77)					
8. Sexual problems	.13	.20	.07	.21	.24	.13	.27	(.90)				
9. Satisfaction with family life	.05	.20	.07	.16	.33	.09	.33	.21	(.93)			
10. Marital functioning	.06	.13	.05	.17	.30	.06	.30	.21	.63	(.82)		
11. Anxiety I	.18	.34	.26	.33	.56	.17	.56	.26	.39	.35	(.92)	
12. Depression/behavioral-emotional control I	.15	.35	.25	.33	.64	.18	.65	.28	.49	.46	.80	(.95)
13. Positive affect I	.19	.42	.22	.35	.56	.18	.61	.28	.56	.49	.71	.83
14. Feelings of belonging	.07	.24	.07	.21	.42	.08	.42	.23	.68	.63	.50	.65
15. Psychological distress I	.17	.36	.26	.34	.63	.18	.64	.28	.45	.42	.91	.97
16. Psychological well-being I	.16	.39	.18	.33	.55	.16	.59	.28	.64	.57	.68	.82
17. Mental health index I	.17	.39	.24	.35	.63	.18	.65	.30	.56	.51	.86	.96
18. Cognitive functioning	.26	.34	.29	.40	.57	.23	.57	.28	.36	.35	.71	.74
19. Current health	.59	.66	.45	.60	.42	.46	.60	.28	.26	.22	.42	.44
20. Prior health	.31	.30	.24	.31	.16	.27	.25	.12	.08	.07	.17	.17
21. Health outlook	.33	.39	.24	.31	.21	.22	.30	.18	.17	.16	.24	.24
22. Health perceptions index III	.57	.66	.49	.63	.50	.46	.67	.29	.28	.24	.52	.56
23. Health distress	.46	.55	.46	.54	.51	.38	.63	.26	.24	.23	.55	.60
24. Energy/fatigue	.54	.63	.42	.63	.49	.37	.60	.23	.28	.24	.49	.52
25. Sleep disturbance	.30	.34	.27	.38	.36	.25	.43	.20	.25	.26	.49	.47
26. Sleep adequacy	.15	.31	.17	.27	.34	.12	.39	.16	.27	.25	.45	.47
27. Sleep somnolence	.36	.36	.34	.45	.30	.29	.37	.19	.15	.16	.32	.33
28. Sleep problems index I	.35	.43	.34	.47	.44	.28	.53	.23	.30	.30	.57	.57
29. Effects of pain	.55	.56	.46	.66	.40	.37	.58	.21	.22	.20	.43	.43
30. Pain severity	.48	.51	.38	.57	.29	.29	.43	.16	.16	.16	.34	.31
31. Pain index	.55	.57	.46	.66	.38	.35	.55	.20	.20	.19	.41	.40
32. Physical/psychophysiologic symptoms	.49	.52	.39	.56	.40	.34	.48	.20	.24	.21	.47	.43

Note: Reliability estimates, where available, are in parentheses on the diagonal. All measures are positively scored.

dimensionality); (2) the validity (e.g., incorporated into the definitions of limitations the person's attribution of those limitations as due to physical or mental health problems); (3) the coarseness of scales (by adding items or response choices to increase the number of possible scale levels); (4) the sensitivity (e.g., by assessing role limitations due to emotional problems; (5) the reliability; and (6) the efficiency of items (e.g., by shortening existing scales with very high reliability to reduce burden without sacrificing reliability).

13.	14.	15.	16.	17.	18.	19.	20.	21.	22.	23.	24.	25.	26.	27.	28.	29.	30.	31.	32.
(.94)																			
.72	(.87)																		
.81	.59	(.97)																	
.97	.87	.79	(.94)																
.92	.74	.96	.92	(.98)															
.61	.48	.76	.60	.73	(.87)														
.49	.30	.45	.46	.48	.42	(.88)													
.17	.10	.17	.16	.18	.17	.47	(.74)												
.31	.20	.24	.29	.28	.22	.54	.28	(.87)											
.55	.35	.57	.52	.58	.51	.93	.45	.50	(.94)										
.53	.34	.61	.50	.60	.53	.67	.33	.35	.89	(.94)									
.59	.37	.53	.55	.57	.49	.68	.29	.37	.70	.60	(.88)								
.44	.33	.49	.43	.49	.43	.41	.20	.21	.45	.42	.44	(.84)							
.50	.36	.48	.48	.51	.38	.36	.14	.20	.39	.36	.46	.51	(.75)						
.29	.19	.34	.27	.33	.39	.42	.22	.23	.45	.42	.49	.35	.30	(.76)					
.55	.40	.59	.53	.60	.53	.52	.24	.27	.57	.52	.59	.88	.74	.61	(.86)				
.43	.26	.44	.40	.45	.41	.58	.29	.28	.62	.57	.56	.44	.36	.38	.53	(.91)			
.33	.19	.33	.30	.34	.30	.51	.28	.23	.53	.44	.48	.36	.30	.32	.44	.79	(.86)		
.40	.24	.42	.38	.42	.38	.58	.30	.27	.62	.54	.55	.43	.35	.37	.52	.95	.93	(.93)	
.42	.29	.47	.40	.46	.46	.57	.30	.27	.60	.53	.58	.45	.39	.40	.57	.63	.66	.68	(.75)

Selecting Measures from the MOS Sets

For those preferring an overall, comprehensive assessment of functioning and well-being, the full 149-item MOSFWBP, which takes 30–37 minutes, is recommended. If this is too long, the 113-item MOSFWBP-C, which takes 23–28 minutes, is recommended. If 113 items is too many, investigators can administer the MOS 20-Item Short-Form General Health Survey, which takes 4–5 minutes. This survey can be augmented with additional measures of interest for the study purpose.

Table 20–8 Characteristics of M O S 6-Item General Health Survey Measures: P A Q Baseline (N = 3,445)

Category/Scale	Observed Range	Mean	S D	Skewness
Physical functioning (+)	0–100	76.5	28.8	− 1.0
Role functioning (+)	0–100	71.3	28.5	− 0.6
Social functioning (+)	0–100	79.5	26.2	− 1.2
Psychological distress (+)	0–100	68.4	27.9	− 0.6
Current health perceptions (+)	0–100	60.7	25.3	− 0.5
Pain (+)	0–100	69.9	26.2	− 0.5

Note: Current health and pain scales recalibrated (see chapter 17).

Table 20–9 Characteristics of M O S 20-Item Short-Form General Health Survey Measures: M O S Screening Sample (N = 11,186)

Category/Scale	# of Items	Mean	S D	Reliability	Skewness
Physical functioning (+)	6	78.5	30.8	.86	− 0.8
Role functioning (+)	2	77.5	38.3	.81	− 1.0
Social functioning (+)	1	87.2	23.6	.67[b]	− 2.0
Mental health index (+)	5	72.6	20.2	.88	− 1.1
Current health perceptions (+)	5	63.0	26.8	.87	− 0.2
Pain (−)	1	31.4	27.7	.76[b]	− 0.3

Note: All measures range from 0–100.
[a] A (+) high score indicates better health; a (−) high score indicates poorer health.
[b] Alternate forms reliability; a lower-bound estimate.

Finally, a subset of measures from the M O S F W B P can be selected to meet the needs of the study.

If the full M O S F W B P is not used, the selection of appropriate concepts and measures is dictated by the purpose of the study. If particular treatment interventions are being studied, appropriateness of a concept can be based on an evaluation of which concepts are likely to be affected by the condition being studied and by potential side effects and benefits of the treatment. For example, pain, the most characteristic feature of angina, is usually brought on by exertion and affects patients' physical and role functioning, causing worry about health. The pain, however, is not likely to interfere with sleep. Similarly, chronic obstructive pulmonary disease, which affects physical and role functioning,

Table 20–10 Comparison of Concepts of Functioning and Well-Being Included in MOS and Other Health Surveys

Concept	MOS MOSFWBP	SF20	SF6	HIE	SIP	DHP	NHP	QWB
Physical functioning[a]	x	x	x	x	x	x	x	x
Mobility/travel	x			x	x			x
Role functioning[b]	x	x	x	x	x	x		x[c]
Social functioning	x	x	x	x	x	x	x	
Family functioning	x							
Sexual functioning	x							
Psychological distress/ well-being	x	x	x	x	x	x	x	
Cognitive functioning	x				x			
Health perceptions	x	x	x	x			x	
Health distress	x							
Energy/fatigue	x			x[d]			x	
Sleep	x				x		x	
Eating					x			
Recreation/hobbies					x			
Communication					x			
Pain	x	x	x				x	
Physical/psycho- physiologic symptoms	x				x		x	x

Note: MOSFWBP = Full MOS 149-item survey; SF20 = MOS 20-item Short-Form General Health Survey; SF6 = MOS 6-item General Health Survey; HIE = Health Insurance Experiment (Brook, Ware, Davies-Avery, et al., 1979); SIP = Sickness Impact Profile (Bergner, Bobbitt, Carter, and Gilson, et al., 1981); DHP = Duke-UNC Health Profile (Parkerson, Gehlbach, Wagner, et al., 1981); NHP = Nottingham Health Profile (Hunt and McEwen, 1980); QWB = Quality of Well-Being Scale (Patrick, Bush, and Chen, 1973a).
[a] Includes self-care, ambulation, and body movements.
[b] Includes home management and work.
[c] QWB measure of social activity is actually a role functioning measure.
[d] The HIE assessed energy/fatigue only in one site at baseline; it was dropped from all follow-up assessments.

will be associated with sleep problems and fatigue. Some studies of hypertension may not need to focus on physical functioning or pain but on health perceptions. In all three cases, a different set of measures is relevant for different conditions and treatments.

In any study, once particular concepts are judged relevant, the selection of particular measures for each can be made. Longer measures are better in a psychometric sense (i.e., they provide the possibility of being more sensitive). For cross-sectional analyses or descriptive studies involving large samples, short-form measures may be adequate. For

Table 20–11 Summary of Main State-of-the-Art Improvements in
the M O S F W B P

Concept	Main Improvements
Physical Functioning	Reduced coarseness of H I E measure on which it is based. Old measure had only 7 scale levels, M O S measure has 20 scale levels and obtains information on the degree of limitation for a broader set of functions. This should improve the sensitivity of the measure. Developed a new measure of satisfaction with physical ability (single item).
Mobility	Added a separate mobility measure (in the H I E, it was incorporated into the physical functioning scale).
Role Functioning	Developed a separate measure of role limitations due to physical health problems and role limitations due to emotional problems, which has never been done. Developed both measures to be appropriate for people with a variety of possible roles such as volunteering, caring for children, and being involved in community activities, in addition to the traditional roles of work, housework, and school. Assessed specific kinds of limitations instead of asking about more general limitations. This greatly improved the sensitivity of the measure of providing scales with more than the 2–3 scale levels of earlier measures.
Social Functioning	Measure of social activity limitations taps limitations in normal social activities due to physical health or emotional problems. This complements prior measures which focus primarily on the number of social contacts. Further, it allows respondents to define what is normal for them. Developed a new measure of sexual problems relevant to heart disease, diabetes, hypertension, or depression, or the treatments for these conditions. Developed a new brief measure of satisfaction with family life and a single-item measure of overall happiness with family life, especially for use as an outcome of care for depression. Developed the measures to allow people to form their own interpretation of "family" to allow for nontraditional families, so that scores can be obtained for more respondents than just those with a nuclear family. Developed a new brief measure of marital functioning, to allow people to form their own interpretation of "spouse" or "partner," to obtain the maximum number of those with nonmissing scores.
Psychological Distress/ Well-Being	Determined that behavioral-emotional control could not be distinguished from depression, thus combined these into one scale. Their distinction in the H I E was somewhat unclear. Shortened all measures so that depression/behavioral-emotional control, anxiety, positive affect, and feelings of belonging can be assessed with 32 items instead of 38 (as in the H I E). Revised response choices to be comparable, to facilitate telephone administration, the 17-item set, of these items. Expanded content of feelings of belonging (previously emotional ties).

Table 20–11 (*Cont.*)

Concept	Main Improvements
Cognitive Functioning	Modified an existing measure of self-reported cognitive dysfunction that shows promise as a supplement to more common observer-rated measures. MOS measure is based on SIP "alertness behavior" items (Bergner, Bobbitt, Carter, et al., 1981) but instead of a yes/no format, items were designed to tap extent of various problems (e.g., poor memory, trouble concentrating) as perceived by respondents.
Health Perceptions	Shortened the current health scale from the HIE scale on which it was based, without sacrificing reliability. Improved the reliability of the HIE measure of health outlook by modifying it slightly. Developed new measure of health concern that focuses on the concern about health, based on the concern items in the HIE health worry/concern measure. Improved the reliability of the HIE measure of resistance to illness by modifying it slightly.
Health Distress	Developed a new measure of distress due to health problems, based on part of the HIE health worry/concern measure. This measure focuses on the psychological distress associated with health problems, thus should be more sensitive to the psychological impact of disease and health care than measures of general psychological distress and well-being (because the latter measures are affected by more than just health).
Energy/Fatigue	Developed a measure of energy/fatigue based on several prior measures, especially the "vitality" measure from Dupuy's General Well-Being Schedule which was piloted in (but later dropped from) the HIE. The items were simplified and developed to be independent of closely related mental health and other items such as sleep problems.
Sleep	Developed a multidimensional battery of sleep problems and perceptions about sleep. No adequate self-report measures of all relevant aspects of sleep problems existed before these were developed. Most studies simply assess the quantity of sleep, which is difficult to interpret in relation to health. Behavioral aspects of sleep (sleep disturbance, sleepiness during the day, quantity of sleep) as well as perceived adequacy are assessed. The measures are based on a strong conceptual framework and were developed to be independent of one another. An overall index is also provided that summarizes sleep problems.
Pain	Developed three new measures of (1) pain severity, (2) effects of pain on daily activities, mood, and life enjoyment, and (3) number of days pain interfered with things. Most prior measures were very lengthy as they were usually designed specifically for pain populations. The MOS measures are intended to be applicable to people with a variety of conditions and are relatively brief.

Table 20–11 (*Cont.*)

Concept	Main Improvements
Physical/Psycho-physiologic Symptoms	Developed new brief measure of 8 general (nondisease-specific) physical symptoms that are fairly common; some of these are physiologic (could be due to physical or emotional problems). This measure is not intended to be an indicator of clinical status, but of physical well-being (i.e., bodily distress or discomfort).

longitudinal studies of change due to treatment interventions, longer measures may be necessary. The extent of change in particular outcomes that is expected due to the treatment can be taken into account in deciding which of the measures would have adequate sensitivity. This process of selection is subjective in nature, and tradeoffs have to be made between the resources available and the level of sensitivity required.

If a particular treatment is expected or known to affect one or two particular aspects of functioning or well-being, selection of the best measure of those aspects is desirable to achieve adequate precision and sensitivity. This decision might result in substituting a full measure for one of the short-form measures but administering the remainder of the short-form battery. The advantage is the increased likelihood of the measure being sensitive to the expected treatment differences.

It is recommended that scales be administered and scored as in the MOS. Further item deletion or construction of scales based on groups of items not tested in the MOS is not recommended without thorough evaluation in terms of scaling, variability, reliability, and validity.

These and other considerations involved in the selection of measures for a particular study have been discussed elsewhere (Bergner and Rothman, 1987; McDowell and Newell, 1987; Ware, Brook, Davies, et al., 1981).

Preparing a Questionnaire

The MOSFWBP (149 items) and the MOS Short-Form General Health Survey (20 items) were administered as part of larger questionnaires. In these questionnaires, items from different scales were often combined on the same page if they had the same response format. Thus, if only certain measures are going to be selected from the questionnaires, the questionnaire items need to be carefully extracted. When a subset of MOS measures is selected, we do not yet know the nature of any changes due to change in the context or the effects of asking questions on one health concept after another. To facilitate selecting all items for a given concept, a guide to the location of items for each measure precedes the actual questionnaires in the appendix.

Future Directions

Extensive prior experience with measures of physical functioning, psychological distress/well-being, and health perceptions in the HIE enabled us to improve them. The MOS measures have retained many of the strengths of earlier measures while solving some known problems. The validity work performed on the earlier versions should apply to the new MOS measures. Other MOS measures—role functioning, sleep, cognitive functioning, pain, physical/psychophysiologic symptoms, and health distress—need further study to confirm their usefulness as part of a comprehensive approach. These measures were developed especially for the MOS to fill in gaps in the overarching framework. The multitrait scaling analyses shoud be replicated and the reliability tested in any new population to assure the adequacy of the scaling decisions.

Several gaps exist in the MOS findings to date. One that stands out is the need to directly assess changes in health over time. Do people perceive that their health is improving, staying the same, or getting worse? Questions about perceived change were included in the annual MOS surveys. A potential pitfall in the use of perceived change items is that people might report a change when none occurred (e.g., due to fear, anxiety, hopefulness, or optimism). Thus, these items need to be validated (e.g., by comparing information on actual change with perceived change). However, a benefit of perceived change over actual change scores is for patients scoring at the extreme end of a scale. In this case, items asking about perceived change would allow assessment of deterioration or improvement that might otherwise be missed (Bindman, Keane, and Lurie, 1990). If many people report change that is not detected in the original scales, this report of change would indicate that the scales might be truncated at that end (i.e., that they need to be revised so that people will not bottom out or top out on them).

Some additional validity studies of MOS health measures are under way. The relationship of these measures to measures of disease status, disease severity, and treatments of hypertension, diabetes, heart disease, and major depression and dysthymia will be evaluated. In addition, the ability of these measures to predict transitions in disease status and severity over time will be evaluated. Although the MOS studied disease status in relation to the measures on the 20-item Short-Form General Health Survey (Stewart, Greenfield, Hays, et al., 1989; Wells, Stewart, Hays, et al., 1989), results need to be replicated for the long-form measures. Comparison of the relative sensitivities of long- and short-form measures will help determine how short a measure can be and still retain needed sensitivity (McHorney, Ware, Rogers, et al., 1992).

The use of the MOS measures in other studies will advance our understanding of the nature of the measures, in addition to providing information on outcomes of various conditions and treatments. When a measure discriminates between treatment, disease, or population groups in anticipated ways, support for the validity of the measures is provided.

Some information on the meaning of score differences or what might be called "effect sizes" has been provided (Stewart, Greenfield, Hays, et al., 1989). For example, we learned that a difference of about ten points (about one-third of a standard deviation in our sample) on the short-form physical functioning scale appears to reflect the impact of having back problems on physical functioning, all other things being equal. However, study features such as study methodology, treatments, settings, or subjects often influence effect sizes (Raudenbush, Becker, and Kalaian, 1988). For example, the standard deviation is related to sample homogeneity and size (smaller standard deviations will be observed in more homogeneous samples and in larger samples; see Mosteller, Ware, and Levine, 1989).

Much remains to be learned regarding what can be considered a meaningful difference for the various measures. Studies in which these measures are used, in addition to other measures with well-established score interpretations, will contribute to this knowledge.

Issues of missing data have not been adequately addressed in the MOS or by others in terms of nonreturned questionnaires and missing items within a survey. Preliminary work indicates that people who are more depressed are less likely to return self-administered instruments and that more data are missing from older people on the short-form survey. Arnold (1989) found that missing data among older persons are explained by poorer health. There is a large literature on estimating missing scores using available data (e.g., Raymond, 1986; Raymond and Roberts, 1987). In the MOS, which relied primarily on multi-item measures, when some items were missing, scores were estimated based on remaining items. However, there are instances when all items are missing and a missing score must be assigned. It is important to understand the exact nature of nonresponse because in multivariate analyses those with missing data on any one measure are usually dropped from the entire analysis. If missing data are more prevalent in one of the important subgroups compared (e.g., older or depressed patients), then biases can be introduced into the conclusions.

The accuracy of a report is another concern. Patients are often asked to report their past functioning and well-being (e.g., prior to the onset of an illness), yet little is known about the validity of their reports. Questions have been administered in subsequent MOS questionnaires asking patients to report on their past functioning and well-being so that their recalled status can be compared with their actual status on the same questions.

We encourage investigators to conduct additional methodological studies to continue to expand our understanding of the measures, especially in the areas of understanding the sensitivity of the scales and the meaning of score differences. However, despite the need to continue to study these measures, we feel confident in recommending them for a variety of applications and population groups.

Appendix

Actual Patient Assessment Questionnaire (PAQ)

(Note: Only questions relating to specific chapters are given here.)

SECTION 1: HEALTH AND DAILY ACTIVITIES

The first part of the Health Questionnaire is about your health and your daily activities. Please try to answer every question as accurately as you can.

13-17/

PLEASE WRITE IN THE TIME YOU STARTED THE QUESTIONNAIRE:_____AM/PM

---

1. What is today's date?

WRITE IN
THE DATE: | | | / | | | / |**8**|**6**| *18-23/*
         MO.   DAY   YEAR

---

2. In general, would you say your health is:

(Circle One)

Excellent............. 1   *24/*

Very good............. 2

Good................. 3

Fair................. 4

Poor................. 5

---

3. In the past 4 weeks, to what extent did health problems limit you in your everyday physical activities (such as walking and climbing stairs)?

(Circle One)

Not at all............ 1   *25/*

Slightly 2

Moderately 3

Quite a bit........... 4

Extremely 5

4. How much <u>bodily</u> pain have you generally had during the <u>past 4 weeks?</u>

                                                 (Circle One)

                    None........................... 1   *26/*

                    Very mild..................... 2

                    Mild.......................... 3

                    Moderate...................... 4

                    Severe........................ 5

                    Very severe................... 6

---

5. During the <u>past 4 weeks,</u> how much have you been bothered by <u>emotional problems</u> (such as feeling anxious, depressed, or irritable)?

                                                 (Circle One)

                    Not at all.................... 1   *27/*

                    Slightly...................... 2

                    Moderately.................... 3

                    Quite a bit................... 4

                    Extremely..................... 5

---

6. During the <u>past 4 weeks,</u> how much difficulty did you have doing your daily work, both inside and outside the house, because of your physical health or emotional problems?

                                                 (Circle One)

                    None at all................... 1   *28/*

                    A little bit.................. 2

                    Some.......................... 3

                    Quite a bit................... 4

                    Could not do daily work....... 5

      6A. If you had difficulty, what was the cause?

                                                 (Circle One)

                    Mostly or entirely physical.... 1   *29/*

                    Mostly or entirely emotional... 2

                    Physical and emotional
                      about equally............... 3

7. During the past 4 weeks, to what extent has your physical health or emotional problems interfered with your normal social activities with family, friends, neighbors, or groups?

(Circle One)

Not at all..................... 1   *30/*

Slightly...................... 2

Moderately.................... 3

Quite a bit.................. 4

Extremely.................... 5

SECTION 2: PHYSICAL HEALTH

These questions are about your physical activities and symptoms.

---

1. The following items are activities you might do during a typical day. Does your health limit you in these activities?

(Circle One Number on Each Line)

ACTIVITIES	Yes, Limited A Lot	Yes, Limited A Little	No, Not Limited At All	
a. Vigorous activities, such as running, lifting heavy objects, participating in strenuous sports	1	2	3	*32/*
b. Moderate activities, such as moving a table, pushing a vacuum cleaner, bowling, or playing golf	1	2	3	*33/*
c. Lifting or carrying groceries	1	2	3	*34/*
d. Climbing several flights of stairs	1	2	3	*35/*
e. Climbing one flight of stairs	1	2	3	*36/*
f. Bending, kneeling or stooping	1	2	3	*37/*
g. Walking more than a mile	1	2	3	*38/*
h. Walking several blocks	1	2	3	*39/*
i. Walking one block	1	2	3	*40/*
j. Bathing or dressing yourself	1	2	3	*41/*

2. How satisfied are you with your physical ability to do what you want to do?

(Circle One)

Completely satisfied.......... 1   *42/*

Very satisfied................ 2

Somewhat satisfied............ 3

Somewhat dissatisfied......... 4

Very dissatisfied............. 5

Completely dissatisfied....... 6

---

3. When you travel around your community, does someone have to assist you because of your health?

(Circle One)

Yes, all of the time.......... 1   *43/*

Yes, most of the time......... 2

Yes, some of the time......... 3

Yes, a little of the time...... 4

No, none of the time.......... 5

---

4. Are you in bed or in a chair <u>most</u> or <u>all</u> of the day because of your health?

(Circle One)

Yes, every day................ 1   *44/*

Yes, most days................ 2

Yes, some days................ 3

Yes, occasionally............. 4

No, never..................... 5

---

5. Are you able to use public transportation?

(Circle One)

No, because of my health....... 1   *45/*

No, for some other reason...... 2

Yes, able to use public
transportation.............. 3

6. How often have you had any of the following symptoms during the <u>past</u> 4 weeks?

(Circle One Number on Each Line)

	Never	Once or Twice	A Few Times	Fairly Often	Very Often	
a. Stiffness, pain, swelling, or soreness of muscles or joints 1		2	3	4	5	*46/*
b. Coughing that produced sputum 1		2	3	4	5	*47/*
c. Backaches or lower back pains 1		2	3	4	5	*48/*
d. Nausea (upset stomach) 1		2	3	4	5	*49/*
e. Acid indigestion, heartburn, or feeling bloated after meals 1		2	3	4	5	*50/*
f. Heavy feelings in arms and legs 1		2	3	4	5	*51/*
g. Headaches or head pains 1		2	3	4	5	*52/*
h. Lump in throat..................... 1		2	3	4	5	*53/*

11. How often during the <u>past 4 weeks</u>...

(Circle One Number on Each Line)

	All of the Time	Most of the Time	A Good Bit of the Time	Some of the Time	A Little of the Time	None of the Time	
a. Did you feel worn out?	1	2	3	4	5	6	*10/*
b. Were you discouraged by your health problems?	1	2	3	4	5	6	*11/*
c. Did you have a lot of energy?	1	2	3	4	5	6	*12/*
d. Did you feel weighed down by your health problems?	1	2	3	4	5	6	*13/*
e. Did you feel full of pep?	1	2	3	4	5	6	*14/*
f. Were you afraid because of your health?	1	2	3	4	5	6	*15/*
g. Did you have enough energy to do the things you wanted to do?	1	2	3	4	5	6	*16/*

h. Was your health a
  worry in your life? 1   2   3   4   5   6   *17*

i. Did you feel tired? 1   2   3   4   5   6   *18*

j. Were you frustrated
  about your health? 1   2   3   4   5   6   *19*

k. Did you feel despair
  over your health
  problems? 1   2   3   4   5   6   *20*

SECTION 3: PAIN

1. Did you experience <u>any</u> bodily pain in the <u>past 4 weeks</u>?

     (Circle One)

       Yes........ 1 ---> Continue with Question 2, Below   *21*

       No......... 2 ---> Skip to SECTION 4,
                            Page 11.

> The following questions are about the pain or pains you experienced in the <u>past 4 weeks</u>. If you had more than one pain, answer the questions by describing your feelings of pain in general.

2. During the <u>past 4 weeks</u>, how often have you had pain or discomfort?

                                     (Circle One)

       Once or twice.................... 1   *22*

       A few times..................... 2

       Fairly often.................... 3

       Very often...................... 4

       Every day or almost every day..... 5

---

3. When you had pain during the <u>past 4 weeks</u>, how long did it usually last?

                                     (Circle One)

       A few minutes................... 1   *23*

       Several minutes to an hour........ 2

       Several hours................... 3

       A day or two.................... 4

       More than two days............... 5

4. During the <u>past 4 weeks</u>, how much did pain interfere with the
   following things?

   (Circle One Number on Each Line)

	Not At All	A Little Bit	Moderately	Quite A Bit	Extremely	
a. Your mood ·············	1	2	3	4	5	*24/*
b. Your ability to walk or move about ··········	1	2	3	4	5	*25/*
c. Your sleep ·············	1	2	3	4	5	*26/*
d. Your normal work (including both work outside the home and housework) ·············	1	2	3	4	5	*27/*
e. Your recreational activities ··············	1	2	3	4	5	*28/*
f. Your enjoyment of life ··················	1	2	3	4	5	*29/*

---

5. During the <u>past 4 weeks</u>, how many days did pain interfere with the
   things you usually do? (Your answer may range from 00 to 28 days.)

   WRITE IN | | | *30-31/*
   # OF DAYS: |_|_|

---

6. Please circle the one number that best describes your pain on the <u>average</u>
   over the <u>past 4 weeks</u>.

   No   Pain As
   Pain   Bad As
                                                You Can
                                                Imagine
                                                             32-33/
   0 1 2 3 4 5 6 7 8 9 10 11 12 13 14 15 16 17 18 19 20

---

7. Please circle the one number that best describes your pain <u>at its worst</u>
   over the <u>past 4 weeks</u>.

   No   Pain As
   Pain   Bad As
                                                You Can
                                                Imagine
                                                             34-35/
   0 1 2 3 4 5 6 7 8 9 10 11 12 13 14 15 16 17 18 19 20

SECTION 4: DAILY ACTIVITIES

The following questions are about your regular daily activities such as
working at a job, keeping house, taking care of children, attending
school, volunteer work, or taking part in community activities.

---

1. During the past 4 weeks, have you had any of the following problems
    with your work or other regular daily activities as a result of
    your physical health? (Please answer YES or NO for each question.)

                                          (Circle One Number on Each Line)

		Yes	No	
a.	Took frequent rests when doing work or other activities	1	2	36
b.	Cut down the amount of time you spent on work or other activities	1	2	37
c.	Accomplished less than you would like	1	2	38
d.	Didn't do work or other activities as carefully as usual	1	2	39
e.	Were limited in the kind of work or other activities	1	2	40
f.	Had difficulty performing the work or other activities (for example, it took extra effort)	1	2	41
g.	Required special assistance (the assistance of others or special devices) to perform these activities	1	2	42

---

2. During the past 4 weeks, have you had any of the following problems
    with your work or other regular daily activities as a result of any
    emotional problems (such as feeling depressed or anxious)?
    (Please answer YES or NO for each question.)

                                          (Circle One Number on Each Line)

		Yes	No	
a.	Cut down the amount of time you spent on work or other activities?	1	2	43
b.	Accomplished less than you would like?	1	2	44
c.	Didn't do work or other activities as carefully as usual?	1	2	45
d.	Acted irritable toward people (for example, snapped at them, gave sharp answers, criticized easily)?	1	2	46

5. Does your health <u>keep you</u> from working around the house?

(Circle One)

Yes.................................... 1   *49/*

No.................................... 2

---

10. Does your health <u>keep you</u> from working at a paying job?

(Circle One)

Yes........................... 1   *54/*

No........................... 2

SECTION 5:   YOUR FEELINGS

These questions are about how you feel and how things have been with you during the past month.

For each question, please circle a number for the one answer that comes closest to the way you have been feeling.

---

1. How happy, satisfied, or pleased have you been with your personal life during the <u>past month</u>?

(Circle One)

Extremely happy, could not have been
   more satisfied or pleased 1   *62/*

Very happy most of the time 2

Generally satisfied, pleased 3

Sometimes fairly satisfied,
   sometimes fairly unhappy.................... 4

Generally dissatisfied, unhappy 5

Very dissatisfied,
   unhappy most of the time.................... 6

2. During the <u>past month,</u> how often did you feel there were people you were close to?

(Circle One)

Always 1

Very often 2

Fairly often 3

Sometimes 4

Almost never 5

Never 6

---

3. During the <u>past month,</u> how often has feeling depressed interfered with what you usually do?

(Circle One)

Always 1

Very often 2

Fairly often 3

Sometimes 4

Almost never 5

Never 6

---

4. How much of the time, during the <u>past month,</u> did you have difficulty reasoning and solving problems; for example, making plans, making decisions, learning new things?

(Circle One)

All of the time 1

Most of the time 2

A good bit of the time 3

Some of the time 4

A little of the time 5

None of the time 6

5. During the <u>past month</u>, how much of the time have you generally enjoyed the things you do?

    (Circle One)

    All of the time 1   *66/*

    Most of the time 2

    A good bit of the time 3

    Some of the time 4

    A little of the time 5

    None of the time 6

---

6. During the <u>past month</u>, have you had any reason to wonder if you were losing your mind, or losing control over the way you act, talk, think, feel or of your memory?

    (Circle One)

    No, not at all 1   *67/*

    Maybe a little 2

    Yes, but not enough to be concerned
       or worried 3

    Yes, and I have been a little concerned 4

    Yes, and I am quite concerned 5

    Yes, and I am very much concerned 6

---

7. How much of the time, during the <u>past month</u>, has your daily life been full of things that were interesting to you?

    (Circle One)

    All of the time 1   *68/*

    Most of the time 2

    A good bit of the time 3

    Some of the time 4

    A little of the time 5

    None of the time 6

---

8. During the past month, how much of the time have you felt loved and
wanted?

(Circle One)

All of the time	1
Most of the time	2
A good bit of the time	3
Some of the time	4
A little of the time	5
None of the time	6

6⁹

---

9. How much of the time, during the past month, have you been a very
nervous person?

(Circle One)

All of the time	1
Most of the time	2
A good bit of the time	3
Some of the time	4
A little of the time	5
None of the time	6

7⬤

---

10. During the past month, how much of the time did you have difficulty
doing activities involving concentration and thinking?

(Circle One)

All of the time	1
Most of the time	2
A good bit of the time	3
Some of the time	4
A little of the time	5
None of the time	6

7⬤

11. During the <u>past month</u>, how much of the time did you feel depressed?

                        (Circle One)

        All of the time 1   *72/*

        Most of the time 2

        A good bit of the time 3

        Some of the time 4

        A little of the time 5

        None of the time 6

12. During the <u>past month</u>, how much of the time have you felt tense or "high-strung"?

                        (Circle One)

        All of the time 1   *73/*

        Most of the time 2

        A good bit of the time 3

        Some of the time 4

        A little of the time 5

        None of the time 6

13. During the <u>past month</u>, how much of the time have you been in firm control of your behavior, thoughts, emotions, feelings?

                        (Circle One)

        All of the time 1   *74/*

        Most of the time 2

        A good bit of the time 3

        Some of the time 4

        A little of the time 5

        None cf the time 6

14. During the past month, how much of the time did you become confused and start several actions at a time?

(Circle One)

All of the time 1   75

Most of the time 2

A good bit of the time 3

Some of the time 4

A little of the time 5

None of the time 6

---

15. During the past month, how much of the time did you feel that you had nothing to look forward to?

(Circle One)

All of the time 1   76

Most of the time 2

A good bit of the time 3

Some of the time 4

A little of the time 5

None of the time 6

---

16. How much of the time, during the past month, have you felt calm and peaceful?

(Circle One)

All of the time 1   77

Most of the time 2

A good bit of the time 3

Some of the time 4

A little of the time 5

None of the time 6

17. How much of the time, during the <u>past month</u>, have you felt emotionally stable?

(Circle One)

All of the time...............	1
Most of the time	2
A good bit of the time	3
Some of the time	4
A little of the time	5
None of the time	6

78/

---

18. How much of the time, during the <u>past month</u>, have you felt downhearted and blue?

(Circle One)

All of the time	1
Most of the time	2
A good bit of the time	3
Some of the time	4
A little of the time	5
None of the time	6

10/

---

19. How often have you felt like crying during the <u>past month?</u>

(Circle One)

Always.........................	1
Very often.....................	2
Fairly often...................	3
Sometimes......................	4
Almost never...................	5
Never..........................	6

11/

20. How much of the time, during the <u>past month,</u> did you feel left out?

(Circle One)

All of the time	1
Most of the time	2
A good bit of the time	3
Some of the time	4
A little of the time	5
None of the time	6

12

---

21. During the <u>past month,</u> how often did you feel that others would be better off if you were dead?

(Circle One)

Always	1
Very often	2
Fairly often	3
Sometimes	4
Almost never	5
Never	6

13

---

22. During the <u>past month,</u> how much of the time did you forget, for example, things that happened recently, where you put things, appointments?

(Circle One)

All of the time	1
Most of the time	2
A good bit of the time	3
Some of the time	4
A little of the time	5
None of the time	6

14

---

23. During the past month, how much of the time did you feel that your love relationships, loving and being loved, were full and complete?

(Circle One)

All of the time 1   *15/*

Most of the time 2

A good bit of the time 3

Some of the time 4

A little of the time 5

None of the time 6

---

24. How much have you been bothered by nervousness, or your "nerves," during the past month?

(Circle One)

Extremely so, to the point where I could
not take care of things 1   *16/*

Very much bothered 2

Bothered quite a bit 3

Bothered some, enough to notice 4

Bothered just a little 5

Not bothered at all 6

---

25. During the past month, how much of the time has living been a wonderful adventure for you?

(Circle One)

All of the time 1   *17/*

Most of the time 2

A good bit of the time 3

Some of the time 4

A little of the time 5

None of the time 6

---

26. How much of the time, during the past month, have you felt so down in the dumps that nothing could cheer you up?

(Circle One)

    All of the time 1   *18*

    Most of the time 2

    A good bit of the time 3

    Some of the time 4

    A little of the time 5

    None of the time 6

27. During the past month, did you ever think about taking your own life?

(Circle One)

    Yes, constantly 1   *1*

    Yes, very often 2

    Yes, fairly often 3

    Yes, a couple of times 4

    Yes, once 5

    No, never 6

28. During the past month, how much of the time have you felt restless, fidgety, or impatient?

(Circle One)

    All of the time 1   *2(*

    Most of the time 2

    A good bit of the time 3

    Some of the time 4

    A little of the time 5

    None of the time 6

29. During the <u>past month</u>, how much of the time have you been moody or brooded about things?

(Circle One)

All of the time 1   *21/*

Most of the time 2

A good bit of the time 3

Some of the time 4

A little of the time 5

None of the time 6

---

30. During the <u>past month</u>, how often did you get rattled, upset, or flustered?

(Circle One)

Always 1   *22/*

Very often 2

Fairly often 3

Sometimes 4

Almost never 5

Never 6

---

31. How much of the time, during the <u>past month</u>, did you have trouble keeping your attention on any activity for long?

(Circle One)

All of the time 1   *23/*

Most of the time 2

A good bit of the time 3

Some of the time 4

A little of the time 5

None of the time 6

---

32. During the <u>past month</u>, how much of the time have you been
    anxious or worried?

                                                          (Circle One)

                          All of the time 1   2.

                          Most of the time 2

                          A good bit of the time 3

                          Some of the time 4

                          A little of the time 5

                          None of the time 6

---

33. During the <u>past month</u>, how much of the time have you been
    a happy person?

                                                          (Circle One)

                          All of the time 1   2

                          Most of the time 2

                          A good bit of the time 3

                          Some of the time 4

                          A little of the time 5

                          None of the time 6

---

34. How often during the <u>past month</u> did you find yourself having
    difficutly trying to calm down?

                                                          (Circle One)

                          Always........................ 1   2(

                          Very often.................... 2

                          Fairly often.................. 3

                          Sometimes..................... 4

                          Almost never.................. 5

                          Never......................... 6

---

35. During the <u>past month</u>, how much of the time have you been in low or very low spirits?

(Circle One)

All of the time.............. 1   *27/*

Most of the time.............. 2

A good bit of the time........ 3

Some of the time.............. 4

A little of the time.......... 5

None of the time.............. 6

36. How much of the time, during the <u>past month</u>, have you felt cheerful, lighthearted?

(Circle One)

All of the time................ 1   *28/*

Most of the time............... 2

A good bit of the time......... 3

Some of the time............... 4

A little of the time........... 5

None of the time............... 6

37. During the <u>past month</u>, how depressed (at its worst) have you felt?

(Circle One)

Extremely depressed............ 1   *29/*

Very depressed................. 2

Quite depressed................ 3

Somewhat depressed............. 4

A little depressed............. 5

Not depressed at all........... 6

38. How much of the time, during the past month, did you react slowly
to things that were said or done?

(Circle One)

All of the time 1   *30*

Most of the time 2

A good bit of the time 3

Some of the time 4

A little of the time 5

None of the time 6

---

39. During the past month, how often did you feel isolated from others?

(Circle One)

Always................ 1   *31*

Very often............ 2

Fairly often.......... 3

Sometimes............. 4

Almost never.......... 5

Never................. 6

SECTION 6: SOCIAL ACTIVITIES

The next questions ask about your social activities.

1. During the past 4 weeks, how much of the time has your physical health
or emotional problems interfered with your social activities
(like visiting with friends, relatives, etc.)?

(Circle One)

All of the time........................ 1   *33/*

Most of the time....................... 2

Some of the time....................... 3

A little of the time................... 4

None of the time....................... 5

2. Compared to your usual level of social activity, has your social activity during the past 6 months decreased, stayed the same, or increased because of a change in your physical or emotional condition?

(Circle One)

Much less socially active
than before............................ 1   *34/*

Somewhat less socially active
than before............................ 2

About as socially active
as before............................ 3

Somewhat more socially active
than before............................ 4

Much more socially active
than before............................ 5

---

3. Compared to others your age, are your social activities more or less limited because of your physical health or emotional problems?

(Circle One)

Much more limited than others.......... 1   *35/*

Somewhat more limited than others...... 2

About the same as others.............. 3

Somewhat less limited than others...... 4

Much less limited than others.......... 5

SECTION 7: YOUR FAMILY

These questions are about your relationship with your family.

---

1. In terms of your satisfaction with your family life, please rate the following:

(Circle One Number on Each Line)

	Poor	Fair	Good	Very Good	Excellent	
a. The amount of togetherness and cohesion you have	1	2	3	4	5	*42/*
b. The support and understanding you give each other	1	2	3	4	5	*43/*
c. The amount you talk things over	1	2	3	4	5	*44/*

2. Overall, how happy are you with your family life?

(Circle One)

Extremely happy............... 1   *45/*

Very happy.................... 2

Somewhat happy................ 3

Not too happy................. 4

Somewhat unhappy.............. 5

Very unhappy.................. 6

---

3. Do you have a spouse or partner?

(Circle One)

Yes........................... 1   *46/*

No............................ 2

---

4. The following statements are about your relationship with your spouse or partner. How TRUE or FALSE has <u>each</u> one been for you during the <u>past 4 weeks?</u> (If you do not have a spouse or partner, please answer these about the person you feel closest to.)

(Circle One Number on Each Line)

	Definitely True	Mostly True	Don't Know	Mostly False	Definitely False	
a. We said anything we wanted to say to each other	1	2	3	4	5	*47/*
b. We often had trouble sharing our personal feelings	1	2	3	4	5	*48/*
c. It was hard to blow off steam with each other	1	2	3	4	5	*49/*
d. I felt close to my spouse or partner	1	2	3	4	5	*50/*
e. My spouse or partner was supportive of me	1	2	3	4	5	*51/*
f. We tended to rely on other people for help rather than on each other	1	2	3	4	5	*52/*

5. These next questions are about the way health problems might interfere
with your sex life. These questions are personal, but your answers
are important in understanding how health problems affect people's lives.

How much of a problem was <u>each</u> of the following during the <u>past 4 weeks</u>?

(Circle One Number on Each Line)

	Not a Problem	Little of a Problem	Somewhat of a Problem	Very Much a Problem	Not Applicable	
a. Lack of sexual interest...	1	2	3	4	5	53/
b. Unable to relax and enjoy sex.................	1	2	3	4	5	54/
c. Difficulty in becoming sexually aroused..........	1	2	3	4	5	55/

MEN ONLY:

d. Difficulty getting or keeping an erection.......	1	2	3	4	5	56/

WOMEN ONLY:

e. Difficulty in having an orgasm................	1	2	3	4	5	57/

SECTION 8: YOUR HEALTH

Next are some general questions about your health and health-related matters.

How TRUE or FALSE is <u>each</u> of the following statements for you?

(Circle One Number on Each Line)

	Definitely True	Mostly True	Don't Know	Mostly False	Definitely False	
1. I am concerned about my health	1	2	3	4	5	58/
2. I am somewhat ill	1	2	3	4	5	59/
5. I have never been seriously ill	1	2	3	4	5	62/
6. I think my health will be worse in the future than it is now ..	1	2	3	4	5	63/

7. I feel about as good
    now as I ever have ...   1   2   3   4   5   *64/*

10. I have never had an
    illness that lasted a
    long period of time 1   2   3   4   5   *67/*

11. I have been feeling
    bad lately   1   2   3   4   5   *68/*

How TRUE or FALSE is <u>each</u> of the following statements for you?

(Circle One Number on Each Line)

	Definitely True	Mostly True	Don't Know	Mostly False	Definitely False	
13. In the future, I expect to have better health than other people I know....	1	2	3	4	5	*11*
15. I have been feeling sickly for a long time..	1	2	3	4	5	*13*
18. I expect to have a very healthy life.......	1	2	3	4	5	*16.*
19. I am in poor health	1	2	3	4	5	*17.*
20. I only think about my health when I go to the doctor for an examination	1	2	3	4	5	*18.*
21. I seem to get sick a little easier than other people	1	2	3	4	5	*19.*

How TRUE or FALSE is <u>each</u> of the following statements for you?

(Circle One Number on Each Line)

	Definitely True	Mostly True	Don't Know	Mostly False	Definitely False	
24. I expect my health to get worse ··········	1	2	3	4	5	*22/*
25. I am usually the last one to catch a cold	1	2	3	4	5	*23/*
26. I often think about my health	1	2	3	4	5	*24/*
27. I am as healthy as anybody I know	1	2	3	4	5	*25/*

28. I was so sick once I thought I might die····	1	2	3	4	5	26/
29. My body seems to resist illness very well ············	1	2	3	4	5	27/
30. My future will be unhealthy ··········	1	2	3	4	5	28/
31. My health is a big concern in my life ·····	1	2	3	4	5	29/
32. When there is an illness going around, I usually catch it······	1	2	3	4	5	30/
33. My health is excellent ··········	1	2	3	4	5	31/
36. Good health is in my future ············	1	2	3	4	5	34/

SECTION 9: YOUR SLEEP

---

1. How long did it usually take for you to <u>fall asleep</u> during the <u>past 4 weeks?</u>

(Circle One)

0-15 minutes·········· 1   35/

16-30 minutes·········· 2

31-45 minutes·········· 3

46-60 minutes·········· 4

More than 60 minutes··· 5

2. On the average, how many hours did you sleep <u>each night</u> during the <u>past 4 weeks?</u>

WRITE IN # OF | | | 36-37/
HOURS PER NIGHT: |_|_|

How often during the past 4 weeks did you...

(Circle One Number on Each Line)

	All of the Time	Most of the Time	A Good Bit of the Time	Some of the Time	A Little of the Time	None of the Time	
3. feel that your sleep was not quiet (moving restlessly, feeling tense, speaking, etc., while sleeping)?	1	2	3	4	5	6	38
4. get enough sleep to feel rested upon waking in the morning?	1	2	3	4	5	6	39
5. awaken short of breath or with a headache?	1	2	3	4	5	6	40
6. feel drowsy or sleepy during the day?	1	2	3	4	5	6	41
7. have trouble falling asleep?	1	2	3	4	5	6	42

How often during the past 4 weeks did you...

(Circle One Number on Each Line)

	All of the Time	Most of the Time	A Good Bit of the Time	Some of the Time	A Little of the Time	None of the Time	
8. awaken during your sleep time and have trouble falling asleep again?	1	2	3	4	5	6	43
9. have trouble staying awake during the day?	1	2	3	4	5	6	44
10. snore during your sleep?	1	2	3	4	5	6	45
11. take naps (5 minutes or longer) during the day?	1	2	3	4	5	6	46
12. get the amount of sleep you needed?	1	2	3	4	5	6	47

MOS 20-Item Short-Form Health Survey (SF-20) *

PATIENT QUESTIONNAIRE

Thank you for filling out this questionnaire.

1. Please start right away and fill out as much of Part 1 as you can <u>before</u> your visit.

2. Keep the questionnaire with you and finish it <u>after</u> your visit, but <u>before</u> you leave the office.

3. When you are finished, seal the questionnaire in the envelope and <u>leave it with the nurse or receptionist</u> on your way out.

STATEMENT OF CONFIDENTIALITY

All information that would permit identification of clinicians or their patients will be regarded as strictly confidential, will be used only for the purposes of operating and evaluation the study, and will not be disclosed or released for any other purposes without prior consent, except as required by law.

```
DIRECTIONS:

●  PLEASE USE A NO. 2 PENCIL ONLY.  Do not use ink, felt-tip
   or ballpoint pen.

●  Fill the circle entirely

●  Erase errors completely.

●  Avoid stray marks or notes.  (There's a space at the end
   for your comments.)

EXAMPLE:

            O O ● O        .O ◑ ◐ O
              RIGHT          WRONG
```

---

2. In general, would you say your health is:

     1-O   Excellent
     2-O   Very Good
     3-O   Good
     4-O   Fair
     5-O   Poor

* Taken from Patient Questionnaire (Screening Form SP2). Questions used in SF-20 are depicted in order as they appeared on the original screener.

16. For how long (if at all) has your <u>health limited you</u> in <u>each</u> of the following activities?

(Mark <u>One</u> Circle on <u>Each</u> Line)

		1 Limited for more than 3 months	2 Limited for 3 months or less	3 Not limited at all
a.	The kinds or amounts of <u>vigorous</u> activities you can do, like lifting heavy objects, running or participating in strenuous sports	0	0	0
b.	The kinds or amounts of <u>moderate</u> activities you can do, like moving a table, carrying groceries or bowling	0	0	0
c.	Walking uphill or climbing a few flights of stairs	0	0	0
d.	Bending, lifting or stooping	0	0	0
e.	Walking one block	0	0	0
f.	Eating, dressing, bathing, or using the toilet	0	0	0

17. How much <u>bodily</u> pain have you had <u>during the past 4 weeks</u>?

1-0   None
2-0   Very mild
3-0   Mild
4-0   Moderate
5-0   Severe
6-0   Very Severe

18. Does your health <u>keep</u> you from working at a job, doing work around the house or going to school?

1-0   YES, for more than 3 months
2-0   YES, for 3 months or less
3-0   NO

19. Have you been unable to do <u>certain kinds or amounts</u> of work, housework or schoolwork because of your health?

1-0   YES, for more than 3 months
2-0   YES, for 3 months or less
3-0   NO

For <u>each</u> of the following questions, please mark the circle for the <u>one</u> answer that comes <u>closest</u> to the way you have been feeling <u>during the past month.</u>

(Mark <u>One</u> Circle on <u>Each</u> Line)	1 All of the Time	2 Most of the Time	3 A Good Bit of the Time	4 Some of the Time	5 A Little of the Time	6 None of the Time
20. How much of the time, during the past month, has your <u>health limited your social activities</u> (like visiting with friends or close relatives)?	O	O	O	O	O	O
21. How much of the time, during the past month, have you been a <u>very nervous person</u>?	O	O	O	O	O	O
22. During the past month, how much of the time have you felt <u>calm and peaceful</u>?	O	O	O	O	O	O
23. How much of the time, during the past month, have you felt <u>downhearted and blue</u>?	O	O	O	O	O	O
24. During the past month, how much of the time have you been a <u>happy person</u>?	O	O	O	O	O	O
25. How often, during the past month, have you felt so <u>down in the dumps that nothing could cheer you up</u>?	O	O	O	O	O	O

26. Please mark the circle that <u>best</u> describes whether <u>each</u> of the following statements is <u>true</u> or <u>false</u> for you.

(Mark <u>One</u> Circle on Each Line)	1 Definitely True	2 Mostly True	3 Not Sure	4 Mostly False	5 Definitely False
a. I am somewhat ill	O	O	O	O	O
b. I am as healthy as anybody I know .	O	O	O	O	O
c. My health is excellent	O	O	O	O	O
d. I have been feeling bad lately . . .	O	O	O	O	O

Glossary

Acquiescent Response Set—the tendency to agree with or to endorse an item regardless of content; a form of response bias.

acute—a temporary state or condition.

affect—emotional or feeling state.

alpha (coefficient)—Cronbach's alpha, an estimate of internal-consistency reliability based on the average interitem correlation and number of items.

assessment—in the case of health assessment, a standardized procedure used to quantify an individual's health.

attribute—a characteristic of an individual.

battery—a collection of measures.

chronic—a state or condition that is persistent or long lasting, usually more than three months.

closed-ended questions—a question that contains specific response options (e.g., yes or no).

coarse—a measure that has relatively fewer possible scale levels.

coefficient of reproducibility (CR)—used to indicate the internal-consistency reliability of Guttman scales. It is the extent to which a correct pattern of item scores can be reproduced from the scale score.

communality—estimate of the proportion of variance shared between one measure and another measure or set of measures.

component—part of a larger concept or construct. For example, anxiety is a component of psychological distress.

concurrent validity—a form of validity in which the measure being tested and the comparison measure are administered at the same point in time.

construct—a variable that is relatively abstract as opposed to concrete and is defined or operationalized in terms of observed indicators. Anxiety is an example of a mental health construct.

construct validity—a process in which validity is evaluated as the extent to which a measure correlates with variables in a manner consistent with theory.

content validity—the extent to which a measure or battery represents the universe of measurement objects or domains (i.e., adequacy of coverage).

convergent validity—strength of association between two methods of measuring the same construct.

convergent-discriminant validity—a form of construct validity in which reliability coefficients, convergent validity coefficients, and discriminant validity evidence are simultaneously interpreted (such as in a multitrait-multimethod matrix of correlations with reliability coefficients in the diagonal).

corrected for overlap—correction of a correlation coefficient for the inflation due to inclusion of the item in the scale score. A correlation corrected for overlap is the correlation of the item with the sum of other items in the same scale (multitrait scaling analysis). When a correlation coefficient is calculated between an item and the scale it is part of (to determine if the item has convergent validity), the scale is scored with the item omitted in order to remove the bias of correlating the item with itself. The item-scale correlation is then said to be corrected for item overlap.

criterion validity—the extent to which a measure corresponds to an accurate or previously validated measure of the same concept.

cross-validation—testing the usefulness of an operational definition derived from one sample on a second sample.

descriptive statistics—indicators that characterize the score distributions for a particular sample such as the mean, standard deviation, range, skewness, and percentage missing.

dimension—a distinct component of a multidimensional construct that can be theoretically or empirically specified; for example, physical and mental health are dimensions of health.

dimensionality—the number and nature of distinct components of a construct.

discriminant validity—an aspect of construct validity in which a measure is shown to correlate higher with concepts it is intended to measure than with concepts it is not intended to measure.

disease-specific—measures of severity, symptoms, or functional limitations pertaining specifically to a particular disease or condition.

dysfunction—a limitation or decrement in the performance of usual or normal activities.

empirical—based on analysis of data.

empirical validity—evidence of validity based on the analysis of data.

empirically distinct—analysis of data yields evidence that two measures do not have the same interpretation.

external validity—representativeness or generalizability of results.

face validity—extent to which a measure "looks like" what it is intended to measure.

factor—a latent (unobserved) variable or theoretical construct operationalized in terms of the associations among the indicators in a factor analysis.

factor analysis—a multivariate analytic method for testing the extent to which underlying hypothetical constructs are defined by a set of measures. Also used to determine whether a set of measures can be reduced to a smaller set without loss of information.

factorial validity—a sophisticated form of construct validity; extent to which the structural relationship among measures corresponds to their underlying theoretical framework.

five percent rule—the rule that factors should only be interpreted if they account for five percent or more of the common variance; suggested by Guertin and Bailey (1970).

frequency distribution—the number of respondents who score at each level of a scale.

functional status—historically used to refer collectively to a variety of concepts of functioning and well-being.

functioning—the ability of individuals to perform their normal or usual behaviors and activities; usually observable; distinct from well-being, which pertains to subjective, internal states that cannot be directly observed.

general population—refers to the population at large, including sick and well persons, rather than a patient population; general population samples are relatively healthier than patient samples.

generic—general as opposed to disease-specific health assessment; applicable to all types of patients as well as general populations.

grid-type format—a series of items in which the response choice labels are presented across the top of the page with numbers corresponding to each response choice repeated for each item. The format saves space by eliminating the need to repeat the response choice labels for each separate item.

Guttman scale—a cumulative scale in which each item consists of increasingly more severe or extreme items (e.g., can you walk a block? can you walk a mile? can you walk several miles?) In a perfect Guttman scale, each person's response to items in the scale can be determined from his or her total scale score.

health dimension—theoretical component of health such as physical or mental.

health framework—systematic and comprehensive way of organizing health constructs; a theoretical model that specifies distinct health concepts and how they relate to one another.

health indicator—an operational definition of health.

HIE—Health Insurance Experiment, a randomized experiment conducted by The RAND Corporation in 1974–1981.

index—an aggregation of two or more distinct health measures into an overall summary measure.

internal-consistency reliability—a method for estimating score reliability from the correlations among the items in the scale. Cronbach's alpha (or coefficient alpha) is an internal-consistency reliability coefficient.

internal validity—refers to research designs, not measures; confidence in conclusions drawn regarding relationships (adequacy of controls).

interval scale—a scale in which the distances between all levels along the scale have known numerical values.

item—a single question or statement and its standardized response scale.

item analysis—evaluation of the psychometric attributes of an item such as its descriptive statistics, correlation with the scale, convergence, and discrimination for the purpose of combining into scales.

408   *Glossary*

item weights—for some scales, items are given differential emphasis in the scoring rules and are thus weighted unequally. When no weights are assigned, equal weights are assumed.

known-groups validity—the usefulness of a measure in distinguishing between (or among) groups of people with "known" characteristics (most often a kind of construct validity).

latent variable—an unobserved construct defined in terms of a weighted linear combination of observed or measured variables.

Likert scale—a scale evaluated and scored according to the method of summated ratings in which items are summed or averaged to obtain an overall score; items shown to be linearly related to the total scale score are included.

limitation—a problem such as having pain, difficulty, or fatigue upon performance of a particular activity.

loading—a correlation between a measure and a factor.

mean—the average calculated by summing the items and dividing by the number of items.

measure—a single-item or multi-item scale or index; can be a nominal, ordinal, interval, or ratio scale.

measurement error—random error occurring in the measurement of an attribute; portion of observed score that is *not* true score.

median—the midpoint of a particular score distribution marking the fiftieth percentile.

modal respondent—hypothetical person who has attributes like the mode or most frequently occurring response.

multiple regression—multivariate analytic procedure that evaluates the relationship between a continuous outcome and the linear combination of two or more predictor variables.

multitrait scaling—a method for evaluating scale items that considers both item convergence (whether each item correlates substantially with the scale it is part of) and item discrimination (whether each item correlates significantly higher with the scale it is part of than with other conceptually similar scales).

nominal scale—a scale in which the numeric values assigned to scale levels are arbitrary and have no numeric meaning. Categories are classifications rather than ordered value (e.g., 1 = male, 2 = female).

ordinal scale—a scale in which the numbers reflect levels ordered from "most" to "least" with respect to some attribute. The relative distances between each level differ throughout the scale, and the number assigned to each level does not reflect an exact quantity. For example, the rating of health as excellent, good, fair, or poor is an ordinal scale.

outcome—a measure of health used specifically as an endpoint or dependent variable, for example, in studies evaluating health care interventions.

PAQ—Patient Assessment Questionnaire.

PAQ baseline sample—an MOS sample of 3,053 patients who completed the baseline Patient Assessment Questionnaire (PAQ). A subset of these were selected to become the M O S panel sample.

Pearson product-moment correlation—an index of association between two continuous variables.

pilot study—small study, usually of a convenience sample, to test preliminary measurement decisions and identify unanticipated problems in fielding the instruments in a study.

precision—extent to which a measure is capable of detecting small differences.

predictive validity—a form of construct validity in which the hypothesis being tested is whether the measure can forecast the probability of another event (e.g., use of services) or future score.

psychometric—the use of tests or scales to measure an attribute of an individual or object.

psychophysiologic symptoms—physical symptoms that can have either a physical health or mental health cause; for example, loss of appetite can be caused by illness or by emotional distress.

ratio scale—a scale with all the properties of an interval scale but that has in addition an absolute zero (i.e., a point at which there is none of the property being measured), so that ratios between values are meaningful.

reliability—the extent to which a measure is free of measurement error; the ratio of true score variance to observed score variance.

respondent—person answering questions or completing a survey.

respondent burden—the amount of time and effort required of those completing questionnaires.

response level—a particular choice or category defined by an item or combination of items.

response scale—the response choices (numbers and their definitions) presented to a respondent with which to answer a particular question (e.g., 1 = yes, 2 = no).

response set—a tendency of respondents to answer questions in patterned ways irrespective of content (e.g., the tendency to present oneself in a favorable light, the tendency to agree with questions regardless of item content).

scale—an item or aggregation of one or more items scored in a manner that satisfies the assumptions underlying an accepted method of scale construction.

scalogram analysis—a method for analyzing the statistical relationships among three or more items to determine whether the items meet properties of Guttman scales—that is, whether the items define a single underlying dimension, whether they are cumulative (i.e., ordered by degree of difficulty), and whether responses to each item are predictable from the total scale score.

scoring rules—numbers assigned to item responses and, if applicable, the formula for their aggregation in a scale or index.

self-administration—respondents read and answer the questions by themselves, without assistance.

self-report—questions are answered by the subjects about themselves, either by self-administration or by responding to an interviewer's questions.

sensitivity—the extent to which a measure detects true differences or changes in the construct being measured.

skewness—the extent of asymmetry in a frequency distribution.

somatic—pertaining to the body.

standard deviation—an indicator of dispersion or variation around the mean. The standard deviation is the square root of the variance, which is the average squared deviation around the mean.

standard error of measurement—determines the confidence interval around an individual score; the standard error of measurement equals the standard deviation times the square root of one minus the score reliability.

standardize—to convert raw scores so that the resulting mean and standard deviation have specific values.

statistical power—the probability of detecting an effect of a given size under the conditions of a particular study.

subscale—a scale within a scale; an analyzable smaller unit of a more inclusive scale or index.

test-retest reliability—a method of estimating reliability by correlating scores from two different administrations, separated by a short time interval.

tracer condition—a medical condition defined in order to have a somewhat homogeneous sample by which to trace the effects of health care interventions. In the MOS, the following tracer conditions were defined: hypertension, diabetes, heart disease (myocardial infarction, congestive heart failure), and depression.

validity—the extent to which a measure measures what it is supposed to and does not measure what it is not supposed to. See content validity, criterion validity, predictive validity, concurrent validity, face validity, construct validity.

variability—the extent to which all possible scale levels are observed.

visual analogue scale—a method for obtaining a response to a question that involves having the respondent mark a line (usually 10 cm) to reflect the psychological distance from the endpoints, which are labeled.

well-being—subjective bodily and emotional states; how an individual feels; a state of mind distinct from functioning which pertains to behaviors and activities.

WHO—World Health Organization.

Bibliography

Aday, L. A. 1989. *Designing and conducting health surveys.* San Francisco: Jossey Bass.

Aday, L. A., and Anderson, R. 1975. *Development of indices of access to medical care.* Ann Arbor, Mich.: Health Administration Press.

Aday, L. A., Anderson, R., and Fleming, G. V. 1980. *Health care in the U.S.: Equitable for whom?* Beverly Hills, Calif.: Sage Publications.

Aiken, L. R. 1982. *Psychological testing and assessment.* 4th ed. Boston: Allyn and Bacon.

Allen, S. J. 1986. "Regression equations of the latent roots of random data correlation matrices with unities on the diagonal." *Multivariate Behavioral Research* 21:393–98.

American College of Physicians. 1988. "Comprehensive functional assessment for elderly patients." *Annals of Internal Medicine* 109:70–72.

American Psychiatric Association, Committee on Nomenclature and Statistics. 1980. *Diagnostic and statistical manual of mental disorders DSM-III.* 3d ed., Washington, D.C.: American Psychiatric Association.

American Psychological Association. 1985. *Standards for education and psychological testing.* Washington, D.C.: American Psychological Association.

Anastasi, A. 1976. *Psychological testing.* 4th ed. New York: Macmillan.

Andrews, F. M. 1984. "Construct validity and error components of survey measures: A structural modeling approach." *Public Opinion Quarterly* 48:409–442.

Andrews, F. M., and Withey, S. B. 1976. *Social indicators of well-being.* New York: Plenum Press.

Angus, R. G., Heslegrave, R. J., and Myles, W. S. 1985. "Effects of prolonged sleep deprivation, with and without chronic physical exercise, on mood and performance." *Psychophysiology* 22:276–82.

Anthony, J. C., LeResche, L., Niaz, U., et al. 1982. "Limits of the mini-mental state as a screening test for dementia and delirium among hospital patients." *Psychological Medicine* 12:397–408.

Armor, D. J. 1974. "Theta reliability and factor scaling." In *Sociological methodology: 1973–74,* edited by H. L. Costner, 17–50. San Francisco: Jossey-Bass.

Arnold, S. 1989. *Aging versus disease: Current health perceptions among the elderly.* Publication no. N–2949. Santa Monica, Calif.: RAND Corporation.

Atkinson, H. 1985. *Women and fatigue.* New York: G. P. Putnam's Sons.

Attanasio, V., Adrasik, F., Blanchard, E. B., et al. 1984. "Psychometric properties of the SUNYA revision of the psychosomatic checklist." *Journal of Behavioral Medicine* 7:247–57.

Beck, A. T. 1967a. *Depression—Cause and treatment*. Philadelphia: University of Pennsylvania Press.

Beck, A. T. 1967b. *Depression: Clinical, experimental and theoretical aspects*. New York: Harper and Row.

Beck, A. T., Weissman, A., Lester, D., and Trexler, L. 1974. "The measurement of pessimism: The hopelessness scale." *Journal of Consulting and Clinical Psychology* 42:861–65.

Becker, M. H. 1974. "The health belief model and personal health behavior." *Health Education Monographs* 2:409–19.

Becker, M. H., and Maiman, L. A. 1975. "Sociobehavioral determinants of compliance with health and medical care recommendations." *Medical Care* 13:10–24.

Becker, M. H., Maiman, L. A., Kirscht, J. P., et al. 1977. "The health belief model and prediction of dietary compliance: A field experiment." *Journal of Health and Social Behavior* 18:348–66.

Belloc, N. B. 1973. "Relationship of health practices and mortality." *Preventive Medicine* 2:67–81.

Belloc, N. B., Breslow, L., and Hochstim, J. R. 1971. "Measurement of physical health in a general population survey." *American Journal of Epidemiology* 93:328–36.

Bentler, P. M., and Eichberg, R. H. 1975. "A social psychological approach to substance abuse construct validity: Prediction of adolescent drug use from independent data source." In *Predicting adolescent drug abuse: A review of issues, methods and correlates,* edited by D. J. Lettieri, 131–46. Washington, D.C.: U.S. Government Printing Office.

Bentler, P. M., Jackson, D. N., and Messick, S. 1971. "Identification of content and style: A two-dimensional interpretation of acquiescence." *Psychological Bulletin* 76:186–204.

Berdit, M., and Williamson, J. W. 1973. "Function limitation scale for measuring health outcomes." In *Health status indexes,* edited by R. L. Berg. Chicago: Hospital Research and Educational Trust.

Berg, R. L. 1973. *Health status indexes*. Proceedings of a conference conducted by Health Service Research. Chicago: Hospital Research and Educational Trust.

Bergner, M. 1985. "Measurement of health status." *Medical Care* 23:696–704.

Bergner, M., and Rothman, M. L. 1987. "Health status measures: An overview and guide for selection." *Annual Review of Public Health* 8:191–210.

Bergner, M., Bobbitt, R. A., Carter, W. B., and Gilson, B. S. 1981. "The Sickness Impact Profile: Development and final revision of a health status measure." *Medical Care* 19:787–805.

Berk, M. L., and Meyers, S. 1980. "Reasons for nonresponse on the physicians practice survey," in American Statistical Association, *Proceedings of the Social Statistics Section,* 202–4.

Berk, M. L., Mathiowetz, N. A., Ward, E. P., and White, A. A. 1987. "The effect of prepaid and promised incentives: Results of a controlled experiment." *Journal of Official Statistics* 3:449–57.

Berki, S. E., and Ashcraft, M. L. 1979. "On the analysis of ambulatory utilization." *Medical Care* 17:1163–1181.

Berkman, L. F., and Breslow, L. 1983. *Health and ways of living: The Alameda county study*. New York: Oxford University Press.

Berman, D. M., Brook, R. H., Lohr, K. N., et al. 1981. *Conceptualization and measurement of physiologic health for adults. Vol. 4: Angina pectoris*. Publication no. R–2262/4–HHS. Santa Monica, Calif.: RAND Corporation.

Berry, S. H., and Kanouse, D. E. 1987. "Physician response to a mailed survey: An experiment in timing of payment." *Public Opinion Quarterly* 51:102–14.

Berwick, D. M., Budman, S., Damico-White, J., et al. 1987. "Assessment of psychological morbidity in primary care: Explorations with General Health Questionnaire." *Journal of Chronic Diseases* 40:71S–79S.

Berwick, D. M., Murphy, J. M., Goldman, P. A., et al. 1991. "Performance of a five-item mental health screening test." *Medical Care* 29:169–76.

Bindman, A. B., Keane, D., and Lurie, N. 1990. "Measuring health changes among severely ill patients: The floor phenomenon." *Medical Care* 28(12):1142–1152.

Birrell, P. C. 1983. "Behavioral, subjective, and electroencephalographic indices of sleep onset." *Journal of Behavioral Assessment* 5:179–90.

Bixler, E. O., Kales, A., Soldatos, C. R., et al. 1979. "Prevalence of sleep disorders in the Los Angeles metropolitan area." *American Journal of Psychiatry* 136:1257–1262.

Bliwise, D. L., Yesavage, J. A., Sink, J., et al. 1986. "Depressive symptoms and impaired respiration in sleep." *Journal of Consulting and Clinical Psychology* 54:734–35.

Bloom, B. L. 1985. "A factor analysis of self-reported measures of family functioning." *Family Process* 24:225–39.

Bollen, K. A., and Barb, K. H. 1986. "Pearson's *R* and coarsely categorized measures." *American Sociological Review* 46:232–39.

Bombardier, C., Ware, J., and Russell, I. J. 1986. "Auranofin therapy and quality of life in patients with rheumatoid arthritis." *The American Journal of Medicine* 4:565–78.

Bradburn, N. M. 1969. *The structure of psychological well-being*. Chicago: Aldine Publishing.

Bradburn, N. M., and Sudman, S. 1980. *Improving interview method and questionnaire design*. San Francisco: Jossey-Bass.

Bradley, L. A., Prokop, W. D., Gentry, L. H., et al. 1981. "Assessment of chronic pain." *Medical psychology contributions to behavioral medicine*, edited by C. Prokop and L. Bradley. New York: Academic Press.

Breslow, L. 1972. "A quantitative approach to the World Health Organization definition of health: Physical, mental and social well-being." *International Journal of Epidemiology* 1:347–55.

414   *Bibliography*

Brodman, K., Erdmann, A. J., Lorge, I., et al. 1949. "The Cornell Medical Index." *Journal of the American Medical Association* 140:530–34.

Brook, R. H., Ware, J. E., Davies-Avery, A., et al. 1979. *Conceptualization and measurement of health for adults in the Health Insurance Study. Volume 8: Overview.* Publication no. R–1987/8–HEW. Santa Monica, Calif.: RAND Corporation.

Brook, R. H., Ware, J. E., Rogers, W. R., et al. 1983. "Does free care improve adults' health? Results from a randomized controlled trial." *New England Journal of Medicine* 309:1426–1434.

Brown, G. W., and Harris, T. O. 1978. *Social origins of depression: A study of psychiatric disorder in women.* New York: Free Press.

Bulpitt, C. J., and Dollery, C. T. 1973. "Side effects of hypotensive agents evaluated by a self-administered questionnaire." *British Medical Journal* 3:585–90.

Burnam, M. A., Wells, K. B., Leake, B., et al. 1988. "Development of a brief screening instrument for detecting depressive disorders." *Medical Care* 26:775–89.

Bush, J. W., Anderson, J. P., Kaplan, R. M., et al. 1982. "Counter-intuitive preferences in health-related quality of life measurement." *Medical Care* 20:516–25.

Cafferata, G. L. 1987. "Marital status, living arrangements, and the use of health services by elderly persons." *Journal of Gerontology* 42(6): 613–18.

Campbell, D. T., and Fiske, D. W. 1959. "Convergent and discriminant validation by the multitraite-multimethod matrix." *Psychological Bulletin* 56:81–105.

Canadian Sickness Survey, 1950–51: Illness and health care in Canada. 1960. Ottawa.

Cantril, H. 1965. *The pattern of human concerns.* New Brunswick, N.J.: Rutgers University Press.

Carskadon, M. A., Dement, W. C., Mitler, M. M., et al. 1976. "Self-reports versus sleep laboratory findings in 122 drug-free subjects with complaints of chronic insomnia." *American Journal of Psychiatry* 133:1382–1388.

Cassileth, B. R., Lusk, E. J., Strouse, T. B., et al. 1984. "Psychosocial status in chronic illness: A comparative analysis of six diagnostic groups." *New England Journal of Medicine* 311:506–511.

Cattell, R. B., ed. 1966. *Handbook of multivariate experimental psychology.* Chicago: Rand-McNally.

Cernovsky, Z. Z. 1984. "Life stress measures and reported frequency of sleep disorder." *Perceptual and Motor Skills* 58:39–49.

Chambers, L. W., MacDonald, L. A., Tugwell, P., et al. 1982. "The McMaster Health Index Questionnaire as a measure of quality of life for patients with rheumatoid disease." *Journal of Rheumatology* 9:780–784.

Chapman, C. R., Casey, K. L., Dubner, R., et al. 1985. "Pain measurement: An overview." *Pain* 22:1–31.

Chen, M. K., and Bryant, B. E. 1975. "The measurement of health—a critical and selective overview." *International Journal of Epidemiology* 4:257–64.

Chesney, M. A., and Rosenman, R. H., eds. 1985. *Anger and hostility in cardiovascular and behavioral disorders*. Washington, D.C.: Hemisphere Publishing.

Chobanian, A. V. 1987. "Antihypertensive therapy in evolution." *New England Journal of Medicine* 314:1701–1702.

Cluff, L. 1981. "Chronic disease, function and the quality of care." *Journal of Chronic Diseases* 34:299–304.

Coates, A., Gebski, V., Bishop, J. F., et al. 1987. "Improving the quality of life during chemotherapy for advanced breast cancer." *New England Journal of Medicine* 317:1490–95.

Coates, T. J., and Thoresen, C. E. 1984. "Assessing daytime thoughts and behavior associated with good and poor sleep: Two exploratory studies." *Behavioral Assessment* 6:153–67.

Coates, T. J., Killen, J. D., George, J., et al. 1982. "Estimating sleep parameters: A multitraite-multimethod analysis." *Journal of Consulting and Clinical Psychology* 50:345–52.

Codman, E. A. 1914. "The product of a hospital." *Surgery, Gynecology and Obstetrics* 18:491–96.

Commission on Chronic Illness. 1957. *Chronic illness in a large city: Chronic illness in the United States—Volume 4*. Cambridge, Mass.: Harvard University Press.

Comrey, A. L. 1970. *Edits manual for the Comrey Personality Scales*. San Diego, Calif.: Educational and Industrial Testing Service.

Connelly, J. E., Philbrick, J. T., Smith, G. R., et al. 1989. "Health perceptions of primary care patients and the influence on health care utilization." *Medical Care* 27, Suppl.:S99–S109.

Conte, H. R. 1986. "Multivariate assessment of sexual dysfunction." *Journal of Consulting and Clinical Psychology* 54:149–57.

Converse, J. M., and Presser, S. 1986. *Survey questions: Handcrafting the standardized questionnaire*. Beverly Hills: Sage Publications.

Costello, C. G., and Comrey, A. 1967. "Scales for measuring depression and anxiety." *Journal of Psychology* 66:303–13.

Cronbach, L. J. 1951. "Coefficient alpha and the internal structure of tests." *Psychometrika* 16:297–334.

Cronbach, L. J. 1970. *Essentials of Psychological Testing*. 3d ed. New York: Harper and Row.

Cronbach, L. J., and Meehl, P. E. 1955. "Construct validity in psychological tests." *Psychological Bulletin* 52:281–302.

Croog, S. H., Levine, S., Testa, M. A., et al. 1986. "The effects of antihypertensive therapy on the quality of life." *New England Journal of Medicine* 314:1657–1702.

Crowne, D. P., and Marlowe, D. 1960. "A new scale of social desirability independent of psychopathology." *Journal of Consulting Psychology* 24:349–54.

Daut, R. L., Cleeland, C. S., and Flanery, R. C. 1983. "Development of the Wisconsin Brief Pain Questionnaire to assess pain in cancer and other diseases." *Pain* 17:197–210.

Davies, A. R., and Ware, J. E. 1981. *Measuring health perceptions in the Health Insurance Experiment*. Publication no. R–2711–HHS. Santa Monica, Calif.: RAND Corporation.

Davies, A. R., Sherbourne, C. D., Peterson, J. R. and Ware, J. E. 1988. *Scoring manual: Adult health status and patient satisfaction measures used in RAND's Health Insurance Experiment*. Publication no. N–2190–HHS. Santa Monica, Calif.: RAND Corporation.

Deniston, O. L., and Jette, A. 1980. "A functional status assessment instrument: Validation in an elderly population." *Health Services Research* 15:21–34.

DePaulo, J. R., and Folstein, M. F. 1978. "Psychiatric disturbances in neurological patients: Detection, recognition, and hospital course." *Annals of Neurology* 4:225–28.

Derogatis, L. R., Lipman, R. S., and Covi, L. 1973. "The SCL-90: An outpatient psychiatric rating scale." *Psychopharmacology Bulletin* 9:13–28.

Derogatis, L. R., Lipman, R. S., Rickels, K., et al. 1974. "The Hopkins Symptom Checklist (HSCL): A self-reported symptom inventory." *Behavioral Science* 19:1–15.

Deyo, R. A., and Centor, R. M. 1986. "Assessing the responsiveness of functional scales to clinical change: An analogy to diagnostic test performance." *Journal of Chronic Disease* 39:897–906.

Deyo, R. A., and Inui, T. S. 1984. "Toward clinical applications of health status measures: Sensitivity of scales to clinically important changes." *Health Services Research* 19:276–89.

Deyo, R. A., and Patrick, D. 1988. "Barriers to the use of health status measures in clinical investigation, patient care, and policy research." *Medical Care* 27, Suppl: S254–S268.

Diamond, E. L. 1982. "The role of anger and hostility in essential hypertension and coronary heart disease." *Psychological Bulletin* 92:410–33.

Dillman, D. A. 1978. *Mail and telephone surveys: The total design method*. New York: Wiley and Sons.

Dohrenwend, B. P., Levav, I., and Shrout, P. E. 1983. "Screening scales from the Psychiatric Epidemiology Research Interview (PERI)." In *Community surveys*, edited by J. K. Myers, M. M. Weissman, and C. Ross. New Brunswick: N.J.: Rutgers University Press.

Dohrenwend, B. P., Shrout, P. E., Egri, G., and Mendelsohn. 1980. "Non-specific psychological distress and other dimensions of psychopathology: Measures for use in general population." *Archives of General Psychiatry* 37:1229–1236.

Dolfman, M. L. 1973. "The concept of health: An historic and analytic examination." *Journal of School Health* 43:491–97.

Dommeyer, C. J. 1988. "How form of mail survey incentive affects mail survey responses." *Journal of the Market Research Society* 30:379–85.

Donald, C. A., and Ware, J. E. 1982. *The quantification of social contacts and resources*. Publication no. R–2937–HHS. Santa Monica, Calif.: RAND Corporation.

Donald, C., Ware, J. E., Brook, R. H., et al. 1978. *Conceptualization and measurement of health for adults in the Health Insurance Study. Volume 4: Social Health*. Publication no. R–1987/4–HEW. Santa Monica, Calif.: RAND Corporation.

Dubos, R. 1965. *Man adapting*. New Haven: Yale University Press.

Dupuy, H. J. 1973. The psychological section of the current Health and Nutrition Examination Survey. *Proceedings of the public health conference on records and statistics meeting jointly with the national conference on mental health statistics, June 12–15, 1972*. U.S. Dept. of Health, Education, and Welfare publication no. (HRA) 74–12–14. Washington, D.C.: U.S. Government Printing Office.

Dupuy, H. J. 1984. "The psychological general well-being (PGWB) Index," in *Assessment of quality of life in clinical trials of cardiovascular therapies*, edited by N. K. Wenger, M. E. Mattson, C. D. Furberg, and J. Elinson. New York: Le Jacq.

Edwards, A. L. 1957. *Techniques of attitude scale construction*. New York: Appleton-Century-Crofts.

Edwards, A. L. 1970. *The measurement of personality traits by scales and inventories*. New York: Holt, Rinehart and Winston.

Eisen, M., Donald, C., Ware, J. E., et al. 1980. *Conceptualization and measurement of health for children in the Health Insurance Study*. Publication no. R–2313. Santa Monica, Calif.: RAND Corporation.

Eisen, S. V., and Grob, M. C. 1979. "Assessing consumer satisfaction from letters to the hospital." *Hospital and Community Psychiatry* 30:344–47.

Eisenstadt, R. K., and Schoenborn, C. A. 1980. *Basic data from Wave II of the National Survey of Personal Health Practices and Consequences: United States*. Working paper series no. 13. National Center for Health Statistics. Washington, D.C.: U.S. Government Printing Office.

Ellis, B. W., Johns, M. W., Lancaster, R., et al. 1981. "The St. Mary's Hospital sleep questionnaire: A study of reliability." *Sleep* 4:93–97.

Ellwood, P. 1988. "Shattuck lecture—Outcomes management: A technology of patient experience." *New England Journal of Medicine* 318:1549–1556.

Endicott, J., Spitzer, R. L., and Fleiss, J. L. 1976. "The Global Assessment Scale: A procedure for measuring overall severity of psychiatric disturbance." *Archives of General Psychiatry* 33:766–71.

Engel, G. L. 1976. "The need for a new medical model: A challenge for biomedicine." *Science* 196:129–36.

Fetter, R. B., Shin, Y., Freeman, J. L., et al. 1980. "Case mix definition by diagnosis-related groups." *Medical Care* 18, Suppl.:1–51.

Finn, S. E. 1986. "Stability of personality self-ratings over 30 years: Evidence for an age/cohort interaction." *Journal of Personality and Social Psychology* 50:813–18.

Fiske, D. W. 1966. "Some hypotheses concerning test adequacy." *Educational and Psychological Measurement* 26:69–88.

Ford, J. K., MacCallum, R. C., and Tait, M. 1986. "The application of exploratory factor analysis in applied psychology: A critical review and analysis." *Personnel Psychology* 39:291–314.

Fowler, F. J. 1984. *Survey research methods.* Beverly Hills: Sage Publications.

Fowler, F. J., Wennberg, J. E., Timothy, R. P., et al. 1988. "Symptom status and quality of life following prostatectomy." *Journal of the American Medical Association* 259:3018–3022.

Frank, E., Anderson, C., and Rubinstein, D. 1978. "Frequency of sexual dysfunction in normal couples." *New England Journal of Medicine* 299:111–15.

Fries, J. F., Spitz, P., Kraines, R. G. 1980. "Measurement of patient outcome in arthritis." *Arthritis and Rheumatism* 23:137–45.

Geigle, R., and Jones, S. B. 1990. "Outcomes measurement: A report for the front." *Inquiry* 27:7–13.

Gilson, B. S., Bergner, M., Bobbitt, R. A., et al. 1975. *Further tests and revisions of the Sickness Impact Profile 1974–75.* Seattle, Wash.: Department of Health Services, School of Public Health and Community Medicine, University of Washington.

Gilson, B. S., Bergner, M., Bobbitt, R. A., and Carter, W. B. 1978. *The Sickness Impact Profile: Final development and testing.* Seattle, Wash.: Department of Health Services, School of Public Health and Community Medicine, University of Washington.

Gilson, B. S., Gilson, J. S., Bergner, M., et al. 1975. "The Sickness Impact Profile: Development of an outcome measure of health care." *American Journal of Public Health* 65:1304–1310.

Givens, J. D. 1979. *Current estimates from the health interview survey.* U.S. Dept. of Health, Education, and Welfare, Vital and Health Statistics series 10, no. 130, DHEW publication no. (PHS) 80–1551. Washington, D.C.: U.S. Government Printing Office.

Goldberg, D. 1978. *Manual of the General Health Questionnaire.* Windsor, England: NFER Publishing.

Goldberg, D. P., and Hillier, V. 1978. "A scaled version of the General Health Questionnaire." *Psychological Medicine* 9:139–45.

Goldman, L., Hashimoto, B., Cook, E. F., et al. 1981. "Comparative reproducibility and validity of systems for assessing cardiovascular functional class: Advantages of a new Specific Activity Scale." *Circulation* 64:1227–1234.

Gonella, J. S., and Goran, M. J. 1975. "Quality of patient care—A measurement of change: The staging concept." *Medical Care* 8:467–73.

Good, M. J., Smilkstein, G., Good, B. J., et al. 1979. "The Family APGAR Index: A study of construct validity." *Journal of Family Practice* 8:577–82.

Greenblatt, H. N. 1976. *Measurement of social well-being in a general population survey.* California State Dept. of Health.

Guerney, B. G. 1977. *Relationship enhancement.* San Francisco: Jossey-Bass.

Guilford, J. P. 1954. *Psychometric methods.* New York: McGraw-Hill.

Gunn, W. J., and Rhodes, I. N. 1981. "Physician response to a telephone survey: Effects of monetary incentives on response level." *Public Opinion Quarterly* 45:109–15.

Gurin, G., Veroff, J., and Field, S. 1960. *Americans view their mental health— A nationwide interview survey.* New York: Basic Books.

Guttman, L. A. 1942. "A basis for scaling qualitative data." *American Sociological Review* 9:139–50.

Guttman, L. A. 1954. "Some necessary conditions for common factor analysis." *Psychometrika* 19:149–61.

Haber, L. D. 1970. "The epidemiology of disability: 2. The measurement of functional capacity limitations." *Social security survey of the disabled: 1966 report no. 10.* Washington, D.C.: Office of Research and Statistics, Social Security Administration, U.S. Department of Health, Education, and Welfare.

Hargreaves, M. 1977. "The fatigue syndrome." *Practitioner* 218:841–43.

Haylock, P. J., and Hart, L. K. 1979. "Fatigue in patients receiving localized radiation." *Cancer Nursing* 461–67.

Hays, R. D. 1985. "LAMBDA: A basic program for calculating random data eigenvalues." *Educational and Psychological Measurement* 45:623–24.

Hays, R. D. 1987. "PARALLEL.EXE: A program for performing parallel analysis." *Applied Psychological Measurement* 11:58.

Hays, R. D., and Hayashi, T. 1990. "Beyond internal consistency reliability: Rationale and user's guide for multitrait analysis: Program on the microcomputer." *Behavior Research Methods, Instruments, Computers* 22:167–75.

Hays, R. D., and Stewart, A. L. 1990. "The structure of self-reported health in chronic disease patients." *Psychological Assessment: A Journal of Consulting and Clinical Psychology* 2:22–30.

Hays, R. D., Hayashi, T., and Stewart, A. L. 1989. "A five-item measure of socially desirable response set." *Educational and Psychological Measurement* 49:629–36.

Hays, R. D., Hayashi, T., Carson, S., and Ware, J. E. 1988. *The Multitrait Analysis Program* (MAP) *user's guide.* (Publication no. N–2786–RC.) Santa Monica, Calif.: RAND Corporation.

Hays, R. D., and Huba, G. J. 1988. "Reliability and validity of drug use items differing in the nature of their response options." *Journal of Consulting and Clinical Psychology* 56:470–72.

Heft, M. W., and Parker, S. R. 1984. "An experimental basis for revising the graphic rating scale for pain." *Pain* 19:153–61.

Helmstadter, G. C. 1964. *Principles of psychological measurement.* New York: Appleton-Century-Crofts.

Hennen, B. K. 1987. "Fatigue." In *Family medicine: A guidebook for practitioners of the art,* by D. B. Shires, B. K. Hennen, and D. I. Rice, 172. New York: McGraw-Hill.

Herzlich, C. 1973. *Health and illness: A social psychological analysis.* London: Academic Press.

Hinkle, L. E. 1961. "Ecologic observations of the relation of physical illness, mental illness, and social environment." *Psychosomatic Medicine* 23:289–90.

Hoelscher, T. J., and Edinger, J. D. 1988. "Treatment of sleep-maintenance insomnia in older adults: Sleep period reduction, sleep education, and modified stimulus control." *Psychology and Aging* 3:258–63.

Hogan, M. J., Wallin, J. D., and Baer, R. M. 1980. "Antihypertensive therapy and male sexual dysfunction." *Psychosomatics* 21:235–37.

Holden, R. R., Longman, R. S., Cota, A. A., and Fekken, G. C. 1989. "PAR: Parallel analysis routine random data eigenvalue estimation." *Applied Psychological Measurement* 13:192.

Horn, S. D., Sharkey, P. D., and Bertram, D. A. 1983. "Measuring severity of illness: Homogeneous case mix groups." *Medical Care* 21:14–30.

House, J. S., and Kahn, R. 1985. "Measures and concepts of social support." In *Social support and health*, edited by S. Cohen and S. L. Syme. Orlando: Academic Press.

Howard, K. I., and Forehand, G. G. 1962. "A method for correcting item-total correlations for the effect of relevant item inclusion." *Educational and Psychological Measurement* 22:731–35.

Hoyt, C. 1941. "Test reliability estimated by analysis of variance." *Psychometrika* 6:153–60.

Humphreys, L. G., and Ilgen, D. R. 1969. "Note on a criterion for the number of common factors." *Educational and Psychological Measurement* 29:571–78.

Hunt, S. M., and McEwen, J. 1980. "The development of a subjective health indicator." *Sociology of Health and Illness* 2:231–46.

Hunt, S. M., McKenna, S. P., McEwen, J., et al. 1981. "The Nottingham Health Profile: Subjective health status and medical consultations." *Social Science and Medicine* 15A:221–29.

International Association for the Study of Pain Subcommittee on Taxonomy. 1979. "Pain terms: A list with definitions and notes on usage." *Pain* 6:249–52.

Institute of Medicine. 1987. *Pain and disability: Clinical, behavioral, and public policy perspectives*, edited by M. Osterweis, A. Kleinman, and D. Mechanic. Washington, D.C.: National Academy Press.

Jackson, A. L. 1973. *Prevalence of selected impairments: United States—July 1963–June 1965*. U.S. Dept. of Health, Education, and Welfare, Vital and Health Statistics series 10, no. 48, DHEW publication no. (HRA) 74–1286. Washington, D.C.: U.S. Government Printing Office.

Jackson, D. N. 1970. "A sequential system for personal scale development." In *Current topics in clinical and community psychology. Volume 2*, edited by C. D. Spielberger, 61–96. New York: Academic Press.

Jacobsen, L. J., Brown, R. F., and Ariza, M. J. 1983. "A revised multidimensional social desirability inventory." *Bulletin of the Psychonomic Society* 21:391–92.

Jahoda, M. 1958. *Current concepts of positive mental health*. New York: Basic Books.

Janz, N. K., and Becker, M. H. 1984. "The health belief model: A decade later." *Health Education Quarterly* 11:1–47.

Jehu, D. 1979. *Sexual dysfunction: A behavioral approach to causation, assessment, and treatment.* New York: John Wiley and Sons.

Jette, A. M. 1980. "Health status indicators: Their utility in chronic-disease evaluation research." *Journal of Chronic Diseases* 33:567–79.

Jette, A. M., Cummings, M., Brock, B. M., et al. 1981. "The structure and reliability of health belief indices." *Health Services Research* 16:81–98.

Jette, A. M., Davies, A. R., Cleary, P. D., et al. 1986. "The functional status questionnaire: Reliability and validity when used in primary care." *Journal of General and Internal Medicine* 1:143–49.

Jette, A. M., and Deniston, O. L. 1978. "Inter-observer reliability of a functional status assessment instrument." *Journal of Chronic Diseases* 31:573–80.

Johns, M. W. 1971. "Methods for assessing human sleep." *Archives of Internal Medicine* 127:484–92.

Johns, M. W. 1975a. "Factor analysis of subjectively reported sleep habits, and the nature of insomnia." *Psychological Medicine* 5:83–88.

Johns, M. W. 1975b. "Factor analysis of objective and subjective characteristics of a night's sleep." *Psychological Medicine* 5:413–18.

Johns, M. W., Bruce, D. W., and Masterton, J. P. 1974. "Psychological correlates of sleep habits reported by healthy young adults: Use of a sleep questionnaire." *British Journal of Medical Psychology* 47:181–87.

Johns, M. W., Egan, P., et al. 1970. "Sleep habits and symptoms in male medical and surgical patients." *British Medical Journal* 2:509–12.

Johns, M. W., Gay, J. A., et al. 1971. "Sleep habits of healthy young adults: Use of a sleep questionnaire." *British Journal of Preventive Social Medicine* 25:236–41.

Johnson, J. A. 1981. "The "self-disclosure" and "self-presentation" views of item response dynamics and personality scale validity." *Journal of Personality and Social Psychology* 40:761–69.

Johnson, D. R., and Creech, J. D. 1983. "Ordinal measures in multiple indicator models: A simulation study of categorization error." *American Sociological Review* 48:398–407.

Johnson, W. L., and Dixon, P. N. 1984. "Response alternatives in Likert scaling." *Educational and Psychological Measurement* 44:563–67.

Johnson, E. H., and Broman, C. L. 1987. "The relationship of anger expression to health problems among black Americans in a national survey." *Journal of Behavioral Medicine* 10:103–16.

Jones, W. H. 1985. "The psychology of loneliness: Some personality issues in the study of social support." In *Social support: Theory, research and applications,* edited by I. G. Sarason and B. R. Sarason. Boston: Nijhoff.

Jones, W. H., Hansson, R. O., and Cutrona, L. 1984. "Helping the lonely: Issues of intervention with young and older adults." In *Personal relationships 5: Repairing personal relationships,* edited by S. Duck. London: Academic Press.

Kales, A., Bixler, E. O., Cadieux, R. J., et al. 1984. "Sleep apnea in a hypertensive population." *Lancet* 2:1005–1008.

Kales, A., Caldwell, A. B., Cadieux, R. J., et al. 1985. "Severe obstructive sleep apnea—2: Associated psychopathology and psychosocial consequences." *Journal of Chronic Diseases* 38:427–34.

Kales, A., Soldatos, C. R., and Kales, J. D. 1987. "Sleep disorders: Insomnia, sleepwalking, night terrors, nightmares, and enuresis." *Annals of Internal Medicine* 106:582–92.

Kales, A., Vela-Bueno, A., and Kales, J. D. 1987. "Sleep disorders: Sleep apnea and narcolepsy." *Annals of Internal Medicine* 106:434–43.

Kane, R. A., and Kane, R. L. 1981. *Assessing the elderly: A practical guide to measurement*. Lexington, Mass.: Lexington Books.

Kane, R. A., Kane, R. L., and Arnold, S. 1985. *Measuring social functioning in mental health studies: Concepts and instruments*. National Institute of Mental Health, series DN, no. 5, DHHS publication no. (ADM) 85–1384. Washington, D.C.: U.S. Government Printing Office.

Kaplan, R. M. 1989. "Health outcome models for policy analysis." *Health Psychology* 8:723–35.

Kaplan, R. M., and Anderson, J. P. 1987. "The quality of well-being scale: Rationale for a single quality of life index." In *Quality of life: Assessment and application,* edited by S. R. Walker and R. M. Rosser. Proceedings of the Centre for Medicine Research Workshop held at the CIBA Foundation, London.

Karacan, I., Thornby, J. I., Anch, M., et al. 1976. "Prevalence of sleep disturbance in a primarily urban Florida county." *Social Science and Medicine* 10:239–44.

Katz, S., ed. 1987. "The Portugal conference measuring quality of life and functional status in clinical and epidemiological research." Special issue, *Journal of Chronic Diseases* 40(6).

Katz, S., Ford, A. B., Moskowitz, R. W., et al. 1963. "Studies of illness in the aged." *Journal of the American Medical Association* 185:914–19.

Keefe, F. J. 1982. "Behavioral assessment and treatment of chronic pain: Current status and future directions." *Journal of Consulting and Clinical Psychology* 50(6):896–911.

Keeler, E. B., Wells, K. B., Manning, W. G., et al. 1986. *The demand for episodes of mental health services*. Publication no. R–3432–NIMH. Santa Monica, Calif.: RAND Corporation.

Kellner, R. 1985. "Functional somatic symptoms and hypochondriasis." *Archives of General Psychiatry* 42:821–33.

Kerlinger, F. N. 1973. *Foundations of behavioral research*. 2d ed. New York: Holt, Rinehart and Winston.

Kerlinger, F. N., and Pedhazur, E. J. 1973. *Multiple regression in behavioral research*. New York: Holt, Rinehart and Winston.

Kerson, T. S., and Kerson, L. A. 1985. *Understanding chronic illness: The medical and psychosocial dimensions of nine diseases*. New York: Free Press.

Kirscht, J. P., Becker, M. H., and Eveland, J. P. 1976. "Psychological and social factors as predictors of medical behavior." *Medical Care* 14:422–31.

Klassen, D., Hornstra, R. K., and Anderson, P. B. 1975. "Influence of social desirability on symptoms and mood reporting in a community survey." *Journal of Consulting and Clinical Psychology* 43:448–52.

Knab, B., and Engel-Sittenfeld, P. 1983. "The many facets of poor sleep." *Neuropsychobiology* 10:141–47.

Knights, E. B., and Folstein, M. F. 1977. "Unsuspected emotional and cognitive disturbance in medical patients." *Annals of Internal Medicine* 87:723–24.

Koskenvuo, M., Kaprio, J., Partinen, M., et al. 1985. "Snoring as a risk factor for hypertension and angina pectoris." *Lancet* 1:893–96.

Kripke, D. F., Simons, R. N., Garfinkle, L., et al. 1979. "Short and long sleep and sleeping pills: Is increased mortality associated?" *Archives of General Psychiatry* 36:103–16.

Kristiansen, C. M., and Harding, C. M. 1984. "The social desirability of preventive health behavior." *Public Health Reports* 99:384–88.

Kroenke, K., Wood, D. R., Manglesdorff, A. D., et al. 1988. "Chronic fatigue in primary care: Prevalence, patient characteristics, and outcome." *Journal of the American Medical Association* 260:929–34.

Lamberg, L. 1985. "Newly awakened interest in sleep research spans many specialties." *Journal of the American Medical Association* 254:1275–1284.

Lau, R. R., Hartman, K., and Ware, J. E. 1986. "Health as value: Methodological and theoretical considerations." *Health Psychology* 5:25–43.

Lavie, P., Ben-Yosef, R., and Rubin, A. E. 1984. "Prevalence of sleep apnea syndrome among patients with essential hypertension." *American Heart Journal* 108:373–76.

Lerner, M. 1973. "Conceptualization of health and social well-being." *Health Services Research* 9:6–12.

Levav, I., Arnon, A., and Portnoy, A. 1977. "Two shortened versions of the Cornell Medical Index—A new test of their validity." *International Journal of Epidemiology* 6:135–41.

Levine, S., and Croog, S. H. 1984. "What constitutes quality of life?" In *Assessment of quality of life in clinical trials of cardiovascular therapies,* edited by N. K. Wenger, M. E. Mattson, C. D. Furberg, and J. Elinson. New York: Le Jacq.

Levine, S., Croog, S. H., Sudilovsky, A., et al. 1987. "Effects of antihypertensive medications on vitality and well-being." *Journal of Family Practice* 25:357–63.

Levy, K. J. 1975. "Some multiple range tests for variances." *Educational and Psychological Measurement* 35:599–604.

Lewis, S. A. 1969. "Subjective estimates of sleep: An EEG evaluation." *British Journal of Psychology* 60:203–8.

Liang, J. 1986. "Self-reported physical health among aged adults." *Journal of Gerontology* 41:248–60.

Liang, M. H., Fossel, A. H., and Larson, M. G. 1990. "Comparisons of five health status instruments for orthopedic evaluation." *Medical Care* 28(7):632–642.

Likert, R. 1932. "A technique for the measurement of attitudes." *Archives of Psychology* 140:1–55.

Lohr, K. N. 1989. "Advances in health status assessment: Conference proceedings." *Medical Care* 27:3.

Lohr, K. N., and Ware, J. E., eds. 1987. "Advances in health assessment conference." *Journal of Chronic Disease* 40, suppl. 1.

Lohr, K. N., Kamberg, C. J., Keeler, E. B., et al. 1986. *Conceptualization and measurement of physiologic health for adults: Overview of chronic disease in a general adult population.* Publication no. R–2262/1–HHS. Santa Monica, Calif.: RAND Corporation.

Long, J. S. 1983. *Confirmatory factor analysis.* Beverly Hills: Sage Publications.

Lugaresi, E., Cirignotta, F., Coccagna, G., et al. 1980. "Some epidemiological data on snoring and cardiocirculatory disturbances." *Sleep* 3:221–24.

Manning, W. G., Leibowitz, A., Goldberg, G. A., et al. 1984. "A controlled trial of the effect of a prepaid group practice on use of services." *New England Journal of Medicine* 310:1505–1510.

Manning, W. G., Newhouse, J. P., and Ware, J. E. "The status of health in demand estimation." In *Economic aspects of health,* edited by V. R. Fuchs, 143–84. Chicago: University of Chicago Press.

Manning, W. G., Wells, K. B., Duan, N., et al. 1984. "Cost-sharing and the use of ambulatory mental health services." *American Psychologist* 39:1077–1089.

Mathews, C. O. 1929. "The effect of the order of printed response words on an interest questionnaire." *Journal of Educational Psychology* 20:128–34.

McDermott, W. 1981. "Absence of indicators of the influence of its physicians on a society's health." *American Journal of Medicine* 70:833–43.

McDowell, I., and Newell, C. 1987. *Measuring health: A guide to rating scales and questionnaires.* New York: Oxford University Press.

McGlynn, E. A. 1991. *Physician job satisfaction: Its measurement and use as an indicator of system performance.* Publication no. N–3247. Santa Monica. Calif.: RAND Corporation.

McHorney, C. A., et al. 1992. "The validity and relative precision of MOS. . . ." *Medical Care,* in press.

McNabb, R. 1983. "Family function and depression." *Journal of Family Practice* 16:169–70.

McNair, D. M., Lorr, M., and Doppleman, L. F. 1971. *Profile of Mood States manual.* San Diego, Calif.: Educational and Industrial Testing Service.

McNair, D. M., Lorr, M., and Doppleman, L. F. 1981. *EITS manual for the Profile of Mood States.* San Diego, Calif.: Educational and Industrial Testing Service.

McWhinney, I. R. 1972. "Beyond diagnosis: An approach to the integration of behavioral science and clinical medicine." *New England Journal of Medicine* 287:384–87.

Mead, B. T. 1974. "Depression: How to recognize it." *Postgraduate Medicine* 55:68–71.

Meenan, R. F. 1986. "New approaches to outcome assessment: The AIMS questionnaire for arthritis." *Advances in Internal Medicine* 31:167–85.

Mellinger, G. D., Balter, M. B., and Uhlenhuth, E. H. 1985. "Insomnia and its treatment: Prevalence and correlates." *Archives of General Psychiatry* 42:225–32.

Melzack, R. 1975. "The McGill Pain Questionnaire: Major properties and scoring methods." *Pain* 1:277–99.

Melzack, R., and Torgerson, W. S. 1971. "On the language of pain." *Anesthesiology* 34:50–59.

Menninger, K. A. 1945. *The human mind.* 3d ed. New York: Alfred Knopf, Inc.

Mizes, J. S., Fleece, E. L., and Roos, C. 1984. "Incentives for increasing return rates: Magnitude levels, response bias, and format." *Public Opinion Quarterly* 48:794–800.

Montag, I., and Comrey, A. L. 1982. "Personality construct similarity in Israel and the United States." *Applied Psychological Measurement* 6:61–67.

Montanelli, R. G., and Humpreys, L. G. 1976. "Latent roots of random data correlation matrices with squared multiple correlations on the diagonal: A Monte Carlo study." *Psychometrika* 41:341–48.

Montgomery, E. A., and Paranjpe, A. V. 1985. *A report card on HMOS 1980– 1984.* Menlo Park, Calif.: Henry J. Kaiser Family Foundation.

Montgomery, L. M., Shadish, W. R., Orwin, R. G., et al. 1987. "Psychometric structure of psychiatric rating scales." *Journal of Abnormal Psychology* 96:167–70.

Moos, R. H. 1974. *The social climate scales: An overview.* Palo Alto, Calif.: Consulting Psychologist Press.

Moos, R. H., and Moos, B. S. 1981. *Family Environment Scale manual.* Palo Alto, Calif.: Consulting Psychologist Press.

Morewitz, J. H. 1988. "Evaluation of excessive daytime sleepiness in the elderly." *Journal of the American Geriatrics Society* 36:324–30.

Morrison, J. D. 1980. "Fatigue as a presenting complaint in family practice." *Journal of Family Practice* 10:795–801.

Mosteller, F., Ware, J. E., and Levine, S. 1989. "Comments on the conference on advances in health status assessment." *Medical Care* 27, suppl.:S282– S294.

Nachmias, C., and Nachmias, D. 1981. *Research methods in the social sciences.* London: St. Martin's Press.

Nagi, S. Z. 1969. "Congruency in medical and self-assessment of disability." *Industrial Medicine* 38:27–36.

Nagi, S. Z. 1976. "Epidemiology of disability among adults in the United States." *Milbank Memorial Fund Quarterly* 54:439–66.

National Center for Health Statistics. 1966. "Conceptual problems in developing an index of health." *Vital and health statistics,* series 10, no. 96, Rockville, Md.: U.S. Dept. of Health, Education, and Welfare.

National Center for Health Statistics. 1974. "Limitation of activity and mobility due to chronic conditions: United States." 1972 DHEW publication no. HRA–75–1523. *Vital and health statistics,* series 10, no. 96, Rockville, Md.: U.S. Dept. of Health, Education, and Welfare.

National Center for Health Statistics. 1981. *Health, United States.* U.S. Dept. of Health and Human Services Publication.

Nelson, E. C., and Berwick, D. M. 1989. "The measurement of health status in clinical practice." *Medical Care* 27, suppl.:S77–S90.

Nelson, E. C., Conger, B., Douglass, R., et al. 1983. "Functional health status levels of primary care patients." *Journal of the American Medical Association* 249:3331–3338.

Nelson, E. C., Landgraf, J. M., Hays, R. D., Kirk, J. W., Wasson, J. H., Keller, A., and Zubkoff, M. 1990. "The COOP function charts: A system to measure patient function in physicians' offices." In *Functional status measurement in primary care,* edited by I. G. Sarason and B. R. Sarason. New York: Springer-Verlag.

Nelson, E. C., Landgraf, J. M., Hays, R. D., et al. 1990a. "The functional status of patients: How can it be measured in physicians' offices?" *Medical Care* 28:1111–1127.

Nelson, E. C., Wasson, J., Kirk, A., et al. 1987. "Assessment of function in routine clinical practice: Description of the COOP chart method and preliminary findings." *Journal of Chronic Diseases* 40:15S–63S.

Newcomb, M. D., and Bentler, P. M. 1987. "The impact of late adolescent substance use on young adult health status and utilization of health services: A structural equation model over four years." *Social Science and Medicine* 24:71–82.

Norcross, J. C., Guadagnoli, E., and Prochaska, J. O. 1984. "Factor structure of the Profile of Mood States (POMS): Two partial replications." *Journal of Clinical Psychology* 40:1270–1277.

Nunnally, J. C. 1978. *Psychometric theory.* 2d ed. New York: McGraw-Hill.

Ohnhaus, E. E., and Adler, R. 1975. "Methodological problems in the measurement of pain: A comparison between the verbal rating scale and the visual analogue scale." *Pain* 1:379–84.

Olson, D. H., Russell, C. S., and Sprenkle, D. H. 1983. "Circumplex model of marital and family systems: 6. Theoretical update." *Family Process* 22:69–83.

Osgood, C., Suci, G., and Tannenbaum, P. 1957. *The measurement of meaning.* Urbana: University of Illinois Press.

Parkerson, G. R., Gehlbach, S. H., Wagner, E. H., et al. 1981. "The Duke-UNC Health Profile: An adult health status instrument for primary care." *Medical Care* 19:806–28.

Partinen, M., and Palomaki, H. 1985. "Snoring and cerebral infarction." *Lancet* 2:1325–1326.

Patrick, D., and Elinson, J. 1984. "Sociomedical approaches to disease and treatment outcomes in cardiovascular care." *Quality of Life and Cardiovascular Care* 1:2, 53–65.

Patrick, D. L., Bush, J. W., and Chen, M. M. 1973a. "Methods for measuring levels of well-being for a health status index." *Health Services Research* 8:228–45.

Patrick, D. L., Bush, J. W., and Chen, M. M. 1973b. "Toward an operational definition of health." *Journal of Health and Social Behavior* 14:6–24.

Pennebaker, J. W. 1982. *The psychology of physical symptoms.* New York: Springer-Verlag.

Pennebaker, J. W., and Epstein, D. 1983. "Implicit psychophysiology: Effects of common beliefs and idiosyncratic physiological responses on symptom reporting." *Journal of Personality* 51:3–30.

Peplau, L. A. 1985. "Loneliness research: Basic concepts and findings." In *Social support: Theory, research, and applications,* edited by I. G. Sarason and B. R. Sarason. Boston: Nijhoff.

Phillips, M. 1980. "Fatigue as an unwanted effect of drugs." *Lancet* 2:540.

Pincus, T., Summey, J. A., Soraci, S. A., et al. 1983. "Assessment of patient satisfaction in activities of daily living using a modified Stanford Health Assessment Questionnaire." *Arthritis and Rheumatism* 26:1346–1353.

Pless, I. B., and Satterwhite, B. 1973. "A measure of family functioning and its application." *Social Science and Medicine,* 7:613–21.

Pless, I. B., and Satterwhite, B. 1975. "Family functioning and family problems." In *Child health and the community,* R. J. Haggarty, K. J. Roghmann, and I. B. Pless. New York: John Wiley and Sons.

Pless, I. B., Roghmann, K., and Haggerty, R. 1972. "Chronic illness, family functioning, and psychological adjustment: A model for the allocation of preventive mental health services." *International Journal of Epidemiology* 1(3):271–277.

Radloff, L. S. 1977. "The CES-D scale; A self-report depression scale for research in the general population." *Applied Psychological Measurement* 1:385–401.

Raudenbush, S. W., Becker, B. J., and Kalaian, H. 1988. "Modeling multivariate effect sizes." *Psychological Bulletin* 103:111–20.

Raymond, M. R. 1986. "Missing data in evaluation research." *Evaluation and the Health Professions* 9:395–420.

Raymond, M. R., and Roberts, D. M. 1987. "A comparison of methods for treating incomplete data in selection research." *Educational and Psychological Measurement* 47:13–26.

Read, L. J., Quinn, R. J., and Hoefer, M. A. 1987. "Measuring overall health: An evaluation of three important approaches." *Journal of Chronic Diseases* 40:7S–22S.

Reddon, J. R., Marceau, R., and Holden, R. R. 1985. "A confirmatory evaluation of the Profile of Mood States: Convergent and discrimination item validity." *Journal of Psychopathology and Behavioral Assessment* 7:243–59.

Reed, W. L. 1983. "Physical health status as a consequence of health practices." *Journal of Community Health* 8:217–28.

Renne, K. 1974. "Measurement of social health in a general population survey." *Social Science Research* 3:25–44.

Reynolds, C. F., Kupfer, D. J., Hoch, C. C., et al. 1987. "Sleep deprivation as a probe in the elderly." *Archives of General Psychiatry* 44:982–90.

Reynolds, C. F., Kupfer, D. J., Taska, L. S., et al. 1985. "Sleep apnea in Alzheimer's dementia: Correlation with mental deterioration." *Journal of Clinical Psychiatry* 46:257–61.

Reynolds, W. J., Rushing, W. A., and Miles, D. L. 1974. "The validation of a function status index." *Journal of Health and Social Behavior* 15:271–88.

Ries, P. W. 1979. "Acute conditions: Incidence and associated disability." U.S. Dept. of Health, Education, and Welfare. *Vital and health statistics* series 10, no. 132, DHEW publication no. (PHS) 79–1560. Washington, D.C.: U.S. Government Printing Office.

Robins, L. N., Helzer, J. E., Croughan, J., and Ratcliff, K. S. 1981. "National Institute of Mental Health Diagnostic Interview Schedule." *Archives of General Psychiatry* 38:381–89.

Roen, S. R., Ottenstein, D., Copper, et al. 1966. "Community adaptation as an evaluative concept in community mental health." *Archives of General Psychiatry* 15:36–44.

Roper, W. L., Winkenwerder, W., Hackbarth, G. M., et al. 1988. "Effectiveness in health care: An initiative to evaluate and improve medical practice." *New England Journal of Medicine* 319:1197–1202.

Rosen, R. C., and Kostis, J. B. 1985. "Biobehavioral sequelae associated with adrenergic-inhibiting antihypertensive agents: A critical review." *Health Psychology* 4:579–604.

Rosenberg, M. 1965. *Society and the adolescent self-image.* Princeton, N.J.: Princeton University Press.

Rosenstock, I. M. 1974. "The health belief model and preventive health behavior." *Health Education Monographs* 2:354–86.

Rummel, R. J. 1970. *Applied factor analysis.* Evanston, Ill.: Northwestern University Press.

Russell, D. 1982. "The measurement of loneliness." In *Loneliness: A sourcebook of current theory and therapy,* edited by L. A. Peplau and D. Perlman. New York: Wiley-Interscience.

Russell, D., Peplau, L. A., and Cutrona, L. E. 1980. "The revised UCLA Loneliness Scale: Concurrent and discriminant validity evidence." *Journal of Personality and Social Psychology* 39:472–80.

Russell, D., Peplau, L. A., and Ferguson, M. L. 1978. "Developing a measure of loneliness." *Journal of Personality Assessment* 42:290–94.

Sanazaro, P. J., and Williamson, J. W. 1986. "End results of patient care: A provisional classification based on reports by internists." *Medical Care* 6:123–30.

Sanders, B. S. 1962. "Have morbidity surveys been oversold?" *American Journal of Public Health* 52:1648–1659.

Saultz, J. W. 1988. "Commentary." *Journal of Family Practice* 26:37–38.

Schroeder, S. A. 1987. "Outcome assessment 70 years later: Are we ready?" *New England Journal of Medicine* 316:160–162.

Schulberg, H. S., McCleland, M., Ganguli, G., Christy, W., and Frank, R. 1985.

"Assessing depression in primary medical and psychiatric practices." *Archives of General Psychiatry* 42:1164–1170.

Sechrest, L. 1967. "Incremental validity." In *Problems in human assessment*, edited by D. N. Jackson and S. Messick. New York: McGraw-Hill.

Shapiro, M., Ware, J. E., and Sherbourne, C. D. 1986. "Effects of cost sharing on seeking care for serious and minor symptoms." *Annals of Internal Medicine* 104:246–51.

Sherbourne, C. D. 1988. *The role of social supports and life stress events in use of mental health services. Social Science and Medicine* 27:1393–1400.

Sherbourne, C. D., and Stewart, A. L. 1991. "The MOS social support survey." *Social Science and Medicine* 32:705–14.

Siegrist, J. 1987. "Impaired quality of life as a risk factor in cardiovascular disease." *Journal of Chronic Diseases* 40:571–78.

Silverstein, A. B. 1987. "Note on the parallel analysis criterion for determining the number of common factors or principal components." *Psychological Reports* 61:351–54.

Simonds, J. F., and Parraga, H. 1982. "Prevalence of sleep disorders and sleep behaviors in children and adolescents." *Journal of the American Academy of Child Psychiatry* 21:383–88.

Simonds, J. F., and Parraga, H. 1984. "Sleep behaviors and disorders in children and adolescents evaluated at psychiatric clinics." *Developmental and Behavioral Pediatrics* 5:6–10.

Smilkstein, G. 1978. "The family APGAR: A proposal for a family function test and its use by physicians." *Journal of Family Practice* 6:1231–1239.

Smilkstein, G., Ashworth, C., and Montano, D. 1982. "Validity and reliability of family APGAR as a test of family function." *Journal of Family Practice* 15:303–11.

Smith, D. H. 1967. "Correcting for social desirability response sets in opinion-attitude survey research." *Public Opinion Quarterly* 31:87–94.

Smith, L. 1987. "Qualms about QALYs." *Lancet* 1:1134–1136.

Snyder, D. K., and Berg, P. 1983. "Determinants of sexual dissatisfaction in sexually distressed couples." *Archives of Sexual Behavior* 12:237–46.

Snyder-Halpern, R., and Verran, J. A. 1987. "Instrumentation to describe subjective sleep characteristics in healthy subjects." *Research in Nursing and Health* 10:155–63.

Social Psychiatry Research Unit. 1984. "Psychiatric Epidemiology Research Interview (PERI) revised." New York: Columbia University Press.

Social Psychiatry Research Unit. 1977. *The Psychiatric Epidemiology Research Interview: A report on twenty-two scales, appendix I to the measurement of psychopathology in the community.* New York: Columbia University Press.

Solberg, L. I. 1984. "Lassitude: A primary care evaluation." *Journal of the American Medical Association* 251:3272–3276.

Spielberger, C. D., Johnson, E. H., Russell, S. F., et al. 1985. "The experience and expression of anger: Construction and validation of an anger expression scale." In *Anger and hostility in cardiovascular and behavioral disorders,* edited by M. A. Chesney and R. J. Rosenman. Washington, D.C.: Hemisphere Publishing.

Spitzer, W. O. 1987. "State of science 1986: Quality of life and functional status as target variable for research." *Journal of Chronic Diseases* 40:465–71.

Spitzer, W. O., Dobson, A. J., Hall, J., et al. 1981. "Measuring the quality of life of cancer patients: A concise QL-index for use by physicians." *Journal of Chronic Diseases* 34:585.

Starfield, B. 1974. "Measurement of outcome: A proposed scheme." *Milbank Memorial Fund Quarterly* 52:39–50.

Sternbach, R. A. 1978. "Clinical aspects of pain." In *The psychology of pain,* edited by R. A. Sternbach. New York: Raven Press.

Stewart, A. L., Greenfield, S., Hays, R. D., et al. 1989. "Functional status and well-being of patients with chronic conditions: Results from the Medical Outcomes Study." *Journal of the American Medical Association* 262:907–13.

Stewart, A. L., Hays, R. D., and Ware, J. E. 1988. "The MOS Short-Form General Health Survey: Reliability and validity in a patient population." *Medical Care* 26:724–35.

Stewart, A. L., Ware, J. E., and Brook, R. H. 1978. *Conceptualization and measurement of health for adults in the Health Insurance Study: Vol. 2, Physical health in terms of functioning.* Publication no. R–1987/2–HEW. Santa Monica, Calif.: RAND Corporation.

Stewart, A. L., Ware, J. E., and Brook, R. H. 1981. "Advances in the measurement of functional status: Construction of aggregate indexes." *Medical Care* 19:473–88.

Stewart, A. L., Ware, J. E., and Brook, R. H. 1982. *Construction and scoring of aggregate functional status measures: Vol. 1.* Publication no. R2551–1–HHS. Santa Monica, Calif.: RAND Corporation.

Sugarman, J. R., and Berg, A. O. 1984. "Evaluation of fatigue in a family practice." *Journal of Family Practice* 19:643–47.

Tarlov, A. R. 1980. *Summary report of the Graduate Medical Education National Advisory Committee, Vol. I.* Washington, D.C.: U.S. Department of Health and Human Services.

Tarlov, A. R. 1983. "Shattuck lecture—The increasing supply of physicians, the changing structure of the health services system, and the future practice of medicine." *New England Journal of Medicine* 308:1235–1244.

Tarlov, A. R., Ware, J. E., Greenfield, S., et al. 1989. "The Medical Outcomes Study: An application of methods for monitoring the results of medical care." *Journal of the American Medical Association* 262:925–30.

Taylor, S. E., and Brown, J. D. 1988. "Illusion and well-being: A social psychological perspective on mental health." *Psychological Bulletin* 103:193–210.

Thompson, J. D., Fetter, R. B., and Shin, Y. 1978. "One strategy for controlling costs in university teaching hospitals." *Journal of Medical Education* 53:167–75.

Thorndike, R. L. 1967a. "The analysis and selection of test items." In *Problems in human assessment,* edited by D. N. Jackson and S. Messick. New York: McGraw-Hill.

Thorndike, R. L. 1967b. "Reliability." In *Problems in human assessment,* edited by D. N. Jackson and S. Messick. New York: McGraw-Hill.

Twaddle, A. C. 1974. "The concept of health status." *Social Science and Medicine* 1:29–38.

Tyler, T. A., and Fiske, D. W. 1968. "Homogeneity indices and test length." *Educational and Psychological Measurement* 28:767–77.

U.S. Dept. of Health and Human Services. 1980. *International classification of diseases, ninth revision, clinical modification.* 2d ed. Publication (PHS) no. 80–1260.

Urponen, H., Vuori, I., Hasan, J., et al. 1988. "Self-evaluations of factors promoting and disturbing sleep: An epidemiological survey in Finland." *Social Science and Medicine* 26:443–50.

Vaillant, G. E. 1977. *Adaptation to life.* Boston: Little, Brown.

Valdez, R. B., Ware, J. E., Manning, W. G., et al. 1989. "Prepaid group practice effects of the utilization of medical services and health outcomes for children: Results from a controlled trial." *Pediatrics* 83:168–80.

Valdini, A. F. 1985. "Fatigue of unknown aetiology—A review." *Family Practice* 2:48–53.

Valdini, A. F., Steinhardt, S., Valicenti, J., et al. 1988. "A one-year follow-up of fatigued patients." *Journal of Family Practice* 26:33–38.

Veit, C. T., and Ware, J. E. 1983. "The structure of psychological distress and well-being in general populations." *Journal of Consulting and Clinical Psychology* 51:730–42.

Verbrugge, L. M., and Ascione, F. J. 1987. "Exploring the iceberg: Common symptoms and how people care for them." *Medical Care* 25:539–63.

Wan, T. T. H., and Livieratos, B. 1978. "Interpreting a general index of subjective well-being." *Millbank Memorial Fund Quarterly* 56:531–57.

Ware, J. E. 1976. "Scales for measuring general health perceptions." *Health Services Research* 11:396–415.

Ware, J. E. 1984. "The General Health Rating Index." In *Assessment of quality of life in clinical trials of cardiovascular therapies,* edited by N. K. Wenger, M. E. Mattson, C. D. Furberg, and J. Elinson, 184–88. New York: Le Jacq.

Ware, J. E. 1986. "The assessment of health status." In *Applications of social science to clinical medicine and health policy,* edited by L. H. Aiken and D. Mechanic, 9th ed. New Brunswick, N.J.: Rutgers University Press.

Ware, J. E. 1987. "Standards for validating health measures: Definition and content." *Journal of Chronic Disease* 40:473–80.

Ware, J. E. 1990. "Outcomes study foresees greater patient input." QA *Review* 5.

Ware, J. E., and Allen, H. M. 1986. "Instruments used in the assessment of health status outcomes." Paper presented at the American Public Health Association annual meeting.

Ware, J. E., and Hays, R. D. 1988. "Methods for measuring patient satisfaction with specific medical encounters." *Medical Care* 26:393–402.

Ware, J. E., and Karmos, A. H. 1976a. *Development and validation of scales to measure perceived health and patient role propensity: Volume 2 of a final report.* NTIS publication no. PB 288–331. Springfield, Va.: National Technical Information Services.

Ware, J. E., and Karmos, A. H. 1976b. "Scales for measuring general health perceptions." *Health Services Research* 11:396–415.

Ware, J. E., Brook, R. H., Davies, A. R., et al. 1981. "Choosing measures of health status for individuals in general populations." *American Journal of Public Health* 71:620–625.

Ware, J. E., Brook, R. H., Davies-Avery, A., et al. 1980. *Conceptualization and measurement of health for adults in the Health Insurance Study: Vol. I Model of health and methodology.* Publication no. R–1987/1–HEW. Santa Monica, Calif.: RAND Corporation.

Ware, J. E., Brook, R. H., Rogers, W. H., et al. 1986. "Comparison of health outcomes at a health maintenance organization with those of fee-for-service care." *Lancet* 1:1017–1022.

Ware, J. E., Davies-Avery, A., and Brook, R. H. 1980. *Conceptualization and measurement of health for adults in the Health Insurance Study: Vol. 6. Analysis of relationships among health status measures.* Publication no. R–1987/6–HEW. Santa Monica, Calif. RAND Corporation.

Ware, J. E., Davies-Avery, A., and Donald, C. 1978. *Conceptualization and measurement of health for adults in the Health Insurance Study: Volume 5: General health perceptions.* Publication no. R–1987/5–HEW. Santa Monica, Calif.: RAND Corporation.

Ware, J. E., Davies-Avery, A., and Stewart, A. L. 1978. "The measurement and meaning of patient satisfaction." *Health and Medical Care Services Review* 1:2–15.

Ware, J. E., Johnston, S. A., Davies-Avery, A., et al. 1979. *Conceptualization and measurement of health for adults in the Health Insurance Study: Volume 3: Mental health.* Publication no. R–1987/3–HEW. Santa Monica, Calif.: RAND Corporation.

Ware, J. E., Manning, W. G., Duan, N., et al. 1984. "Health status and the use of outpatient mental health services." *American Psychologist* 39:1090–1100.

Ware, J. E., and Sherbourne, C. D., 1992. "A 36-item short form health survey (SF-36)." *Medical Care,* in press.

Ware, J. E., Snyder, M. R., Wright, R., et al. 1983. "Defining and measuring patient satisfaction with medical care." *Evaluation and Program Planning* 6:247–63.

Ware, J. E., Veit, C., and Sherbourne, C. D. 1985. *Refinements in the measurement of mental health for adults in the Health Insurance Study.* Publication no. WD–2618–HHS. Santa Monica, Calif.: RAND Corporation.

Weber, S. J., Wycoff, M. L., and Adamson, D. R. 1982. "The impact of two clinical trials on physician knowledge and practice." *Market Facts, Inc.* Arlington, Va.

Weinberger, M., Darnell, J., Therney, W., Martz, B., Hiner, S., Barker, J., and

Neill, P. 1986. "Self-rated health as a predictor of hospital admission and nursing home placement in elderly public housing tenants." *American Journal of Public Health* 76:457–59.

Weinstein, M. C. 1980. "Estrogen use in postmenopausal women—Costs, risks, and benefits." *New England Journal of Medicine* 303:308–16.

Weinstein, M. C., and Stason, W. B. 1977. "Foundations of cost-effectiveness analysis for health and medical practices." *New England Journal of Medicine* 296:716–21.

Weinstein, M. C., Berwick, D. M., Goldman, P. A., et al. 1989. "A comparison of three psychiatric screening tests using Receiver Operating Characteristic (ROC) analysis." *Medical Care* 27:593–607.

Weissfeld, J. L., Brock, B. M., Kirscht, J. P., et al. 1987. "Reliability of health belief indexes: Confirmatory factor analysis in sex, race, and age subgroups. *Health Service Research* 21:777–93.

Weissman, M. M., and Bothwell, S. 1976. "Assessment of social adjustment by patient self-report." *Archives of General Psychiatry* 33:1111–1115.

Weissman, M. M., Sholomskas, D., and John, K. 1981. "The assessment of social adjustment: An update." *Archives of General Psychiatry* 38:1250–1258.

Wells, K. B. 1985. *Depression as a tracer condition for the National Study of Medical Care Outcomes: Background review.* Publication no. R–3293–RWJ/HJK. Santa Monica, Calif.: RAND Corporation.

Wells, K. B., Burnam, M. A., Leake, B., et al. 1988. "Agreement between face-to-face and telephone-administered versions of the depression section of the NIMH Diagnostic Interview Schedule." *Journal of Psychiatric Research* 22:207–20.

Wells, K. B., Manning, W. G., Duan, N., et al. 1982. *Cost sharing and the demand for ambulatory mental health services.* Publication no. R–2960–HHS. Santa Monica, Calif.: RAND Corporation.

Wells, K. B., Manning, W. G., Duan, N., et al. 1984. "The sensitivity of mental health care use and cost estimates to methods effects." *Medical Care* 22:783–88.

Wells, K. B., Stewart, A., Hays, R. D., et al. 1989. "The functioning and well-being of depressed patients: Results from the Medical Outcomes Study." *Journal of the American Medical Association* 262:914–19.

Wells, L. E., and Marwell, G. 1976. *Self-esteem: Its conceptualization and measurement.* Madison: University of Wisconsin Press.

Wenger, N. K., Mattson, M. E., Furberg, C. D., and Elison, J. 1984. *Assessment of quality of life in clinical trials of cardiovascular therapies.* New York: Le Jacq.

Werts, C., Linn, R. L., and Jöreskog, K. G. 1978. "Reliability of college grades from longitudinal data." *Educational and Psychological Measurement* 38:89–95.

Wetzler, H. P., and Cruess, D. F. 1975. "Self-reported physical health practices and health care utilization: Findings from the National Health Interview Survey." *American Journal of Public Health* 75:1329–1330.

Wheaton, B., Muthen, B., Alwin, D. F., and Summers, G. F. 1977. "Assessing reliability and validity in panel models." In *Sociological methodology, 1972*, edited by D. R. Heise, 84–136. San Francisco: Jossey-Bass.

Wiley, D. E., and Wiley, J. A. 1970. "The estimation of measurement error in panel data." *American Sociological Review* 35:112–17.

Wiley, J. A., and Camacho, T. C. 1980. "Life-style and future health: Evidence from Alameda County study." *Preventive Medicine* 9:1–21.

Williams, A. W., Ware, J. E., and Donald, C. A. 1981. "A model of mental health, life events, and social circumstances applicable to general populations." *Journal of Health and Social Behavior* 22:324–36.

Williams, J. D., and Lindem, A. C. 1976. *A computer program for two-way analysis of variance with multiple covariates* (ANCOVA2). Grand Forks: Computer Center, University of North Dakota.

Williamson, J., Stokoe, I. H., Gray, S., et al. 1964. "Old people at home: their unreported needs." *Lancet* 1:1117–1120.

Wingard, D. C., and Berkman, L. F. 1983. "Mortality risk associated with sleeping patterns among adults." *Sleep* 6:102–7.

World Health Organization. 1948. "World Health Organization constitution." In *Basic documents*. Geneva: World Health Organization.

World Health Organization. 1980. *International classification of impairments, disabilities and handicaps: A manual classification relating to the consequences of disease.* Geneva: World Health Organization.

Yoshitake, H. 1971. "Relations between the symptoms and the feelings of fatigue." *Ergonomics* 14:175–86.

Zung, W. W. K. 1965. "A self-rating depression scale." *Archives of General Psychiatry* 12:63–70.

Contributors

Anita L. Stewart, PH.D., is Associate Professor in Residence at the University of California–San Francisco, Institute for Health & Aging, Department of Social and Behavioral Sciences, and School of Nursing. She participated in the planning, implementation, measurement development, and analyses of the Medical Outcomes Study while at RAND. Anita Stewart's current work focuses on evaluating the benefits of physical activity for older adults as well as for the chronically ill. She is conducting a community-based intervention to encourage older adults to increase their levels of physical activity as well as a study comparing quality of life outcomes of smokers who successfully quit to smokers who are unable to quit.

John E. Ware, Jr., PH.D., is Senior Scientist in The Health Institute at the New England Medical Center Hospitals (NEMCH) and Director of the International Resource Center for Health Care Assessment at NEMCH in Boston. He is also Principal Investigator for the Medical Outcomes Study, and for the Child Health Assessment Project at NEMCH. Formerly Senior Research Psychologist at The RAND Corporation, he was the principal architect of the health status and patient satisfaction surveys used in the Health Insurance Experiment. John Ware's current activities include research in the U.S. and other countries designed to develop and validate more practical patient-based measures of the quality of services and medical care outcomes for use in health policy evaluation, health care management, clinical research, and medical practice.

Sandra H. Berry, Director of the RAND Survey Research Group, is a sociologist who specializes in health-related data collection and in implementation of complex research designs. She currently conducts methodological research on data collection in the health area as well as substantive research on HIV-related risk and prevention behaviors, self-reported health outcomes in HIV clinical trials, and related measurement issues.

Ron D. Hays, PH.D., is a social policy analyst at RAND specializing in drug use and health outcome measurement. Current research includes an NIAAA-sponsored study to develop a microcomputer system for assessing alcohol use at impaired driver treatment programs, and a study of adherence among chronic disease patients. Dr. Hays serves on the editorial board of the journal *Quality of Life Research*. He received the UC–Riverside Outstanding Young Alumnus award in 1989.

William H. Rogers, PH.D., is a senior statistician at RAND with fifteen years of experience in health policy research. Dr. Rogers was a key analyst for the Health Insurance Experiment and the PPS Quality of Care Study, as well as the Medical Outcomes Study. He is also a software designer and contributor to the STATA statistics package.

Cathy Donald Sherbourne, PH.D., is Associate Social Scientist in the Social Policy Department at RAND. She is a medical sociologist specializing in health outcome measurement for adults and children for several of RAND's large-scale health policy evaluations. Current projects examine the ability of psychologic and social factors to explain individual variations in functional status and well-being; a study of adherence among chronic disease patients; and the impact of comorbid alcoholism in depression.

Harris M. Allen, Jr., PH.D., is Scientist at The Health Institute, and on the senior staff of the International Resource Center for Health Care Assessment, New England Medical Center Hospitals, Boston.

Sharon B. Arnold, PH.D., is Senior Policy Analyst at the Prospective Payment Assessment Commission, Washington, D.C.

Allyson Ross Davies, PH.D., is Director of the Department of Quality Assessment at New England Medical Center Hospitals and a Research Scientist at The Health Institute, Boston.

Sheldon Greenfield, M.D., is Senior Scientist at The Health Institute, New England Medical Center Hospitals, Boston; Professor of Medicine and Chief Division of Health Services Research, Department of Medicine, Tufts University School of Medicine, Medford; and Adjunct Professor of Public Health, Harvard School of Public Health, Cambridge.

Caren J. Kamberg, M.S.P.H., is Research Administrator for the health program at RAND.

Elizabeth A. McGlynn, PH.D., is Health Policy Analyst at RAND.

Eugene C. Nelson, D.SC., is Director of Quality of Care Research, Hospital Corporation of America, Nashville.

Edward B. Perrin, PH.D., is Chairman at the Department of Health Services, University of Washington, Seattle.

Kenneth B. Wells, M.D., M.P.H., is Senior Researcher, RAND, and Associate Professor, Department of Psychiatry and Biomedical Sciences, UCLA School of Medicine, Los Angeles.

Michael Zubkoff, PH.D., is Professor & Chairman, Department of Community and Family Medicine, Dartmouth Medical School, and Professor of Economy and Management, Amos Tuck School of Business, Dartmouth College, Hanover.

Index

(GHRI), MOS health perceptions index developed to be similar to GHRI, 157–162, 171, predictor of mortality, 146; generic health status instrument, 5; health perceptions items as basis for MOS Short-Form General Health Survey, 279; Health Perceptions Questionnaire (HPQ), 143–145, 279; health perceptions items compared to MOS final items, 152 (Table 8–1); mental health items as basis for MOS Short-Form General Health Survey, 279; mental health items compared to MOS items, 112–115 (Table 7–2); Mental Health Inventory (MHI), 104; mobility items as basis for MOS mobility scale, 91; physical functioning items as basis for MOS Short-Form General Health Survey, 278; role functioning items as basis for MOS Short-Form General Health Survey, 278; sleep item, 240; vitality scale, 147–148

Health Insurance Experiment Symptoms List, 262

Health perceptions (Chapter 8): characteristics of measures, 163; construction of scales, 157, of summary index, 157; content and measurement strategy, 149; correlations among subscales, 170 (Table 8–10); correlations between subscales and validity variables, 160–161; definition and issues, 143; descriptive statistics, 163 (Table 8–9); factor analysis of energy/fatigue, health perceptions, health distress, 170 (Table 8–11); final questionnaire items, 150, 373, 397–399; future directions, 170; issue resolution and future directions, 170; item-scale correlation matrix, 158 (Table 8–4); item variability, 154, 155 (Table 8–3); MOS single item, 298; NCHS single item, 291; pilot studies, 149; reliability, 163 (Table 8–9); scale characteristics, *see* characteristics of measures, 163; scale construction, *see* construction of subscales, 157, summary index, 157; scoring rules,

162, 164 (Table 8–8); short-form, 273, 278; single items, MOS item, 298, NCHS item, 291; summary index, analysis plan, 151, construction and evaluation of indexes, 157, correlations between indexes and validity variables, 161, hypothesized indexes, 151; validity, 160–163; variability of items, 154, 155 (Table 8–3); variability of scale scores, 163

Health Perceptions Questionnaire (HPQ), 143–145, 279

Health status. *See* Health

Health surveys, uses of, 9–11; clinical decision making in medical practice, 9, 10; clinical trials, 9, 10; health care policy studies, 9; monitoring health of the general population, 9, 10

Heft, M. W., 222
Helmstadter, G. C., 81
Hennen, B. K., 145
Herzlich, C., 20, 145
HIE. *See* Health Insurance Experiment
Heart disease, definition of MOS tracer condition, 39
HIE Vitality Scale, 147
Hinkle, L. E., 20
Hoelscher, T. J., 252
Hogan, M. J., 196
Holden, R. R., 79
Hopkins Symptom Checklist, 262
Horn, S. D., 17
House, J. S., 175
Howard, K. I., 75, 77, 280, 326
Hoyt, C., 82
Human Population Laboratory, 13
Humphreys, L. G., 79
Hunt, S. M., 235, 361, 365
Hypertension, definition of MOS tracer condition, 39

IASP, 220
Incentives for participation, 61–63
Institute of Medicine, 220, 221
Instruments: description, 48–50; overview, 50 (Table 4–2)
Internal-consistency reliability, 81–83
International Classification of Diseases, 16
Interpretability of scale scores, 317–319:

Radloff, L. S., 40, 262
Raudenbush, S. W., 370
Raymond, M. R., 370
Read, L. J., 301
Recall period, 71
Record management system, 62
Reddon, J. R., 149
Reed, W. L., 238
Reliability: estimates for specific measures. See Chapters 6–17; single-item vs. multi-item scales, 301
Reliability methods: estimating reliability for single items, 83–84; internal-consistency, 81–83; in disadvantaged groups, 84; methods, 81–85
Renne, K., 12
Respondent burden, 55–56; reduction of, 288
Respondent cooperation, 56–58; incentives for study participation, 53, 61–63; maintaining cooperation over time, 62; patients, 56, 61–63; providers, 56–61
Respondent incentives, 61–63
Response bias, 320–322; acquiescent response set, 321. *See also* Socially desirable response set
Response options, 68
Response rates: of clinicians, 30–33; of patients in baseline sample, 42–45; of patients in cross-sectional sample, 36
Responsiveness of scale scores, 318–319
Restricted activity days. *See* Bed days, 281, 284
Reynolds, C. F., 238, 239
Reynolds, W. J., 86, 205–207
Rheumatology Rehabilitation Questionnaire, as basis for MOS mobility scale, 91
Ries, P. W., 16
Robins, L. N., 40
Roen, S. R., 162
Role functioning (Chapter 12): characteristics of measures, 216; content and measurement strategy, 208; correlations with validity variables, 215; definition and issues, 205; descriptive statistics, 216 (Table 12–5); final questionnaire items, 212, 380; future directions, 217; issue resolu-

tion and future directions, 217; item-scale correlation matrix, 214 (Table 12–3); item variability, 212 (Table 12–2); pilot study, 208; reliability, 214, 216 (Table 12–5); scale characteristics, *see* characteristics of measures, 214; scale construction, 211; scoring rules, 213, 215 (Table 12–4); single item measure, 294; short form measure, 273, 277; validity, 214; variability of items, *see* item variability, 212, 213 (Table 12–2); variability of scale scores, 214
Roper, W. L., 9
Rosen, R. C., 239, 258
Rosenberg, M., 141
Rosenstock, I. M., 145
Rummel, R. J., 78, 79
Russell, D., 107, 108

Sample bias, baseline sample, 44–45
Sample characteristics: of clinicians, 34–35; of patients in baseline sample, 45–47 (Table 3–17, 3–18); of patients in cross-sectional study, 37 (Table 3–9)
Sample size: patients, 45–46; providers, 45–46
Sampling clinicians: incentives for participation, 61; procedures for approaching clinicians, 58; procedures for selecting clinicians, 58, 60
Sampling patients: for cross-sectional study, 35–37; for longitudinal study, 37–41, 61
Sampling procedures (Chapter 3): clinicians, 29–35, 58–60; goals of sampling, 27; Health Maintenance Organizations (HMOs), 29–31; multispecialty group practices (MSGs), 29, 30; overview of sampling methods, 27–28; patients for cross-sectional study, 35–37; patients for longitudinal study, 37, 61; providers, 29–35, 58–60; sites and group practices, 28–29; solo and small group practitioners, 29–33
Sanazaro, P. J., 13
Sanders, B. S., 22
Satisfaction with health, 19–20

Library of Congress Cataloging-in-Publication Data

Measuring functioning and well-being—the medical outcomes study approach / Anita L. Stewart and John E. Ware, Jr. (editors) ; with a foreword by Alvin R. Tarlov.
p. cm.
Includes bibliographical references and index.
ISBN 0–8223–1212–3 (alk. paper)
1. Health surveys—Statistical methods. 2. Medical care—Evaluation. 3. Health status indicators. I. Stewart, Anita L. II. Ware, John E.
RA408.5.M43   1992
362.1′021—dc20
DNLM/DLC
for Library of Congress   91–34579
                                                                                                          CIP